Facing the Finish

Sheri L. Samotin

Facing the Finish

A Road Map for
Aging Parents *and* Adult Children

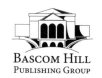

BASCOM HILL
PUBLISHING GROUP

MINNEAPOLIS, MN

Bascom Hill Publishing Group
322 First Avenue N, 5th floor
Minneapolis, MN 55401
612.455.2294
www.bascomhillbooks.com

ISBN-13: 978-1-62652-441-5

Distributed by Itasca Books

Cover Design by Alan Pranke
Typeset by Mary Kristin Ross

Printed in the United States of America

CONTENTS

DEDICATION

This book is dedicated with love and affection to my Mom and Dad, Bob and Johann Lesser, who gave my sister Susie and me so many gifts—including Dad's "black book," his version of a Life Transition Plan—and to my own two sons, Sacha and Noah, who will be the Adult Children to my Older Adult persona! I only hope I can give you "the best gift" too!

INTRODUCTION

EARLIER THIS WEEK, I was with a new client, Deborah. Her eighty-four-year-old father, Saul, has lived alone about fifteen minutes from Deborah and her family ever since Deborah's mother died seven years ago. Saul suffers from moderate memory impairment, which often leaves him frustrated, and he lashes out at Deborah whenever she tries to help. Saul insists on driving but often can't find his way home and calls Deborah in a rage. He leaves the lights on in the car, so the battery is dead several mornings each month and, you guessed it, he calls Deborah in a rage. Deborah and her three brothers, who live in other states, have talked with Saul about moving to a senior living community or getting some help at home. Saul won't hear of it. Deborah is at her wit's end, but her brothers have told her to "deal with it."

In my work, stories like Deborah's are my daily diet, and I've learned that when it comes to our parents, it's only a matter of time before we Adult Children will need to become more involved in their day-to-day lives.

Family caregiving is a life stage, often called "the other midlife crisis." Since I myself am an Adult Child (and not yet an Older Adult), I do tend to empathize with my own generation's struggle with this reality. However, as a life transition coach practicing in

Florida, I spend a lot of my time working with Older Adults and have grown to see things much more clearly from their vantage point.

This book was born to fill a specific need, to create a foundation for dialogue between the two generations. It seems that the many other books out there are either from the vantage point of the Adult Child or directed at family caregivers in a general way. When clients would ask me to recommend a book that would guide them in preparing for their future (as either an Older Adult *or* Adult Child) in a way that treated both generations with equal time and equal respect, I couldn't find one. My clients asked me to write it, and so I have.

As you will see as you dive in, this book is not meant to be an encyclopedic guide to aging or caregiving. There are many other sources for that. At the same time, it is not merely a series of stories about the struggles of growing older or caring for your parents. Rather, I have incorporated real-life examples to illustrate the challenges and opportunities along with conversation starters, tips, and tricks from the field. The book is designed to be read as a whole, but each chapter stands on its own, so if you want to jump in to a particular section, you will be able to. I also anticipate that you will return to certain sections over time as things change in your real-life situation.

The one point I make over and over again is the importance of planning. I advocate creating a Life Transition Plan and include an appendix covering everything that should be included. In addition, readers are invited to visit www.FacingTheFinish.com, where I provide other materials you will find helpful. I've also included a resources section at the end of this book (and will continue to add to it and update it on the website mentioned above).

When I started my practice, LifeBridge Solutions, LLC in 2009, I had no idea how rich and rewarding my life would become through sharing transitions with so many families—families no doubt like yours. I am passionate about my work and appreciate the opportunity to help you through one of life's most challenging transitions. I also welcome your stories, insights, questions, and suggestions. Some of the most important tips and tricks I share in this book have resulted from ideas that started with my clients. Please keep them coming.

1

THE BEST GIFT YOU CAN GIVE: MAKING DECISIONS

EIGHTY-TWO-YEAR-OLD Betty has determined her "final exit" strategy. She plans to live life to the fullest for the next five years, throw a grand party, and call it a life. She has documented her wishes and much more in her Life Transition Plan and has held a family meeting to tell her children what she has asset-wise, where her assets are, and how she has arranged for them to be distributed upon her death. Her children have thanked her for giving them the best gift ever—decisions they won't have to anguish over.

Getting Older: It's Not a Question of "If" but "When"

It can be tough for you Older Adults to face the fact that when you look down the road of your days, more miles are behind you than in front of you. It seems like just yesterday that your kids were young or you ran your company as a corporate giant or you knew you had many more stops to make along your journey. Now, despite your fervent wish that the sand would empty more slowly from the hourglass, time *is* rushing by. It is the moment to plan your last act and get ready to vacate the stage, surrendering it to a new troupe of players. But facing one's own mortality isn't for the faint of heart. It takes courage to look life—and death—squarely in the eye and say, "When you come for me, I'll be ready."

It's also the time to admit you may need help, and your Adult Children may be the people who will provide it. Reconciling that need with the automatic reaction you undoubtedly have, that you "don't want to be a burden," is part of the wrangling you'll have to do to get through this last rodeo.

For Adult Children, facing the issues of your parents' aging takes a different brand of courage. First, face the fact that your folks aren't going to live forever, and that takes acknowledging that, at last, you really must be an adult. They very probably will require your help, and you may feel some guilt along the way. Let's face it: You have a life, perhaps a family of your own, and not a second, or cent, to spare. And the idea of helping care for your parents comes with an internal groan of "Why me?" Therein lies the guilt. It's okay if that is your first thought (you'll never get above being human), but it's not okay if it's your last thought.

It will be time to step up and pitch in, just as your parents pitched in to help you. How many times do you think your Dad didn't want to throw that ball to you one more time or your Mom didn't want to get out of bed to comfort you during a nightmare? Consider it payback, and the first step is accepting that the time will come when your help is needed.

It is possible that your Older Adult will live to be one hundred, financially and physically independent, and die quietly in his sleep with all of his affairs in order. Adult Children, you may be lucky enough to inherit such good genes and feel only a small sadness when your very aged parent dies that way—having kept their championship tennis score and their mental faculties right till the end. You'll attend the perfectly arranged funeral or memorial service and go on about living your own life.

But you can't bet on it . . .

For the rest of us, we need to be prepared for the inevitable time when either we need our Adult Children's help or when our parents need that help from us. It makes sense to sit down to think about how you'll handle things before the need to do so becomes apparent because of a crisis. After all, these are not easy issues to think about—much less discuss—and being able to consider them over a period of time is preferable to making decisions during a time of extreme stress.

According to the National Clearinghouse for Long-Term Care Information, "The definition of 'Long-Term Care' is a variety of services and supports to meet health or personal care needs over an extended period of time. Most long-term care is nonskilled personal care assistance, such as help performing everyday 'activities of daily living' such as bathing, dressing, and eating."

If you don't think this topic concerns you, consider that at least 70 percent of people over age sixty-five will require some long-term-care services at some point in their lives. More than 40 percent will need care in a nursing home. The proportion of Adult Children providing assistance to a parent has more than tripled over the past fifteen years. Currently, a quarter of Adult Children assist a parent. A "caregiver" is typically a family member, partner, friend, or neighbor who helps care for an Older Adult or person with a disability who lives at home. About 80 percent of care at home is provided by these unpaid caregivers.

Approximately two-thirds of caregivers are women. Fourteen percent of caregivers caring for Older Adults are themselves aged sixty-five or over. The typical caregiver is a forty-six-year-old woman who is married and employed, and is caring for her widowed mother who does not live with her. On average, unpaid caregivers spend twenty hours a week providing care. If you're interested in learning more, check out the National Clearinghouse for Long-Term Care Information at www.longtermcare.gov and download their very informative planning guide.

Don't Delay Planning

Due to medical and other technological breakthroughs, people are living longer these days. Because of this, many people wrongly assume that they can put off getting their affairs in order for a few more years. However, exactly the opposite is true.

Why?

While living in a time with wonderful medical advances means that many of us can expect to live to a ripe old age, the scary reality is that we often didn't plan for that long life. The nest egg that we put away for our retirement years ago was probably designed to last for twenty years or so, taking us from the historical retirement age of sixty-five to our mid-eighties, if we were lucky.

The reality is that for many such people, their planning will have them come up short since they may live well into their nineties. Making matters worse, many Older Adults assumed that the equity in their homes would cover their final years, but with the collapse of the residential real estate market over the past few years, that may no longer by true.

Everyone is also aware of the roller coaster that is the financial marketplace. The best time to start planning is when you are young enough to take steps that can have a positive impact on the outcome, but many of us don't.

Here's what we are facing: As was mentioned previously, statistics tell us that at least 70 percent of people over sixty-five years of age will require assistance with activities of daily living at some point during their lives, and typically this will continue for three years, including one year of full-time or nursing home care. One year of paid care at home, assuming you need periodic personal-care help from a home health aide (the average is about eighteen hours a week) will cost almost $20,000 per year, based on current national statistics. Multiply that by two years, and you are looking at $40,000 just for this one expense. The current average cost for a semi-private room in a nursing home is $75,000 per year, bringing the average expected total bill for care up to nearly $125,000 per person. (You Adult Children in your fifties and sixties would benefit by exploring purchasing long-term-care insurance while you are still young enough and healthy enough to obtain it for a reasonable premium.)

Planning ahead might also help you decide when to stop working and when to begin taking your Social Security benefits. This is a complicated decision and depends a lot on your income while you've been working, the lifestyle you envision in retirement, and the assets and insurance you have to draw upon in your later years. Doing a little analysis might help you determine that it is prudent to continue working a bit longer than you might otherwise have planned.

Finally, living longer might mean that you are living without your spouse for many years. If you've assumed you will have two Social Security payments and perhaps two pensions, you might be surprised at how dramatically things change (and how immediately) when you lose your spouse. I always advise clients to plan a budget that is comfortable on one retirement income to protect the surviving partner from a significant change in lifestyle following the death of the other spouse. Of course, one way to plan to mitigate this is through the use of life insurance or the accumulation of assets that can be liquidated to help pay living expenses.

Planning ahead is always a good idea, but even more so now that we have to plan for longer and longer periods of time.

Execute Your Plans

We've all met that person who carries on about how worried he is about the future or who talks about being afraid of what will happen to her. How often do we find ourselves thinking (or saying), "Why don't you stop talking about it and *do* something?"

Why is it so hard to overcome worry and fear, make a plan, and then act on it?

Some people seem to need to have something to worry about. We can call them the "worry warts." They seem wired to worry, and if there isn't something worth worrying about, they'll create something.

But let's assume that we are talking about the rest of the population, those who don't want to worry about their future but can't seem to figure out how to stop.

As I said in the previous section, the most important thing that each of us needs to do is to start planning. Making a plan is a huge step in reducing worry because the simple process of thinking through what you will do if this or that happens can make the unknowns feel less daunting. But once you've made the plan, you need *to put it into motion*. This is where so many get stopped in their tracks. The plans are made and neatly bound and placed in the file cabinet or bookshelf, never to be looked at again.

Let's say that part of your plan is to slowly go through and streamline your belongings, because you have given a deposit to move to a senior living community and you realize you will have a smaller home with less storage space. With good intentions, you tell yourself that you will get the clean-out done over the next few months. You try, really you do, but you're just so busy with the grandchildren, a cruise, and your book group. Suddenly months have gone by and you're in a panic, staying up at night worried about where everything will fit in your new home when you move in just a few days.

Consider Hiring a Professional

The easiest way to guarantee that you implement your plan is to build in some accountability. Set deadlines and milestones for yourself, and then enlist someone to make sure that you accomplish them.

For example, in this case, if you had hired a professional organizer or a senior move manager, that person would have kept you on track. You did the first part by setting a deadline, but you weren't able to hold yourself accountable.

A good professional will make sure that you execute your plans and achieve your milestones. He or she might have to engage in some tough love at times, but you'll be glad in the end. There's a reason why weight-loss programs that require you to weigh in post consistently good results, and why working with a personal trainer helps most people who engage the services of one to stay with their exercise plans.

Dealing with the business of life is no different. If you want to worry less, make a Life Transition Plan (I'll discuss how to do this later in this book) and implement it. And if you want *that* to happen, hold yourself accountable.

Taking the time to plan ahead for your own or your parent's long-term-care needs will reduce the inevitable stress when the time comes. You will have an idea of the resources that are available to help yourself or your parents, and you will have prepared for how to pay for it. If you as an Adult Child have siblings, it helps if you are all on the same page regarding how each of you will contribute to your parents' care, whether it is financially or by providing hands-on care.

So where do you begin?

No matter if you are the Older Adult or the Adult Child, you must both begin at the same place—acknowledging the fact that time is passing and soon enough you will be facing the finish of what has hopefully been a long and fulfilling life for you or a life well-lived for your parents.

Accepting Aging

Advancing age is often frustrating for both generations as you face the new limitations age imposes on a person's body and mind; turning over control of even little things to others might make any Older Adult feel insecure. A loss of control is always frightening, but acknowledging that your own (or your parent's) situation is changing is not about a *loss of control*—it is actually about *taking control* of how things will go from now on.

According to a recent study by Home Instead Senior Care, more than half of Older Adults resist asking for help, even from their Adult Children, fearing it signals a neediness that could land them in a nursing home. Similarly, the survey indicates that 51 percent of Adult Children acting as caregivers say their aging relatives can be so reluctant to accept help that the caregiver fears for their safety. Don't let this be you. As an Older Adult, you may benefit by accepting help.

In her classic book *On Death and Dying,* Elisabeth Kübler-Ross put forth her now widely applied model for the grieving process. Since its publication, this model has been adapted to explain the feelings associated with many types of transition or personal loss. The stages include: denial, anger, bargaining, depression, and, finally, acceptance.

In my work, I have noticed that the individuals who seem to "age well" and capture the attention and admiration of others are those who reach the stage of acceptance long before the ravages of advancing age take over in a profound way. They are also the people who continue to believe that their lives have meaning and purpose.

Adult Children go through a similar progression. It takes time for you to adjust your vision of your parent's reality. We tend to place people, in our mind's eye, as though they were frozen in time. We see them in a way we saw them once, like a snapshot taken long ago, and see them just that way for a very long time—long after the reality has changed. That's why we are so shocked at our high school reunion when we can't quite believe how our old flame, once young and handsome, is now bald and pot-bellied or that goddess we took to the prom is now a middle-aged matron with a thick waist. It is harder still to see our parents not as the providers of comfort they were when we were young children, but as older, perhaps frailer, versions of those people.

The sooner you can advance through the stages and reach acceptance of your reality, the better—though it does take some time to adjust. This is true whether you are the Older Adult or the Adult Child watching the changes in your parents. Once you are able to accept that you are indeed getting older, be willing to ask for help and evaluate and prioritize what you most need help with.

A story by an anonymous author illustrates this point well:

A poised and proud ninety-two-year-old lady, who was known for being fully dressed each morning by eight o-clock—including her hair fashionably coifed and her make-up perfectly applied, even though she was legally blind—moved to a nursing home. Her husband of seventy years had recently passed away, making the move necessary. After many hours of waiting patiently in the lobby of the nursing home, she smiled sweetly when told her room was ready.

As she maneuvered her walker to the elevator, I had the opportunity to provide her with a visual description of her tiny room, including the eyelet curtains that had been hung on her window.

"I love it," she stated, with the enthusiasm of an eight-year-old having just received a new puppy.

"But, Mrs. Jones, you haven't even seen the room yet."

"That doesn't have anything to do with it," she replied. "Happiness is something you decide ahead of time. Whether I like my room or not doesn't depend on how the furniture is arranged—it's how I arrange my mind. I already decided to love it. . . . It's a decision I make every morning when I wake up. I have a choice: I can spend the day in bed recounting the difficulty I have with the parts of my body that no longer work, or get out of bed and be thankful for the ones that do. Each day is a gift, and as long as my eyes open, I'll focus on the new day and all the happy memories I've stored away . . . just for this time in my life. Old age is like a bank account. You withdraw from what you've put in. So, my advice to you would be to deposit a lot of happiness in the bank account of memories. Thank you for your part in filling my memory bank. I am still depositing."*

Getting Your Affairs in Order

To prove it is (almost) never too late to begin transition planning, here is a story from my case files:

John and Jane Smith are a lovely couple who at the time were in their mid-seventies and had retired to Florida. When I met them, the Smiths were both healthy and engaged in an active lifestyle. Their

---

*"Happiness is something you decide ahead of time," Matt Townsend, accessed July 17, 2013, http://matttownsend.com/happiness-is-something-you-decide-ahead-of-time/.

two adult daughters lived in Connecticut and Ohio and led busy lives with careers and families of their own. The elder Smiths had always been highly independent and determined never to become a burden on their children. They had consulted with an estate-planning attorney and had a financial advisor they trusted.

Mr. Smith had always handled the bulk of the family finances, and it was the Smiths' financial advisor who suggested that they consult with me regarding putting all of their day-to-day affairs in order, so that if something happened to John, Jane would be able to take over. As it turned out, that advice was incredibly important.

When I first met with the Smiths, they weren't sure exactly why their financial advisor had suggested the meeting, since John was confident that all of their financial details were under control.

But during that first meeting, we discovered that while John knew all of those details, Jane had only a vague idea of what their financial picture looked like. She was unsure what investments they had and had no idea what the password was for their online banking service, which John used to pay most of their bills. She also didn't know where the insurance policy papers were kept or much about what they covered. Finally, we discovered that Jane did not have a credit card in her own name.

The Smiths, who assumed they had taken all the necessary steps in case of John's incapacity or death, were truly only partially prepared. Jane would have faced fear and bewilderment, on top of the shock of the crisis, had anything happened to John.

During that first meeting, we discussed the various things that needed to be done so that Jane could take care of the family finances in the event of John's incapacity. By the end of that first meeting, the Smiths agreed that their financial advisor was right and they needed some help getting their affairs organized.

I used my usual detailed approach to help the Smiths organize their affairs, with the goal of assembling all their critical information in one place for easy access when it was needed. I refer to this as the "owner's manual" for your life.

As we worked through the various topics, we made a list of all of the things that had to be done, the documents that had to be found, the bills that had to be paid, and the decisions that had to be made. Over the next several weeks, I worked with John and Jane to make sure that they stayed on track.

The end product of our work together was a computer flash drive that contained all of the critical information, including scanned copies of important documents. I also prepared one hard-copy version of the information in a binder since Jane was more comfortable with holding things in her hands than with accessing them on the computer. In addition to the things you'd expect to find, like account numbers, passwords, and copies of military records, this repository also listed important vendors like the air-conditioning company with which the Smiths had a service contract and the name and phone number of the dog walker for their beloved schnauzer, Sam. The idea was that if something happened, the Smiths' daughters (or another trusted person) could quickly take over.

In the Smiths' case, we needed to have Jane apply for a credit card in her own name so she would have access to credit if something happened to John.

We also discussed the Smiths' end-of-life wishes, and they decided to meet with a funeral director to make pre-need arrangements so that no one would have to guess what they would have wanted.

Finally, we prepared documents that permitted the Smiths' daughters to have access to information about their various accounts in the event that was necessary.

As the final step in our process, I facilitated a conference call between the Smiths and their daughters. The stated objective of the conference call was to bring the girls up-to-speed in the event that both of their parents became incapacitated at the same time. While John and Jane did not want to turn the flash drive containing all of the information over to their daughters immediately, they did want them to know that this resource existed and where to find it.

As luck would have it, within several months of completing this effort, John suffered a stroke. While John was recovering, Jane was able to easily step in and take care of the day-to-day matters that had previously been John's domain. The fact that the Smiths had prepared for this in advance meant that both were less stressed than they would have been during an otherwise difficult period.

Older Adults, don't just prepare your will, file it with your attorney, and figure you have done everything needed to get your affairs in order. Make a detailed plan like the one I described and execute it *now*, while you are alive and well. Details of the plan should be updated regularly. I recommend every six months unless acceleration is needed due to something like a rapidly deteriorating health condition, and then new information—like a new home health care worker's contact information—may need to be added more often.

Share the information with your Adult Children and/or caregivers or, if you are not comfortable doing that, at least be sure that they know that the information exists and how to access it when the need arises, sort of like an "In Case of Emergency, Break Glass" instruction.

Adult Children, if you don't have it already, it is up to you to ask for such information about your Older Adult parents, and to keep it updated and accessible. When a crisis hits is *not* the time to be searching for information or paperwork. Keep a paper or electronic file on your hard drive—or better yet, an up-to-date flash drive—with all your Older Adult's information to help make everyone's life easier.

Emergencies and big life changes are tough on everyone. Anything that can be done to smooth the rocky path will be much appreciated—by you and your loved ones.

So many people would rather avoid any discussion or planning for the inevitable. I've seen firsthand that there can be positive results from grabbing the bull by the horns and acknowledging one's mortality. Creating your Life Transition Plan is of vital importance to both generations—and who knows? Perhaps you will create some positive unintended results of your own by doing so.

Older Adults and Adult Children may work together on creating the Life Transition Plan. Having talked over and worked out who does what to whom and where everything necessary can be found will help make that moment of crisis—caused by an unexpected illness, accident, incapacitation, or even death—easier to deal with whether you are the Older Adult or the Adult Child involved. Or the Older Adult can create the plan and inform their Adult Children after its formulation. Either way works, but the important thing is to *begin* the plan.

Age isn't something to fear—it's something to prepare for, and by being prepared ahead of time, it can be a comforting chapter at the end of a long, full life.

Address Tough Questions

The actress Bette Davis was right when she said, "Old age isn't for sissies."

If you've made it through enough years to be called an Older Adult, you have reached such maturity slowly and against many obstacles. It may take ten years for us to realize how old we really are.

You've had a life of making, investing, losing, and saving money. You may have married (maybe more than once) and learned to listen and compromise along the way. You may have been blessed with children—a blessing that comes with much joy, sleepless nights, incandescent memories, dashed hopes, and constant expectation.

You've been sick and well, fit and unfit, suffered broken bones, and had brief periods where you felt on top of the world. You have taken risks and won or lost many a bet. You have laughed with friends, felt despair, and buried people you love.

Your age, formed by threads of desire, regret, hope, love, and things even long forgotten, is a rich tapestry of experiences and memories—and your final years are just more threads to be woven into it. The spinning of those threads, though, necessitates some tough decisions.

Here's the thing: Nobody gets out of life without dying. If we could beat the house on this bet, we would, but the house always wins, so we have a choice. We can close our eyes to the advancing changes coming our way and just react when the inevitable happens, or we can plan for what's coming and respond appropriately—to be as ready as we can be for what is headed our way.

Even though the Welsh poet Dylan Thomas made much hay with his lines, "Rage, rage against the dying of the light . . . do not go softly into that good night," I think he was wrong. Being prepared and going softly is exactly what can make it a "good" night for you and your family.

So, what decisions need to be made by you Older Adults? **Here are some questions we'll explore in more depth throughout this book:**

- Where should I live (and die)? In my home or elsewhere?

- What if I need memory care or custodial care? How do I feel about memory-care units or nursing homes?

- Who should I choose to make decisions for me if/when I can't make them for myself, and who should act as backup for my first choice?

- What will happen to my "stuff"?

- What needs to be discussed and decided about money?

- Do I want to leave an inheritance for my family or my favorite causes vs. spending my money while I'm still here to enjoy it?

- How do I feel about surrendering some of my independence? Am I willing to accept certain changes, like giving up driving myself or setting my own schedule?

- Am I prepared to deal with dementia in my spouse or myself?

- Who will care for me if I can't care for myself?

- Will I know when I can no longer make my own decisions without help? Is there someone besides me watching out for this?

- What health care decisions need to be made? How do I feel about hospice care?

- What are my "final wishes"? What kind of funeral do I want? Shall I donate my organs or my entire body to science? Where shall I be buried?

- How do I define a meaningful life? What do I see as my purpose?

The answers to these questions should be considered long and thoroughly and then added to the plans being made for your future. One of the hardest decisions may be to ask someone else (other than your own Adult Children) to help you formulate your plans for the future, including those concerning any necessary care, illnesses and hospitalizations, eventual death, and settling of your final affairs.

Perhaps your oldest son assumes it will be him you ask, but you may not have faith in his ability to carry out your wishes. Or you may not want to burden your daughter with such weighty matters when she is raising three kids of her own as a single mom and working a full-time job.

Helpers to Aid You in Navigating the Transition

Let me introduce you here to some people who are available to help you through this life transition, in addition to your trusted advisors—such as your attorney, financial planner, and accountant—with whom you are already familiar. Throughout this book, their titles may be substituted for those of your Adult Children or any other relevant caregiver.

Life Transition Coach: A life transition coach is an objective third party who helps provide focus and will have experience with others who have gone through similar transitions so that you don't have to start from scratch. A life transition coach will be knowledge-able about the many resources that are available and, like any other type of coach, will guide you to your best performance. The coach will ask the powerful questions that help you get unstuck and may also be able to point out areas where you need more practice or where you need to build your skills, and can help you figure out how to do that. The coach can serve as a resource to family members and facilitate difficult but necessary conversations and decisions. Life transition coaches are not therapists or counselors. The role of the coach is to empower, mentor, encourage, and motivate *you* to identify, develop, and continue on the path toward managing life's transitions. You will become skilled at planning ahead, anticipating situations, and solving problems. A successful coaching experience creates sustainable results during the coaching process, and for years to come.

Patient Advocate: Patient advocates come from the broad spectrum of professional disciplines that make up today's health care team. They include professionals such as case managers, nurses, disability management specialists, physicians, pharmacists, nurse practitioners, physician assistants, psychologists, nurse navigators, geriatric care managers, life-care planners, rehabilitation nurses, financial/insurance/billing advocates, behavioral health specialists, and social workers and other professionals who have a health-related degree and possess the skills to assist patients and families in navigating the complex health care system. The patient advocate is viewed as a professional who can objectively assist consumers in understanding and making sense of their health care needs.

Geriatric Care Manager: Geriatric care managers (GCMs) provide assessment and monitoring, planning and problem solving, education and advocacy, and family caregiver coaching, bringing a holistic approach to caring for Older Adults or disabled persons. The geriatric care manager is educated and experienced in any of several fields related to care management, including but not limited to nursing, gerontology, social work, or psychology, with a specialized focus on issues related to aging and elder care.

Professional Fiduciary: A professional fiduciary is a person who assumes a position of trust and responsibility, serving an individual by private arrangement or court appointment. A fiduciary as trustee has the responsibility of carrying out the terms of a trust. A fiduciary as conservator or guardian is the person who is legally appointed to manage the conservatee's estate and/or person. A conservatorship or guardianship is a legal tool designed to provide management for the financial and/or personal affairs of individuals deemed by the court to be physically or mentally incapacitated. A fiduciary can also act as agent under a power of attorney, health care surrogate, or executor/personal representative of an estate.

Daily Money Manager: Daily money managers (DMMs) provide personal business assistance to clients who have difficulty in managing their personal monetary affairs. The services meet a continuum of needs, from organizing and keeping track of financial and medical insurance papers, to assisting with check writing, maintaining bank accounts, and preparing and tracking budgets.

These professionals are available to help, should you wish to settle everything yourself and just inform your children of your choices, or to lend a hand in helping you clarify what's needed to create a comprehensive plan that includes your children.

Adult Children: Prepare for the Challenge

When you pause in your own busy lives long enough to notice Mother or Father are getting older, you may notice only the physical signs of aging—more silver in their hair, more wrinkles on their face, a slower step. But what I am asking you to notice is much less readily seen—the internal changes your parents are experiencing. They may be wrestling with the difficult choices and tough decisions referenced above and may be feeling a little tenuous, uncertain, and possibly frightened.

So what should your role be as navigation begins through potentially choppy waters for both yourself and your parents?

You need to begin to make some tough decisions on your own or, if you are one of several children, with your siblings.

Unless your parent suffers from dementia or some other mental incapacity or is unsafe in any way, I am not advocating that you jump in and take over the decisions your parents need to face as they age. It is not your job to "parent" your parents. They have managed their own lives for many decades and have done a pretty good job of it. They're still standing.

Your parents may eventually need help, and later sections of this book urge them to assess what help they need and then to ask for it. They may ask you. Until they do, I urge you to work on answering your own *internal questions* and make your own tough decisions so you are ready to help when that day arrives.

Once you have decided how you feel about future situations that may arise around your Older Adult parents, you can discuss them with your spouse or perhaps even your own children. But I urge you to keep these discussions private in your own little family. No need to rush to discuss what you've decided with your parents. Just be ready when and if they ask for help, unless your parent's safety is an issue. If that's the case—act! Dignity and independence are important, but safety comes first.

No need either to expand the conversation to your siblings, as that can end badly without proper preparation on your part (and theirs). There really is a time for every purpose under heaven. Bide your time.

While considering the questions I've outlined below, created to help you make your own "tough decisions," try to keep yourself in a calm and present state. By that, I mean don't anticipate trouble, problems, and dire circumstances that may never occur and get yourself all riled up ahead of time.

Questions like the ones I propose do tend to stir your emotions and can trigger a flood of memories, as well as half-remembered resentments and family feuds. Now is not the time to bring them up. Now is very probably the time to let them go, but, if you are unable to do that, set them aside in your thinking process.

Questions to Ask Yourself

If you are the Adult Child of an aging parent, you have probably asked yourself, "How do I know what type of help my aging parent needs?" Unless you are a senior resource professional, sorting this out can often seem overwhelming.

- What is my parent's physical condition?

- What is my parent's emotional condition?

- What is my parent's cognitive level?

- What financial resources are available to pay for help?

- What human resources are available to provide help?

- What input has my parent given on the entire topic?

Your parent's physical condition will help you determine such things as whether your parent needs help with ADLs, the activities of daily living (e.g., toileting, dressing, feeding, mobility), with medication management, or with managing medical conditions such as diabetes or using supplemental oxygen.

Your answers will help you decide whether your parent's physical condition allows them to be safe in their current living environment without extra help, or whether you need to arrange for in-home help or possible transfer to an independent or assisted living setting.

If your parent's debilitating physical condition is likely to be short term, (like when Mom is recovering from surgery), you have other options to consider—such as having physical or occupational therapists come to the home, or perhaps a short stay in a rehab setting.

Sometimes your parent is physically capable of taking care of himself, but he has become isolated and is not engaging in social interaction with others. This might be simply because he can no longer see well enough to drive or because many of his friends have passed away and he lacks someone to "hang out" with. Whatever the reason, social isolation can often lead to depression or other emotional difficulties. If this is the situation, you might decide to look into available senior centers, adult day care, or companion services for your parent.

Depending upon your answers to the other questions, you might also consider an independent or assisted living arrangement, since these environments generally offer a great deal of social interaction and stimulating activities.

Some of the toughest decisions come when your parent is memory impaired. If your parent wanders outside of the house and gets lost, or leaves the stove on overnight, he or she needs closer supervision. If Mom becomes agitated due to the cognitive impairment, she may require someone around all of the time to keep her calm. If your parent suffers from Alzheimer's disease, there are often physical considerations as well, especially in the later stages of the disease. As is always the case, safety should be your first concern.

Considering Finances

When it's time to figure out what help to put in place, there is no way to escape thinking about the financial side of the decision. While some home care is covered by health insurance such as Medicare, most care related to the activities of daily living is not. If your parent has long-term-care insurance, it will generally begin paying for services once your parent meets the policy guidelines. These typically state that a physician must certify that the individual has difficulty with two or more activities of daily living (ADLs) and that this state is expected to continue for at least three months. Some long-term-care policies provide for "first day" coverage for in-home assistance or services within an assisted living facility. You need to know whether Medicare will cover the care you seek, and if so, you must use a Medicare-certified home health agency.

If you are paying privately, then you have the flexibility to use any agency or to use a private caregiver who is not associated with an agency. Be sure to take the time to decipher your parent's insurance policies *in advance* so that you have some idea about what will be covered. Your parent may also be eligible for public benefits, such as Medicaid and Veterans Administration programs. The National Council on Aging's website (www.benefitscheckup.org) is very helpful.

Who Will Provide the Care?

Many families are able to take care of their aging parents themselves. This is especially true when many Adult Children live nearby and can take turns or divide up the duties. If this is the case with your family, it is helpful to sit down before a crisis strikes to figure out who has the capabilities and the time to do which tasks. In this way, the entire family will function as a team and, if supplemental resources need to be hired, everyone on that team will understand why that needs to happen. Some families set up care contracts so that the family caregiver is paid by the parent for whom they are providing the care.

Last but not least, if your parent is able to provide input to this discussion, it is a good idea for them to do so. It is helpful to understand what your parent's desires are and, if practical, to honor at least some of them. This is not always possible, but when it is, it is an important step in the process of a smooth transition.

In any event, try to stay with what is before you *now*—the circumstances in which you find yourself at present. Be as generous and big hearted as you can be. You will never regret having been too kind to your aging parents when they are gone—but the reverse will not be true.

Prepare Yourself Mentally

Spend some time allowing yourself to adjust to reality. Children often hold on to the fantasy that their parents will live forever. When we are small, our parents are large and all-powerful. Then, for much of our childhood and adolescence, our parents are the epicenter of our world. They make our decisions, feed and shelter us, and act as the final arbiters of all that we do. As adults, their influence starts to fade, but we really only relegate them to the background of our lives—like a soundtrack faintly heard, but always there.

Then suddenly (it seems), it's time to consider what we will do when they are no longer there, and that realization can be painful and hard to accept. Give yourself time to think about this big change. Nothing can totally prepare you for that inevitable loss, but mental preparation can take some of the gut-wrenching shock away.

Ask yourself these questions to prepare to be ready to help your parents:

- Do I consider it my duty to help take care of my parents?

- Am I willing and able to do the hands-on caregiving, or am I more comfortable with arranging, coordinating, and/or paying for someone else to do this?

- How much extra time do I have, or could I divert from other activities, to help my parents?

- What disposable income am I able to set aside for their care each month?

- Am I willing to make room in my household to have my parent or parents move in with me?

- Are my teenagers willing and able to help with their grandparents' care?

- Should I consider asking my parents to move closer to me or consider moving closer to them?

- Am I able to fund such a move?

- Have I talked over with my spouse/partner what to do in the event his/her parents need help also?

- Am I willing to accompany my parents to doctor's visits and acquaint myself with their medical state and the care they require and might require in the future?

- Am I willing to do the research to find which home health resources, community centers, adult day centers, nursing homes, and hospitals might best suit my parents?

- Do I feel emotionally ready for this?

- Do I have a support structure for myself? How can I build one or enhance the one I have?

- What skills and resources do I bring to this role (time, money, specialized knowledge)?

- Which skills do I lack?

- Do I understand that my parent may be able to make his or her own decisions and that he or she is entitled to make "bad" ones, and that doesn't mean I get to take over?

When you have asked and answered these questions for yourself, you can either wait to be asked for help by your parents or let it be known, in a general way, that when your parents are ready to discuss their next steps in aging, you are ready and willing to have that conversation. Tell them that you have thought over how you may be able to help make their lives easier and that you stand ready to do so. Then, do what you said and sit back to wait. Never make your parents feel rushed, stupid, inadequate, or bullied.

Older Adults: Know When It's Time

You didn't reach the age of silver hair without having been through some tough times and coming out the other side still standing. You have bucked up, knuckled down, pitched in, shut up, spoken your piece, and maybe even said your prayers. What you probably haven't done much of is ask for help.

You've worked hard for your independence and you value it, but independence is not always the best course of action when dealing with aging. The time has come to rethink not going it alone and asking for help, but I know it will be a hard sell. Older Adults like you don't like asking for help and may even fear it.

You've been told your whole lives that winning, succeeding, and pushing on through adversity until you overcome it is the right way to go. You may have been told to never complain, that men don't cry, that not being able to stand alone on your own two feet is a type of weakness.

But there comes a time when we all need help—no man is really an island after all—and it takes a certain type of strength to reach past your pride to ask for what you need. You'll be surprised how quickly people offer to help once they are asked—even your own kids.

Showing vulnerability doesn't come easily, especially to you parents who have spent most of your life shielding your kids from harm and protecting and helping them, but start accepting the idea that now the shoe is on the other foot. That doesn't mean you are now consigned to sit back in a rocking chair keeping silent while all decisions are made for you, but it does mean you need to admit that you have to start the dialogue with your kids or caregivers so that you can help steer the course for this last journey.

In a recent survey, more than half of Adult Children caregivers said they worry constantly about their aging relatives. They worry that, in a misguided bid to maintain their independence, their parents are forgetting to eat meals or take medications—placing their very safety at risk.

Those stubborn Older Adults cited in the survey truly have a bad case of biting off their own nose to spite their face. Don't let this be you.

Realize When You Need Help and Learn to Ask for It

Here's where to start:

Acceptance: Older Adults, look in the mirror and stop wishing you were younger or thinner, and start accepting who you are today. You have a body that has served you well (more or less—after all, you are still ticking) for many years and your eyes have seen a thing or two. You are a sum of all those experiences, and each one has made you stronger and more full of character. Old age is no different. It is a new experience—a journey upon which you are now embarked—for better or worse. So commit to wringing out of this new experience every ounce of joy you can get. Aging is something that comes to us all, so make the most of it. Accept where you stand, and you'll stand in a better place.

Admission: So, like Popeye, once you get past the "I yam what I yam" attitude about aging, admit that your body can't—and never will again—perform like it did when you were younger. But that doesn't mean it doesn't perform at all. A one-hundred-year-old tennis player recently beat athletes decades younger than himself in the Florida Senior Games, and if you haven't seen the YouTube video of Johanna Quaas, an eighty-six-year-old former member of the East German Handball Team who still does a routine on the parallel bars that will quicken your pulse, it's worth viewing. But whether you are in great shape or not-so-great shape, admit the limitations of your body. (If you are looking for something to improve, remember your body has no spiritual limitations.) No matter how self-reliant you were in your youth, realize that you now need the help of others and that such help puts you more in touch with your fellow man.

You could struggle alone, but by sharing with others, especially your Adult Children, you get stronger and learn a little humility along the way. Others can now do some things better than you could in your younger days (playing basketball and putting on a roof are two things that spring immediately to mind), but that doesn't mean you are useless. You've got your brain, your wit, and your experience, and it is age's prerogative to give advice to the younger generations.

Willingness: You need the help. People (and your Adult Children among them) may notice you need the help but may be too fearful of injuring your pride to ask if they can help you. Request their help if you need it. Tap into the fact that we are all social animals and that most people are perfectly willing to lend a hand. Many people even feel blessed by the opportunity to serve others.

Evaluate: What type of help do you need? Start with the basics. Do you need help paying for your mortgage or rent? Or perhaps your utility bills are too high? How about your medications? Are they too expensive or complex? Could you use a hand driving, shopping, fixing your meals, dressing, bathing? Are you spending too much time alone and could use a little companionship, or maybe you just need to get out to lunch or a movie every now and again?

Consider These Areas Where You Might Need Help

Make a list and then prioritize it. Start with one thing at a time and ask for help. Here are a few categories to consider:

Finances: If you are an Older Adult, you are of a generation that was taught it was impolite to talk about money. Couple that with feelings of shame you may have for ending up without enough money (perhaps you mismanaged your financial affairs, perhaps they were mismanaged for you, perhaps you outlived your capital), and you have a recipe for disaster. You must bite the bullet and communicate your problem so the problem can be solved—with a little help, of course. Perhaps your Adult Children can help, or an appointment can be arranged with a CPA or daily money manager, but the first step is admitting there may be a problem. If there is no problem, good for you, but meeting with a financial advisor may optimize your gains and help you arrange trusts, charitable donations, and bequests for your kids and grandkids so you don't leave a mess behind when you die.

Utility Bills: These can often be negotiated downward—all it takes is a phone call from one of your kids (and a little patience on their part), or perhaps services can be combined (as in a phone/cable/Internet package). Or maybe green energy solutions can be implemented in your home. Solar panels or retrofit insulation or new fuel-less water or gas heaters might be able to save you lots of money. Ask your kids to arrange a consultation. (And always remember to check a contractor's references. Some make it a habit of bilking older people.)

Medications: Again your family members can do a service for you and contact the pharmacy first—perhaps a medication comes in a cheaper generic form that you are unaware of. Then get in touch with the pharmaceutical company itself to negotiate a cheaper price or sign up for one of the company's special programs. A call to your doctor might allow you to discontinue a medication, or maybe a new, less expensive, version has come out. Ask your Adult Child to search the Medicare website (www.medicare.gov), and research which medications are completely covered under your Medicare plan. If you don't understand your medications, an appointment can be set up for you with your pharmacist. Compile a list of your questions beforehand so you can discuss your questions and concerns. Ask if anything out there might affect you that you may not be aware of. Ask about any drug interactions with the prescriptions you take. Or ask how a new medicine might affect your glaucoma, diabetes, or blood pressure.

Driving/Shopping: Perhaps you can set up a schedule with one of your Adult Children that suits everybody's available free time where they could pick you up, take you shopping, and help carry in your purchases (a great reason to invite your teenage grandkids along). Or, failing that, maybe your helper can figure out the schedule of your community's ride-on transportation for seniors. Many communities sponsor this service for free, where they pick you up and drop you off at popular shopping locations on certain days. Get on the bus! No more worrying about parking or bad weather, and you can leave the driving to someone else (and perhaps also ditch those high auto insurance and maintenance rates).

Bathing/Dressing/Fixing Meals: The home health aide industry is booming. A few times a week, or even every day, a health aide will come to help you bathe and dress and cook a simple meal. Also, if you've got the funds, have your Adult Children investigate products—and contractors to install them—like step-in bathtubs and sill-less showers with built-in benches so that bathing yourself is safer. Also, Meals on Wheels is a community-sponsored service that brings complete hot meals to your door. Many volunteers will stop in for a cup of coffee and a bit of gossip, too. Or ask your kids to bake an extra casserole or meal for you on the weekends and set it in your freezer—with cooking instructions printed right on it—when they come to visit.

Companionship: Don't suffer in silence. If your kids get lost in their own over-busy lives and forget to visit or forget to let you see the grandkids, speak up! Being a martyr only breeds resentment. Request reinstituting the grand old tradition of Sunday dinner at Grandma's (even if everyone brings a dish), or ask that you go out to lunch together several times a month. If your grandkids are old enough to be independent, issue them an open invitation to visit your home with or without their parents. Seek ways to fit into your kids' busy lives. Ask to go to the grandkids' soccer games or to hang out at their house for an evening and watch TV. If you live far away, arrange visits to your family several times a year (have your kids help foot the bill if you are unable to do so yourself). Staying connected is part of staying alive.

Also, have your Adult Children investigate nearby community or senior centers. Get out of your mind the mental picture of a bunch of old codgers sitting around in wheelchairs. Hot poker games, sizzling line dancing, and lots of romantic opportunities are available among the like-minded Older Adults you will meet there. Join a book club or church group, volunteer at a soup kitchen, sign up for day bus trips to nearby places of interest, or take up a new sport. Expand your social circles and you'll extend your life. You'll also have a new set of people to rely on for help if you need it, and more sets of eyes keeping a watch over you.

Memory Loss: Misplacing your glasses or sometimes forgetting what you were looking for when you entered a room can most often result from mild age-related memory loss. Other reasons for memory loss can be a vitamin B12 deficiency, a side effect from new medication, depression over the loss of a spouse, or the emotional ramifications of having finally retired after working for a lifetime. Often the memory loss is mild and temporary. Try staying sharp with Sudoku or crossword puzzles, or play Words With Friends or Crusader Kings online. Have your grandchildren show you how.

Be sure to closely monitor your memory loss. If it is getting worse, go see your doctor. Liver, kidney, and thyroid problems can cause memory loss, as can blood clots and clinical depression. Most memory loss can be treated with medication and/or counseling, so don't immediately assume you have dementia. But if your trouble with remembering things persists, ask for help. A calendar—with alarms to remind you of events—can be programmed in a cell phone by one of your Adult Children to tell you where to be at a certain time or when to take a medication. Your kids can parcel out medications themselves into day-planner pill holders. An at-home monitoring system can be set up to make sure all the stove burners are off at night. A computer can set the temperature of your home day and night. Your teenage granddaughter can make beaded holders so you can wear your glasses around your neck.

Together the problem of age-related memory loss needn't prove an insurmountable problem. Just ask for help.

Asking for Help

Who to ask for help? Start with your Adult Children and other family members, but in a pinch, ask neighbors or acquaintances as well. No one person has to do everything for you. Split up the favors and ask several people to help with one task if need be. Check if your homeowner's association or neighborhood watch has an intranet (where emails are shared with the whole group) and put your name on the list. It always helps to have lots of people looking out for you.

Check with the local area agency on aging, which might offer certain support services like phone trees, transportation, shopping trips, and home meal delivery.

Be careful of asking strangers, like those you might meet online or on Craigslist. Ask for—or have your Adult Children ask for—references, and check them. A background check—another thing your computer-savvy family members can arrange online—is also vital for anyone you are designating as your helper or caregiver.

***How* to ask for help?** Make sure you have the person's attention when you ask for help. Interrupting the monologue about their troubles that they are pouring on to you (a lifelong habit for some kids) to ask for help is not the optimum time. Wait for a pause, or even set an appointment with time to have a discussion. Today's over-scheduled people appreciate the thoughtfulness you show by trying to accommodate their schedules.

Don't beat around the bush. Now that you know exactly what you need help with (and please keep abreast of changes in your own situation) and who you'll approach, be direct. Ask specifically: "I need a ride to go shopping one weekday morning or afternoon every week. Are you available to help me?" If you receive a yes, then follow up with, "What day and time works with your schedule?"

Realize that anyone you ask has the right to say no. That doesn't mean it's easy to hear, but sticks and stones really won't break your bones. Don't get resentful about it. Perhaps they really do have a good reason to refuse you at the moment. Don't let that stop you from asking later and/or asking someone else.

Don't feel too beholden. Sure, they are doing you a favor now, but you've done plenty of favors for them in the past and, no doubt, will in the future. But do be sure to thank them for their help—every time—and with courtesy. The Golden Rule is still in effect, even if it's with your own children. You really do want them to treat you the way you treat them.

Adult Children: Pay Attention to Signs

As for you Adult Children, you shouldn't just sit back and wait to see if your parents ask for help; you've got to pay attention.

If you are the Adult Child of aging parents, you have probably asked yourself how you would know if they needed more help. If you live many miles away from your parents and don't see them very often, you may worry about this every day. If you aren't worried yet, stick around. You will be in the thick of it one day when "something" happens. If that "something" hasn't hit you personally yet, then I'll bet you have friends or colleagues who are dealing with it right now, up close and personal. There's that moment when you just know that it's all about to become *your* responsibility.

Since dealing with a crisis is always more stressful than planning ahead, it pays to take some time to figure out if Mom or Dad can use some help; then make sure they get it. The best way to do this is to go and see the situation yourself. You need to look for signs about what Mom or Dad are doing *and* for the things they are not doing.

At first, these signs might be subtle. It's easy to ignore them. Who wants to acknowledge that your parents are getting older? Who wants to confront the reality that they aren't going to live forever? Do yourself a favor and be honest with yourself and your siblings about what you see, and then make the commitment to get involved.

Signs Your Parents Need Help

Here are some questions to help you know what to look for in assessing your Older Adult's needs:

Health:
- Has your parent lost weight?
- When you visit, do you find an empty refrigerator and the pantry in pretty much the same state that you last saw it, with now-expired canned goods?
- Have there been recent emergency room visits?
- Is Mom's vision failing?
- Is Dad reluctant to drive at night although he used to think nothing of it?
- Do you have to repeat yourself often?

Safety:

- Has your parent told you about falling?

- Do you notice any unexplained bruises on their body?

- Did they mention they left the teakettle on all night? Or did they leave the cat out?

- Has your Mom or Dad become lost?

Mobility:

- Is your Older Adult having trouble negotiating a curb on the street?

- Do you notice your Mom or Dad can't climb the stairs to their bedroom?

- Is Dad having trouble bending over to pick up something he has dropped?

- Is Mom struggling to make her bed?

- Is the shower or bathtub dirty at your parent's house because they can't reach to clean it?

Financial:

- Have you noticed a pile of unopened mail?

- Are bills being paid late or never?

- Are some bills being paid twice?

- Are donations to charities showing up on their bank statements that you've never heard your parent talk about?

Household:

- Does your parent's home look different than it has in the past?

- Is there a lot of clutter?

- Does the front yard look unkempt?

- Is garbage piling up?

- Is the house being properly maintained?

- Is it clean?

Confusion or irritability:

- Does your Dad forget to call you every Monday evening like he has done for years?

- When you talk to Mom, is she more impatient than usual?

- Do your parents easily lose track of things or time?

Social:

- Has your Mom stopped participating in the knitting circle or volunteering as a reading mentor at the local school?

- Has Dad stopped taking care of the garden, even though that has been his pride and joy for as long as you can remember?

If you can answer yes to more than two or three of these questions above, it's a good bet that your parent needs more help. If you don't already have a Life Transition Plan in place, now would be a good time to create one. If you do already have such a plan, now is the time to start implementing what you planned for. Many excellent resources are available to assist you as you do. (See resources in the back of this book.)

Just a word of caution: Proceed with a light touch. According to Mara Osis, the founder of Elderwise, Inc., a big part of the problem between Older Adults and their Adult Children is children who feel the overwhelming need to "parent their parents."

"You are not your parent's parent. You need to see each other as two adults of different generations trying to work out a problem," stresses Osis. "Boomers are used to being very much in control of everything in their lives and being able to effect change, so when they see that they are getting pushback from their parents, it's an unfamiliar role. Sometimes the Adult Child creates their own problems by saying, 'I'm just going to fix Mom and Dad and their situation because the solution is very simple from my point of view.'"

Remember, it's not that simple from your parent's point of view. Losing their independence and often much of their privacy is a huge thing (walk a mile in their shoes and think how you would feel), and you need to be cognizant of their feelings.

Be sensitive and go slowly. Perhaps your mother or father will accept a home health aide for a couple of hours once a week at first and later (slowly), after they realize the person can be trusted and is a help, they may agree to a few more hours a week or maybe another few days of help. But realize you are asking them to accept a stranger in their home, so allow them time to get used to the idea. Always talk every decision over with your parents before making a *mutual* decision (no emotional bullying!) and allow them to feel in control of their own lives. It can't hurt to reassure them you are not trying to turn them out of their home. The nursing home doesn't loom (unless it does—don't lie, or the trust between you will be irrevocably broken). Help, from you and professionals, can ease their burdens in their own home.

And try to be patient. Your parents didn't kill you during your adolescence when you were often impossible. Now that shoe is on your foot.

It might help you to understand another point made by Kübler-Ross—that what aging means to your parents is that time passing so swiftly means there is less time for your parents to reinvent themselves. The *limitless* possibilities available in the future that one has when one is younger are now *limited*. The Older Adult can now see the end of their life (and it must seem like it is rushing toward them). Kübler-Ross calls each realization of this encroaching end a series of "mini-deaths," and death, in any form, is a scary thing to face. So give your Older Adults a break and time to adjust.

Choose the Right Helpers

Whether you are an Older Adult yourself or an Adult Child, you probably know an Older Adult who is all alone. Perhaps this person is single, widowed, or divorced. Maybe he never had children or is estranged from them. Possibly her siblings have all passed away. Maybe her husband suffers from dementia. Whatever the reason, it is often difficult for individuals in this situation to decide who to appoint as the agent holding their power of attorney or as health care surrogate in the event they can't make decisions for themselves. All too often, these folks simply avoid completing appropriate documents and then are stuck if they lose capacity.

In other cases, plenty of family members could take over if needed, but these folks live far away or are fully committed to their own professional and personal responsibilities. Often, family is willing but not able to help. That is, they would not be a good choice to step into the needed shoes due to the lack of appropriate skills or the potential for conflict with siblings or other relatives. Perhaps a wife is concerned about her husband being the successor trustee to her trust because he is a wonderful artist but not interested in finance. Maybe a parent is concerned that his daughter has a substance abuse issue.

Choosing a Fiduciary

A **fiduciary** is a person who assumes responsibility for a position of trust. Fiduciaries can serve by court appointment or by private agreement. Court-appointed fiduciaries are known as guardians or conservators. In addition, executors (known as personal representatives in some areas) are appointed by the court, typically based on the directions you provided in your will. Fiduciaries can also serve by agreement as daily money managers, trustees, representative payees, or as agents under financial or health care powers of attorney. A fiduciary can be an individual or a corporate entity like a bank's trust department.

But wherever they come from, fiduciaries share one invaluable asset—they hold a position of trust. Restrictions vary by state regarding who may serve as a professional agent or trustee. The responsibility of the fiduciary, in these situations, is to carry out the instructions in any written documents (e.g., trust, power of attorney, Advance Health Care Directive, etc.) or, where appropriate and allowed by law, to use substituted judgment or the best-interest standards to handle the incapacitated person's affairs.

Professional fiduciary services range from those that are less restrictive to those that essentially have the professional step-into-the-shoes of an incapacitated person. It is almost always best to start with the least restrictive alternative, allowing the Older Adult to retain as much independence and decision-making authority as possible.

The most informal fiduciary is, obviously, a spouse, Adult Child, or other family member who can help with management of the Older Adult's financial or health affairs. Sometimes appointing a friend makes sense.

Next up the ladder would be to choose a professional fiduciary. The least restrictive choice here would be to choose a daily money manager (DMM) whose services can be retained by either you, the Older Adult, or the Adult Child acting in their parent's stead. DMMs handle day-to-day finances and can be retained by the person who needs the assistance or by a family member serving as agent under a power of attorney. DMMs often serve as the eyes, ears, hands, and feet of the Older Adult, allowing them to retain maximum control of their own affairs. Sometimes an Older Adult will retain the DMM while their Adult Child will pay the fees.

Next along the continuum are professional fiduciaries who serve as agents under a power of attorney or health care surrogate document, or who serve as trustee under a trust. These arrangements must be made in writing while an Older Adult has the legal capacity to make such an appointment, even if the services of the fiduciary will not begin until the individual lacks capacity. An attorney should always be engaged to draft the appointing documents.

The most restrictive fiduciary arrangement is **guardianship,** known as "conservatorship" in some states. Guardianship is a legal tool to provide management for the financial and/or personal affairs of individuals deemed by the court to be physically or mentally inca-pacitated. The guardian or conservator is legally appointed to manage the incapacitated person's (or ward's) property and/or person. The court oversees all aspects of the guardianship. Avoid court-appointed fiduciaries whenever possible, as they can be both expensive and invasive. Make sure you (or, if you are the Adult Child helping make such arrangements, your parents) have written legal appointments while you still have the capacity to appoint fiduciaries of your choosing. Include legal backups, in case the person you choose can't or won't serve when the time comes, to inoculate yourself from ever facing a court-appointed fiduciary—saving both money and trouble for you and your family.

As I have pointed out throughout this book, the best way to ensure that an Older Adult's affairs will be handled the way you prefer is to work with an attorney to draft appropriate documents and then keep them up-to-date. In the event you find yourself or a loved one in a situation where this hasn't been done or where those named in the documents are unable or unwilling to serve, it is wise to consider engaging a professional fiduciary.

Attributes to Look for in a Fiduciary

Whether you are searching for a family member, friend, or professional to appoint as your fiduciary, I suggest choosing people who possess the five "A" attributes:

Able: Has the skills and knowledge to do the job, exhibits attention to detail, and is resourceful.

Affable: Possesses good people skills, is easy to get along with, and is able to deal with stress.

Available: Is willing to invest the time, is geographically proximate or able to travel, and has the right attitude.

Aboveboard: Is trustworthy, straightforward, honest, and professional.

Anchored: Is stable and has a level head.

Once you have chosen the fiduciary, you must also be sure to not tie their hands. Reveal what they need to know and hold nothing back. Empower them to make judgments for you, should you be unable to make them yourself. Start searching *now* so you will be prepared for that day in the future when the fiduciary's invaluable skills are needed.

Understanding Elder Law

Many Older Adults or their Adult Children can benefit from consulting an attorney who specializes in "elder law" early in the process of planning for later life and possible incapacity. As with so many other aspects of planning, the earlier you do so, the more options you have. I'm often asked why the longstanding family attorney cannot provide this advice. Sometimes they can, depending on their expertise and the particular situation. However, often it is best to consult with an expert who is current on the many nuances within this field.

So what exactly is an "elder law" attorney, and where do you find one? Elder law encompasses many different fields of law, and its practitioners specialize in applying the law to the needs of Older Adults. Most elder law specialists employ a holistic approach that considers the many issues faced by those who are aging, including those related to housing, finances, health, and securing and coordinating private and public resources to finance long-term care. In addition, they typically are concerned with estate planning, minimizing estate tax, and planning for incapacity. Some elder law specialists have additional expertise in guardianship and/or conservatorship matters, asset protection, probate, estate administration, or elder abuse and fraud recovery. A further advantage of working with an elder law specialist is that he or she will be well connected with a network of elder care professionals who can be helpful to you.

As you can probably imagine, elder law specialists must be up-to-date and well versed in a variety of technical disciplines. For example, they must be aware of the many nuances associated with planning for public benefits to pay for long-term care, such as Medicaid and Veterans Administration Aid and Attendance benefits. At the same time, they should have a good understanding of the availability and cost of private long-term-care insurance and how such policies do (or do not) support a particular individual's estate-planning goals.

The best place to find an elder law attorney is through the National Academy of Elder Law Attorneys (NAELA) at www.naela.org. Members of NAELA are experienced and trained in working with the legal problems of aging and have agreed to adopt aspirational standards of professional practice as a condition of membership in the organization.

Create a Life Transition Plan

Whether you are an Older Adult making arrangements for your own final chapters of life or an Adult Child of aging parents trying to ease your parents' (and your own) transition, I advocate creating a Life Transition Plan.

Older Adults: You will be able to use this plan to organize all of your affairs in an "owner's manual" to make it easy for your Adult Children (and even your own spouse) to carry on when you can no longer do so for yourself.

Adult Children: Such a plan will give you great peace of mind by knowing who is responsible for the many tasks that will crop up immediately when there is an emergency. You will be certain of interim decisions your parents have made (and documented) about situations such as where they plan to live if they can no longer live alone, and important end-of-life matters such as how they feel about hospice care and organ donation. The Life Transition Plan will allow you to step into your loved one's shoes when making decisions for them (or that impact them), using the principle of "substituted judgment"—where you act on what your parent has specified he or she wants as opposed to guessing at what you think is "in their best interest."

With everyone in the family's responsibilities decided beforehand and all documents in one place and at hand, when an emergency hits, everyone swings into action, and the designated health care surrogate grabs the document folder and runs. Nothing gets forgotten, overlooked, or misplaced. You may all rest assured that the Older Adult's decisions and interests are clear and that the Adult Child is prepared to carry out those decisions. On both sides of the equation, you'll be as ready as you can be. This book's appendix provides an outline of what should be included in a Life Transition Plan. You can also visit www.FacingtheFinish.com and download the most up-to-date version that I use with my clients.

In my practice, I've worked with many clients to prepare their Life Transition Plans, and, over the years, I've noticed often positive, but unintended, consequences of creating such a plan.

One of my clients, Rhonda, is a long-distance caregiver for her mother and had engaged me to work with her on getting both her own and her mother's affairs in order. As part of the process, we documented the family's biographical details. Rhonda wasn't sure where one of her siblings was born, so she asked her Mom, who suffers from memory impairment. Mom couldn't remember either, and hadn't spoken with that child in many years. Rhonda checked with another sibling who said, "Why doesn't Mom just call [the sister in question] and ask her?" In fact, that's what happened, and now the two are talking again for the first time in many years.

David, another client, took ill and was rushed to the hospital during the weeks that we were working on his Life Transition Plan. Since he didn't have a spouse, sibling, or children, he found the entire episode to be a huge wake-up call. As a result, David and a group of friends in a similar situation got together to talk about how they could support one another as they aged. From these discussions, they've created a phone tree so that each of them has one person who they are supposed to call daily. If that call doesn't arrive, the person who was supposed to receive it calls the next person in the tree, and the two of them work together to try to find out if something has happened to their friend. They've created a "family" for themselves who will help them through any transition.

Another Older Adult couple I worked with finally completed their Life Transition Plan and decided it would be a good idea to convene a family meeting with their Adult Children to share it. Mr. and Mrs. Clark decided to make this event into a fun family vacation and took their kids and grandkids on a weeklong cruise. Their only stipulation was that, during the cruise, the Older Adults and the Adult Children would take a couple of hours to have a very important family discussion. Not only were the Clarks' Adult Children pleased to learn of the actions their parents had taken to make things easier for the kids in the future, but the extended family had a wonderful time together and they've decided to make it an annual tradition.

Naturally, for every happy ending surrounding a comprehensive Life Transition Plan is a sadder story for another Older Adult and his or her family who didn't create one.

One of her close friends referred Mrs. Babbitt, an eighty-year-old woman, because she was concerned that her affairs were not in order. Mr. Babbitt, slightly older than his wife, had recently suffered a fall, leading to a series of medical problems from which he was not expected to recover. This couple had no children and only a few living relatives on the husband's side. After canceling several appointments, Mrs. Babbitt and I were able to meet on a Sunday morning. It very quickly became obvious that the meeting was long overdue, as mail and papers piled up on every surface.

The immediate concern from Mrs. Babbitt's point of view was to know which bills she had to pay and what money she had to pay them with. In other words, we needed to determine her assets and liabilities and her income and expenses, since her husband had always handled these matters.

While this was important, I was more concerned with determining who needed to be contacted if (when) something happened to Mrs. Babbitt or her husband, whether the couple had valid end-of-life documents and where to find the originals, and what their after-death wishes were and whether they had prearranged or prepaid for these arrangements.

While I was working with Mrs. Babbitt on these matters, and before we had made much headway, the phone rang. It was the nursing home calling to inform Mrs. Babbitt that her husband had passed away.

This touched off a whirlwind of activity.

At Mrs. Babbitt's request, I remained in the home searching for documents while a neighbor took her to the nursing home. While there, Mrs. Babbitt herself fell ill and was transported to the hospital where she was admitted.

Now the trouble truly began.

While I was able to find certain documents like Mr. Babbitt's will, I could not find a valid health care surrogate appointment or power of attorney document naming anyone other than Mrs. Babbitt's deceased husband to make financial and medical decisions for her. I also couldn't locate any prearrangements or evidence of prepayment for a funeral.

Fortunately, the attorney who had drafted the husband's will ten years earlier had a working phone number, so I was able to leave a voice mail at his office alerting him to Mr. Babbitt's death. I was also able to contact the few remaining members of Mr. Babbitt's family, since I had been able to get their names from Mrs. Babbitt before she received the fateful call. Armed with the names, I was able to locate contact information in the couple's phone book, which I located buried under a mountain of junk mail on the kitchen table.

Here's where the situation became really challenging.

Mrs. Babbitt was in the hospital, unable to make decisions for her own care or her husband's funeral and burial. Mr. Babbitt's family wanted to proceed with laying him to rest, not knowing how long it would be before Mrs. Babbitt could act on her own.

However, in the absence of Mrs. Babbitt's power of attorney and health care proxy documents naming someone other than her husband as her legal representative, the funeral home would not allow arrangements to proceed.

The only option was for Mr. Babbitt's family to petition the court for the appointment of a guardian for Mrs. Babbitt. The guardian would then be able to proceed with arrangements.

My part of the job was done and I had to remove myself from the case, but I did so with a heavy heart.

The sad part about this real-life case study is that it could have been avoided. If only the couple had prearranged and/or prepaid for their funerals. If only there had been valid end-of-life documents in place for the wife. If only the wife hadn't cancelled those appointments with me and we'd started the process sooner.

"If only"—two little words that can mean the difference between a peaceful transition at the end of life or chaos that can only accentuate the pain. Please begin your planning today. You have no guarantees about tomorrow.

Have the Talk

Sometimes it seems easier to talk to strangers than our own families, and when the topic is the all-important one about how the family is going to face the aging and inevitable death of the parents, the silence can become deafening. If you've created your Life Transition Plan, it is time to communicate that plan—or at least its existence—to your family. If you are an Adult Child and you don't think your parents have done any planning, what do you do?

No one knows how to take the first step.

One of the questions I'm asked most often by Adult Children is, "How do I start talking with my aging parent about the end of their life?" On the flip side, I have been asked by Older Adults, "How do I talk with my Adult Children about the inevitable?" Why then, when the subject is much on everyone's mind, is it so hard for so many families to have this important conversation?

For some, death and dying is a taboo subject. We just don't talk about it, even though we all know intellectually that it will happen to each of us.

In other cases, it's talking about money that's taboo. People of a certain generation were raised to keep their financial life a secret even from those closest to them. Many Adult Children are afraid to bring up the subject because they fear that their parent will assume that they are just after the inheritance.

Still others worry that they will depress their parents by raising the topic. On the other side of the coin, many parents don't want to burden their children or think that it will upset them if the parent brings up his or her own end-of-life wishes.

From either vantage point, having "the talk" isn't the easiest thing to do, but there are ways to approach it that get the job done with as little stress as possible. So, for all of you Adult Children and Older Adult parents, here are some guidelines to get you started. Beware! Since I'm writing for both sides of the equation, I'll be letting you all in on the dirty little secrets the other generation might use on you.

My first suggestion is to simply encourage you to talk to each other.

Adult Children, ask your parents about their plans and preferences for where and how they want to age and the documents and resources they've put in place to allow them to do so. Since communication is a two-way street, feel free to express your opinions about your parents' future.

Older Adults, express your preferences clearly and share any information your Adult Children need to have. Clear, honest, and thorough discussions are the best and allow much less room for misunderstandings.

However, if that's just too difficult for your family or it's not the way things are approached in your family group, then you might have to resort to some more roundabout approaches. While it is best for this conversation to be open and straightforward, I've been doing this long enough to know that's often just not reality.

Adult Children, one way to start the conversation with your parent might be to ask for advice. If you are doing some of your own planning about your *own* future, then you can ask for your Mom or Dad's input and suggestions. As a part of this conversation you will have a natural opportunity to ask what plans they have made for themselves.

Perhaps you've seen your friends struggle with the role of caregiver or financial supporter and you'd like to avoid some of that stress. Talk with your parent about what your friends are experiencing. Ask them if they have any suggestions that you can pass along, and then be sure that you make note of those suggestions for future reference.

For you Older Adults, sit your kids down and share the plans you've made. If you have your affairs in order, let them know this. If you don't feel comfortable sharing all of the details, at least let your Adult Children know where to find such documents and information in the event you are incapacitated or die suddenly.

If you don't know how to start the conversation, consider asking someone from outside the family to facilitate. I've found that it is much easier for many families when I, as a third party, ask the tough questions and make notes regarding the answers, than when they attempt to do this on their own. You will likely find that your Adult Children thank you for preparing them for their future responsibilities.

As the old saying goes, the only sure thing is death and taxes. The earlier you take on the task of talking with your family about these matters, the less likely the topic will become the elephant in the room every time you get together. When the day comes that you need more help with day-to-day activities, your Adult Children will have an idea about what you'd like to have happen, and they will better understand the resources you have available to make things turn out the way you'd like.

2

DEALING WITH FAMILY

*TWO SIXTY-SOMETHING SISTERS agree on one thing: They want to take the best possible care of their ninety-two-year-old mother who suffers from Alzheimer's disease. But that's the problem! It's the **only** thing they agree about. One sister wants to hire caregivers, while the other feels that Mother should be cared for by her family. One sister wants their mother to have aggressive treatment for her newly diagnosed cancer, while the other feels that only comfort care should be provided. Of course, the subject of all this angst, their mother, cannot contribute to the conversation because of her dementia, and she never discussed such matters with her daughters when she was well.*

I Don't Want to Be a Burden

Aging parents seem to come in two different types—those who are determined never to be a burden on their families and who make appropriate plans for their changing situation, and those who are in denial about the reality of their changing condition and make no arrangements at all.

One would think that the first type of Older Adult makes things easier on their families, and on the surface, this is certainly true, but let's look a little deeper to detect an often overlooked part of the dynamic between Older Adult parents and their Adult Children.

The parent who fears being a burden is the parent who plans ahead for his or her old age. He usually has his affairs in order and has written a will and designated a power of attorney and a health care proxy. She might even have one place where all of her important papers are kept, including a list of her medications, doctors' contact information, and other important phone numbers that will be needed should she become incapacitated. This Older Adult Parent has often entered into an arrangement for a prepaid funeral and might have purchased long-term-care insurance or moved to a continuing-care retirement community. This parent has typically taken much of the financial and decision-making burden off of her children, and most Adult Children will agree that this is appreciated.

But is it possible that the Older Adult who is determined never to become a burden has actually cheated herself out of some mean-ingful experiences with her kids? Might this mother and grandmother one day regret that she has done such a good job putting all the plans in place that her kids don't have "reasons" to come around, and so they don't come around very often? Is there a positive benefit that comes from Adult Children participating in their Older Adult parent's later years?

Like so much else in life, it's all about balance. Perhaps the ideal situation is when the Older Adult parents have put the pieces in place so that they won't be a financial burden, but they have also shared with their Adult Children the details about the kind of life they hope to lead when their circumstances change. They have even allowed their Adult Children to help them think through some of these potentially difficult situations in advance. Later, when their health or memory begin to fail, the time you Adult Children spend with Mom or Dad can be about keeping them company, making them comfortable, and allowing them to participate (to the extent that they can) in your life and your children's lives.

Adult Children, consider this: Don't let your parents do such a good job of not being a "burden" to you that you forget that they need you on an emotional level. Don't thank them for all of their planning and preparation by being a stranger. Thank them for making your caregiving job so much easier through your presence and emotional support.

Denial Gets in the Way

What to do if one family member, be it Older Adult or Adult Child, just won't participate in these vital discussions?

Recently, my client Sam asked me to help him develop a strategy for dealing with his adult daughter Annie, who simply refused to engage in the transition planning process he was trying so hard to complete.

Sam was a model of planning. He had carefully gathered all of his important documents and information into one place, and we had worked together to assemble his Life Transition Plan. We had worked through tough questions, like where he would like to age if he could no longer care for himself and how he would pay for the care he needed. We were down to the home stretch—bringing his only child, Annie, into the conversation.

And that's where we came to a screeching halt.

Annie refused to participate in the conversation. First, Sam tried taking his daughter out for dinner when she was in town visiting him and discussing the process he had undertaken and his wishes in that informal setting.

She said, "Dad, why are you telling me this? Are you sick?"

When Sam said that he was not ill but just wanted her to be prepared, Annie said that she was superstitious and didn't want to talk about the subject for fear that something bad would happen to Sam.

So we went to Plan B—a family meeting. Sam told Annie that the two of them were coming to meet with me so that I could explain the process we had undertaken and let her know that there were resources available to her when the time came. Sam and I had crafted an agenda for the meeting and agreed that I would facilitate. Annie did accompany Sam to the meeting but sat with her arms crossed and didn't say a word other than "hello" the whole time. Needless to say, this session was more of a lecture than a conversation.

Annie went back to her home while her father and I brainstormed about next steps. On the one hand, we had accomplished the goal of making Annie aware that the tools she would one day need were available to her. She knew where they were located, and had met me and had my contact information. However, we had not accomplished the very important objective of father and daughter having the important (and often difficult) conversation about his wishes in the event he could no longer make decisions or care for himself.

It seemed that Sam had three tasks on his "to-do" list: Put his thoughts in writing and send them to his daughter, and also include them in his Life Transition Plan; attempt another conversation with Annie at a point when she might be more receptive; and consider naming someone else as either the primary or backup person to make decisions for him in his end-of-life documents, since it seemed that Annie might be unwilling to step into this role.

It is absolutely crucial that you choose people to act on your behalf who are both willing and able to step into your shoes. In this case, Annie was certainly able to do so, but it was not at all clear that she was willing.

Entrusting another person to be your agent for decision making in the event of your incapacity is a big deal. They need not only the facts and figures that will allow them to do their best for you, but also the knowledge of what you would have done if you could have done it for yourself. This requires communication, and a potential agent who is not ready to engage in that communication is very likely not "the one."

Breaking up such a logjam or helping pull together the family meeting both may be facilitated by working with a life transition coach.

I am often asked to describe the benefits derived by Adult Children of aging parents when they elect to work with just such a professional. Such coaches can prove invaluable during a health crisis, but can also prove to be a great asset when Older Adults want to communicate life transition decisions they've made to their Adult Children.

They are also valuable to Adult Children, who may be at different levels of acceptance when it comes to their parents' aging, when they are called together as a group to listen to (and accept) those decisions.

But perhaps the best way to answer the questions about the value of a life transition coach is by using an example from my practice.

Jennifer, an Adult Child, found me by reading an article I had published about life transition coaching in a senior resource publication. I was in a meeting when she initially called, so she left a voice mail message that began, "I really need help, and I need it fast!"

When I called Jennifer back, she told me that she was one of four siblings and the long-distance caregiver for her mother, Nancy. Nancy lived in Southwest Florida and Jennifer lived in Michigan. Jennifer's siblings were scattered across several states, but none lived near their mother.

Nancy was eighty-four and suffered from memory loss and some confusion. She was otherwise in good health and remained fairly active. Ever since her husband died six years ago, Nancy had been managing by herself. She continued to live in the condo that she and Jennifer's dad moved to in 1995 when they first relocated to Florida and, until recently, had maintained an active social life with her friends from church.

Jennifer usually visited Nancy a few times each year. Her siblings visited less frequently. Several months ago when Jennifer came to visit, she noticed that Nancy seemed confused and somewhat withdrawn. Jennifer accompanied Nancy to her doctor's appointment and learned that Nancy's condition was considered to be "age-related memory impairment." It was explained that this was a "normal part of aging" and that "there was nothing to worry about." Nancy assured Jennifer that she was fine and still able to manage on her own.

Several weeks after returning home from that visit, Jennifer called Nancy for her regular check-in and found her agitated and confused.

She became extremely concerned and called Nancy's neighbor, asking her to check on Nancy. When the neighbor called back, she told Jennifer that Nancy seemed okay. The next morning, Nancy didn't answer the phone when Jennifer called, and she didn't respond to a knock on the door by the same neighbor who Jennifer had called previously. Fearing the worst, Jennifer called 911, who responded and took Nancy to the hospital. It turned out that Nancy had suffered a stroke.

Jennifer immediately jumped on a plane to come to be with Nancy. She had taken on the role of primary long-distance caregiver by default. The family had never discussed Nancy's situation as a group.

That's when Jennifer called me. She knew that she had to return home to her job and her family within a few days and was in a panic about what would happen to Nancy when she did. At the same time, she was getting frustrated trying to convey information to her siblings, each of whom offered lots of input, but none of whom offered to come and take over so that she could get home. Jennifer was under extreme stress.

The first thing I helped Jennifer do was to get organized and get her siblings involved. We started by making a list of all the things that had to be done, the documents that had to be found, the bills that had to be paid, and the decisions that had to be made. We then scheduled a conference call among the siblings, which I facilitated. The stated objective of the conference call was to identify Nancy's needs and the resources that could be provided by the family working as a team. These resources included knowledge, time, and money. Once we had an exhaustive list of what needed to be accomplished, we matched the available resources. By the end of that first call, each of the siblings had their assignments and was committed to working as a team. Within a few hours of Jennifer's initial call to me, she was feeling as though she was back in control of the situation and didn't need to carry the burden on her own shoulders.

Over the next several days, I worked with each of the siblings on their piece of the puzzle, making sure that everyone stayed on track.

The family had one very important decision to make, and that was where Nancy was going to go upon her discharge from the hospital. We worked with a geriatric care manager to identify the options and concluded that she could return to her condo safely as long as she had appropriate in-home care.

Nancy's family then needed to address whether this was a sustainable solution given the financial realities, and each sibling arranged to come visit Nancy at the same time within the next month. During that visit, they planned to go and look at several assisted living facilities and determine if that might be a better solution for Nancy.

In preparation for their visit, Jennifer asked me to help her identify several alternative facilities and to gather all of the necessary information so she could share that with her siblings before their visit and make the most of their time together.

Well done on the part of Jennifer and her siblings, particularly as a last-minute response to an emergency situation, but now let's look at the situation from Nancy's point-of-view as the Older Adult.

It is easy to let things drift in life. Once Nancy and her husband had bought the Florida condo and were settled in their new life—surrounded by friends, church activities, and a supportive community—there really was no reason for immediate concern about the future, or so they thought. But life is made up of a collection of curveballs, and nothing remains static for long.

When Nancy's husband died, the transition to widowhood was wrenching, but she was able to stay in the condo, so her living space remained the same. Some social changes became apparent as friends of the couple drifted away, as people do when they were friends with the "unit," as opposed to the individual, and it was harder for Nancy to stay as involved as she had been when her husband was alive.

But the one thing Nancy hadn't counted on, and had trouble accepting when it did happen, was the memory impairment. It is hard to admit when you might be suffering from something other than simply age-related memory issues and, if such a condition rapidly progresses, it may be impossible for you, the Older Adult, to first recognize and then make good decisions about what should be done for yourself as your condition worsens.

In both instances—those of Jennifer and her siblings as Adult Children and for Nancy as the Older Adult—pre-planning for such contingencies would have been helpful. But, the reality is that most people avoid thinking about the inevitable issues that will arise as they themselves or their parents age.

Either as the Older Adult or the Adult Child, *before* you find yourself in the midst of a crisis is the time to reach out to a life transition coach. They can be a great help.

Family Challenges

As an Adult Child, you can probably remember back to the time when you and your siblings were all children under your parents' roof. During that time, you assumed roles and settled into certain patterns within your family.

For example, in a family of three brothers, there was the elder who had his act together, the middle one who was the clown, and the youngest who was Mom's favorite. (Admit it, Mom—he really *was* your favorite.)

Why should it be a surprise that now, forty years later, these three brothers are dealing with their aging mother and the same patterns play out?

The oldest brother, the "responsible" one, takes charge of the nuts and bolts, and at some point he probably feels put upon because his siblings aren't helping enough. The middle brother is always there for the fun and happy times, but he seems to disappear when the going gets tough. He might even feel, though it's his actions that precipitated it, that he's not being kept in the loop. And the baby, Mom's favorite, announces that he is coming to visit, and Mom talks about nothing else for weeks before and after. It's likely that he's unaware that both of his brothers are annoyed with—and a little jealous of— him. This vignette is an example of siblings who, despite the adults they have become, revert to their childhood roles when confronting the aging of their parent and of a parent who sees these adults only as her "children."

Besides historical family patterns, gender roles also often come to the forefront in family caregiving situations. Why is it that women so often take on the caregiver role for the Older Adult? Is it because they expect it of themselves or because their families expect it of them? Is there truth to the old saying that, "A daughter is a daughter for all of her life, but a son's a son until he takes a wife?" Is it because caregiving is often still considered to be "women's work"? While many families certainly have men who play leading and significant roles in the care of their parents, many surveys show that sons most often write checks while daughters (and daughters-in-law) provide more of the hands-on caregiving. Perhaps consciously or unconsciously, the Older Adult assumes that men are the moneymakers and women the homemakers. It was often so in the Older Adult's generation.

Whatever might be the situation in your family, it helps to be aware of gender roles and to think about whether you as an Older Adult are making unfair gender assumptions or if you, as Adult Children, are falling into the default positions of childhood roles, as opposed to really sharing the load of helping to care for your parents.

Proximity and distance also become factors in the family care-giving dynamic and deciding "what to do about Mom and Dad." In many families, one sibling lives near their parents while others don't.

The one who is nearby will tend to see the parents more often and may not notice subtle changes in a parent's ability or behavior. Then, one of the out-of-town Adult Children comes for a visit and begins pointing these things out. If not handled with care, the in-town sibling might take this personally, thinking that the sibling is saying that he or she isn't doing a good enough job of looking after Mom and Dad. At the same time, the distant siblings might take it for granted that their in-town brother or sister is willing to take on the caregiver role, leaving that "caregiver by default" to feel taken advantage of, as though they had no choice in the matter.

Complicating the family dynamic, each of us has different needs.

The Older Adult needs to be cared for, and who better to assume the responsibility than their own children? Perhaps the Older Adult cared for their own parents and just *assumes* their children will benefit from their examples and naturally take on the task now that they are aging. They might not understand, and perhaps be terribly hurt, if their Adult Child finds themselves unable or unwilling to make such a choice.

When it comes to the Adult Children, all may not be as it first appears.

We all know someone who needs to be needed. Or worse, someone who may come to enjoy what they see as their martyrdom in accepting the caregiving role. Perhaps they use this "duty" to avoid addressing problems in their own life. This person will often have great difficulty when their caregiver role naturally comes to an end with the death of a parent. Maybe they devoted themselves solely to the care of the Older Adult and built no life for themselves. In fact, maybe their siblings let them do so, with only a twinge of guilt.

Or what about the personality type who needs to fight fires, and who might even set a few in order to be able to save the day? Without even realizing it, this person might make the caregiving more complicated than it needs to be. Much end-of-life drama created by just such a person is played out in nursing homes and hospital corridors every day.

What about "Diamond Jim," the brother who needs to be seen as the Big Spender? This person is likely to feel that money is the answer to every caregiving challenge and will look for opportunities to show how generous he is. When that generosity isn't sufficiently acknowledged, he's likely to get angry, take his ball (and bankroll), and go home, leaving the dutiful sibling to stay behind and clean up the financial mess.

Finally, do you know anyone who has a need to be the "good" girl? This person will take actions based on how she appears to others, and will look down on siblings who aren't as "good" as she is. He may think himself a saint, but his self-righteousness, harsh judgment, and criticism of his siblings—expressed to their faces and, behind their backs to her parents—may seem more like a sin.

Money, competing responsibilities, and disparate skills rear their heads as well. It is all too easy for families to fall into roles when they don't take the time to discuss these things out loud. The best family caregiving situations arise when everyone is working together. Everyone can play a role, even those who live far away. All it takes is some good ongoing communication and a plan.

Consider Hiring a Life Transition Coach to Help with Family Dynamics

If you're not sure how to get started, you might consider hiring a life transition coach to help. As an objective third party, your coach can help provide focus and will have experience with others who have gone through similar transitions so you don't have to start from scratch.

In addition, a life transition coach will be knowledgeable about the many resources that are available to you and can facilitate necessary, but difficult, conversations and decisions. If you can anticipate the challenges you may face with your Adult Children or you, as an Adult Child, may see coming with your siblings in these circumstances, it is likely that you can avoid some of the pitfalls. You may end up with a functioning and happy family, with both the Older Adults and the Adult Children all having grown from participating in a truly fulfilling caregiving and care getting experience.

Obviously the whole situation would be improved if everyone involved was informed and involved and a frank discussion (or several) were arranged, but first it is helpful for everyone to arm themselves with some current and realistic information about the day-to-day reality of their Older Adult's situation.

Assess the Situation

With children's school schedules, work commitments, geographic distance, and even Older Adults' travel or social schedules, most modern families don't gather for Sunday dinners anymore. In fact, families may be able to get together only rarely, perhaps once or twice a year, and, as evidenced by the jammed highways and crammed airports, those times are often over the holidays.

Whether gathering around a Thanksgiving table, lighting a menorah and spinning the dreidel on Chanukah, or hanging ornaments on a Christmas tree, such events should be considered precious and well-spent times creating memories.

Older Adults, you have had a long life and know from experience that tomorrow is not guaranteed. Life throws out many curveballs. So take this time to resurrect old traditions and maybe even create new ones. Maybe you and your Adult Children used to make cookies when they were small. Now you, your Adult Children, and *their* children can all work together on some delicious creations. Or perhaps you never made that gingerbread house or homemade chocolate *gelt* for your own kids. Now is the time to do so for the grandkids. Use the time spent creating together to recall some family stories to pass on to the latest generation. Adult Children, you may want to videotape the retelling so as to have a permanent memory for when your parents are no longer there to share the tales.

But you Adult Children shouldn't just make memories. You should also make some time during your visits to help your parents with some tasks that have gone undone in your absence. It will not only make you feel good to be helpful, but it will also allow you to spend time with and observe your parents' needs.

Perhaps Dad needs help cleaning out the garage, or Mom could use some new clothes and could use help arranging the shopping trip. Maybe it would be helpful for you to accompany your parent to a doctor's appointment or to take care of some banking. Whatever the task, handling some ordinary activities with your parent will give you a good idea of how he or she functions on a daily basis when you're not around.

It is critical that you are a careful observer of both your parent and his or her surroundings. Observe both what Mom is doing and what she's *not* doing. Sometimes your best clue as to your Older Adult's status is noticing the things they used to do with ease that they're not doing now at all. For example, if Dad used to love to garden and the yard is a mess, that's worthy of your attention. Perhaps the home looks different than it has in the past, with lots of clutter or maintenance and repairs ignored. Those are red flags, begging your attention.

Look for signs of deteriorating health, such as weight loss (check for an empty refrigerator and freezer) and failing vision or hearing. Notice if your parent is sleeping downstairs, perhaps on the couch, when their bedroom is upstairs. Maybe Dad is having trouble climbing the stairs to his bedroom?

Look for safety or mobility problems that might be evidenced by unexplained bruises or scabs on the skin or scalp. Listen carefully for Mom's mention of leaving the back door open all night or Dad recalling his medication mishaps. Notice if your Mom wears her cane like a bracelet or if her walker is going unused in a corner.

Financial issues might be revealed by piles of unopened mail, past-due notices, or medical paperwork unopened or in piles. Look to see if any visits to the emergency room might have gone unmentioned.

Set aside time during your visit to engage in dialogue about these matters with your parents, siblings, or other family members, but make sure you choose the right time and approach. The right time is *not* at the dinner table on Christmas Eve or in the middle of making latkes on Chanukah.

Rather, look for a quieter time or create an opportunity for such a talk. A car ride or long walk can be a great time to talk, as can a mother-daughter visit to the nail salon or spa.

Older Adults, be open to such a talk with your Adult Children. They love you, are concerned about you, and want to help. The fact that you need such help does not mean you are being a burden. You are, in fact, lightening the load by talking freely about what help you might need and giving your Adult Children an opportunity to provide or engage such help.

Work Together

When it comes time to arrange care for yourself as you age or to help set up care for your parent, it works out best for everyone if family members can set aside their differences. Easier said than done, I understand, but a useful goal to set for everyone involved in this often-delicate subject.

Older Adults have to overcome their belief that (above all things) they don't want to become a burden, and Adult Children have to put away the niggling guilt that they should really be taking care of Mom or Dad themselves. These preconceptions need to be set aside before any useful discussion about aging and caregiving decisions can be made. With such heightened emotions in play, both sides are super-sensitive, tension is exacerbated, and flare-ups can occur. While this is understandable, it is not very useful.

When a family first approaches me in search of life transition or caregiver coaching, I try to get a handle on where each family member is coming from to better understand points of agreement and disagreement.

At first, everyone is on "good behavior" and tries hard to come across as agreeable. However, when I talk with each family member individually, I often learn about underlying tensions that already are, or may soon be, in the way of optimal caregiving and decision making. Interestingly, when I talk with the care recipient privately, it is not at all atypical for the Older Adult to bring up this tension that their children think they are doing such a good job of hiding, and to point to it as one of the most stressful aspects of the situation.

The one point that siblings can generally agree on is their objective to make sure that Mom or Dad receives the best care possible; interestingly, this sentiment is mouthed only by the Adult Children—too often, the Older Adult wants to do whatever is easiest or the least trouble for their Adult Children. However, figuring out just how to achieve this is where the trouble often starts. For example, what if one sibling believes that hands-on care for Dad should be provided only by family members, while his sister feels just as strongly that professional caregivers should be employed, thus allowing the family members to be there for the social and emotional support that Dad needs?

Or what if the Older Adult is sticking to their well-meant, but not particularly helpful, just go-along-to-get-along attitude and wants the cheapest care or that which is most convenient for their children, sticking to their lifelong role as the parent who sacrifices for their kids, instead of contributing their two cents about what kind of care they need, really want, and truly deserve?

How to resolve such diametrically opposed opinions?

Start with what is in front of you—not what *should* be or *might* be in the future—but where do you, as a family, stand right now? What options are available to you? Take a dispassionate inventory, just like you were counting cans on your pantry shelf.

Older Adults: Speak your mind and give your opinion of what type of care you believe you need and would like to see arranged. Hiding your desires is, in the end, no help to your Adult Children. If they help set up a caregiving system for you and you are unhappy with it, the arrangement won't last and the whole situation will have to be reworked, costing time and money. Decide what you need and would like, and add your conclusions to the family inventory. It is your responsibility to be a contributing member of the family—especially in a situation that so directly affects your future health and happiness. Martyrdom wins no halos here.

Adult Children: Work together to decide who in the family can provide what. Is one sister great at organizing a schedule of caregivers and people to drive Mom to her appointments? Maybe your brother is a physician and will be the best resource to go to for future medical issues. Perhaps there is a sibling who lives far away and doesn't have much time, but who will volunteer to be the communications director and set up a system for keeping everyone in the family in the information loop.

Talk to each other—and your parent—and reason things out. This may take several discussions, as people have trouble arriving at final reasoned decisions over such emotional issues. Allow each other time to think things over and speak again. This is one of the benefits of discussing such situations before the conversations have to be held in emergency mode, during a crisis.

Take stock of other kinds of resources, too—namely time and money. If each family member can find some way to contribute to the effort that is within his or her skills, time constraints, and financial ability, then things will flow more smoothly. Money isn't called the root of all evil for nothing. It is often at the core of the tension among families, even though no one likes to admit it.

As the Older Adult, you may feel you should be paying for your own care with no help from your children. You may, for example, be trying to honor your husband's wish that each child receive a certain amount of money at your death. But what if, due to stock market fluctuations, your nest egg has shrunk considerably? Or rising costs mean you are no longer able to afford the care you need? Or perhaps you have outlived your savings or fear you will? Speak to your financial advisor, daily money manager, or banker if you are unclear about your financial situation. Taking stock of your own situation is important so that you will be able to convey the proper information for use in the family inventory. You have to accurately count the number of cans on your own shelf to get a clear picture.

Adult Children: You need to assess your own strengths and weaknesses and bring those to the table for discussion about this as well. Perhaps you may feel that Mom or Dad's resources should be used to pay for care, while your brother may feel that he is "entitled" to their money as his future inheritance. He would prefer that the family provide the care so that there is something left for distribution in the will after the parent passes away. One sibling may have more money so she can afford to contribute to care and would prefer to do that rather than providing the hands-on care herself.

These are all valid points, and everyone should be allowed to share their opinions with each other, though the discussions may, at least initially, be tough ones. No one likes to come right out and admit their hang-ups and foibles about money (we still are secretive about finances), and such tensions are often hidden away under other, often petty, issues. If you find yourselves arguing about whether Mom's home health care worker should come on Tuesdays rather than Thursdays or whether a wheelchair ramp should be the fold-away variety or permanently installed, you might consider if you are skirting the important core issues. Take a break and return to just compiling an inventory of what you've got to work with in your family. Details can be hashed out more fully in future family meetings. A discussion of how to best arrange a truly productive family meeting follows later in this chapter.

Sometimes family caregivers simply get stuck in their roles or attitudes and don't know how to change things. In these cases, it is often important to get someone involved who can serve as the objective third party. This person doesn't have a stake in the game and isn't aware of the baggage that accompanies every family. He or she can ask the tough questions right along with the obvious ones. Sometimes, simply having an outsider scratch her head and ask why something is the way it is can be enough to get things unstuck. Consider making use of a life transition coach or a geriatric care manager.

Families and Finances

Ah, money. It is still a sticky wicket even (or especially) among family members. When it comes to arranging who is going to handle your money—or your parent's money—things can get mighty ugly and feelings mighty hurt. Let's look at how you can avoid the quicksand that is families and finances.

As we saw in our discussion of choosing fiduciaries, very often Older Adults empower one of their Adult Children with the responsibility of handling finances when they can no longer do so. In other cases, one of the Adult Children will step forward to take over, sometimes without consulting with his or her siblings. What happens if the other siblings don't agree with how Mom or Dad's finances are being handled?

The answer to this question is "it depends." It depends on who is legally in charge. It depends on whether the siblings were on the same page before Dad couldn't handle the finances any longer. It depends on whether there is underlying trust or distrust among the family members. And, it depends upon whether Mom made a plan before she became incapacitated and shared that plan with the kids.

If you are an Adult Child and your parent has made you or one of your siblings the agent under his or her power of attorney, then you or that named sibling has the responsibility and authority to handle the actions and decisions that are covered by the document.

While the agent is not required to consult with her siblings, it might be a good idea to do so, especially if there may be disagreement. While the ultimate decision belongs to the agent, obtaining the input of siblings and discussing the options will help the others feel involved with the decision even if they don't ultimately agree with it.

On the other hand, if one of you stepped in and took over "helping" your parent with his finances without the benefit of having been designated the agent, you're on shaky ground. The helper doesn't have the "right" to make the decisions, and it isn't unusual for the others to feel angry or frustrated when they try to do so.

As with so many things, communication is really the core solution.

If your parent has named you agent, it's a good idea to have periodic family meetings in person or by phone or video chat to discuss important decisions or changes. Likewise, sending a budget and periodic accounting of your parent's finances to your siblings will help them feel like they know what is going on.

Yet, as agent, there will be times when you simply need to make a decision and act on it quickly, and it is important that your family doesn't miss out on deadlines or opportunities because of "analysis paralysis."

If you aren't the agent but have stepped into the role of "chief financial officer" for your parent, then it is even more critical that you communicate with your siblings, since you don't have any legal authority to take action. The last thing any family needs is to be fighting with each other in court. The only winners in this case are the lawyers who represent each of you.

Let's look at things from the perspective of the sibling who *isn't* in charge. Why is she disagreeing with your management of your parents' affairs? Perhaps it is because she has a different point of view. Or maybe she's hurt or frustrated that you haven't asked for her opinion. Could it be as simple as feeling left out or in the dark? Often, the unknown makes us assume that something is being hidden from us. Whatever the motivation, finding a way to act as a team with your siblings will always make things less stressful for all of you.

As for you Older Adults, the last legacy you want to leave your children is dissension and chaos. You may not be able or even around to undo the harm you may have inadvertently caused among your children. The responsible—and ultimately, most loving—thing you can do is to decide which of your children is best able (emotionally and perhaps geographically) to carry out your wishes and can be counted on to act responsibly and equitably during what can be a tumultuous time. Rarely do we really get to just slip away quietly into the good night. Our passing will cause ripples.

Don't assume that the right person to designate as agent is your eldest Adult Child. Don't automatically assume it must be your son (daughters are most often the caregivers and being an agent is a form of care), and don't assume the Adult Child you choose *wants* the job. Ask them first. Explain to them what responsibilities being an agent entails; if you don't know, ask your life transition coach or your attorney to explain it to them. You should have a backup "go-to" person in any event in case something happens to the one who has agreed to be the agent. And remember, you don't have to name a family member or friend to this important role. You always have the option of naming a professional or corporate fiduciary.

Once the choice is made and agreed to between you and the agent, *do* announce it to your other family members so that, when the time comes, everyone is clear about who has the decision-making power. Keep a copy of the appointing document in your papers, give one to the agent, another to your attorney, and yet another to the assisted living or nursing home if you are a resident.

The agent should have a copy available for any hospital you enter as well.

Planning ahead for the time when you (Older Adult) or your parent (Adult Children) can no longer handle financial affairs is a multistep process, one that most people would rather avoid. Yet taking this important step will often mean the difference between family harmony and fireworks and is a necessary part of any discussion you will have at the all-important family meeting.

Have a Family Meeting

If life were like *The Waltons,* families would all pull up a chair 'round the hand-hewn table and lovingly decide what to do about Grandpa, who would be cheerfully smiling at his brood as they all figured out together how he would best spend his golden years, surrounded by his descendants and the busy bustle of a happy family.

Life, however, is rarely as tidy as programs on television.

Families can be fractious, distant, resentful, clueless, easily offended, or downright uncooperative, with the various personalities barely able to hold a civil discussion about what kind of pie to serve on Thanksgiving, much less able to discuss the Older Adult's Life Transition Plan and their own roles in carrying that out.

So, Older Adult, how do you avoid World War III from breaking out, while still getting your decisions out on the table and having a reasonable expectation at the end that not only will your wishes be carried out, but your family members might be left still speaking to each other?

Whether you are the Matriarch or Patriarch of the family or the Adult Children "youngsters" of the clan, a bit of thoughtful planning can prevent hurt feelings that can grow into grudges; prevent blowups, arguments, and misunderstandings; and go a long way toward enlightening all family members about the important issues that really *do* need discussing. Find ways to arrange a family meeting that makes sure what needs to get accomplished does and has everyone involved still amiable at the end of it.

Tips to Guide Your Family Meeting

Set the stage: Never spring a family meeting on unsuspecting family members. People will feel blindsided (or ambushed) and unprepared. They are much more likely to "react" rather than "respond," and a lot of emotional toads will spring from their mouths rather than pearls of considered wisdom. The person convening the meeting must clearly articulate the time and place of the meeting, the expected length, and the objective. Start by sending an invitation to those who will attend. This invitation can be transmitted in a phone conversation, via email, or even by snail mail.

If you are one of the Older Adult parents and the one convening the meeting, you might say something like, "Mom and I would like for all you kids and your spouses to sit down with us over brunch on Saturday so that we can share what we've been thinking about where and how we'd like to age." If you are one of the Adult Children—maybe the one who lives locally or the one the Older Adult turns to for helping with all forms of communication—make it clear that *you* are not the one convening the meeting (no need to start resentments ahead of time) but rather that Mom or Dad asked your help in letting everyone know that they would like to hold a meeting to discuss important issues weighing on their minds. Be clear that this meeting is about *their* wishes for end-of-life decisions regarding health and long-term-care issues. Don't make everyone think it will be a meeting to distribute any wealth or to go over a will. A who-gets-what fight is the last thing you want. Give everyone time to mentally prepare.

Choose the right time: It is not unusual for families to try to make the most of visits when the whole family is gathered—the holidays, a milestone birthday, christening, *bris*, or wedding—by having those all-important what-to-do-about-Mom-or-Dad discussions while far-flung family members are together. This is all too often the case of the road to hell being paved with good intentions. Such attempts often backfire and can permanently damage familial relationships. No bride wants her special time impinged on by talk of home health aides, and taking the spotlight off the Bar Mitzvah boy to talk over retirement homes is not a good idea. Neither is Christmas Day when kids (and parents) are often overexcited and exhausted. Pick the time reasonably and plan thoroughly to lay the groundwork prior to the family meeting for the best results.

Create an agenda: What do you want to cover at the meeting? How long do you plan to spend in the meeting? Do you plan to send the agenda ahead of time for review by the participants or will you distribute it at the meeting? Try to limit your agenda to no more than three major topics and no more than two hours in length. If you have more material to cover, use the initial meeting to set the stage and provide a framework for future discussions. Arrange for future meetings (either in person or virtually, via Skype or conference call) to delve into various topics more deeply. Depending on the family dynamics, you might consider sharing the agenda with the participants ahead of time, or you might decide to wait until the beginning of the meeting.

Define clear endpoints: For example, as the Older Adult, is your goal to share information with your family about your end-of-life wishes? Or, as one of the Adult Children, is the objective to brainstorm with your siblings about Mom's increasing cognitive impairment and reach a conclusion regarding what will happen if she can no longer care for herself? Participants need to understand whether they are attending a presentation or a discussion. Likewise, they must know if the objective is to reach consensus about a topic or simply to allow each person the opportunity to voice his or her opinion.

Lay some ground rules: At the very beginning of the meeting, it is helpful to establish guidelines. For example, if confidential matters will be discussed, you might ask everyone to agree to keep the discussion within the group. If you have a boisterous family, you might have to ask for each person to allow others to finish and not to talk over one another.

Maintain order: Don't let people just ramble on. In every family is the one who goes on and on, monopolizing all the time and seemingly all the hot air in the room, too. Everyone needs a chance to speak. One way to regulate this is to pass around some object—a knickknack or candle—and have a rule that the only person who is allowed to talk at a given moment is the person holding that object. Or designate someone as timekeeper. Have them hold up a yellow "caution" sign when two minutes have passed and a red "stop" sign at three. Allow everyone two or three go-rounds of the circle to voice their opinions. Ask that everyone try not to raise their voices; having no alcohol served might be useful. Because family meetings can often become emotional and tense—even falling back into traditional patterns ingrained from childhood—whoever "runs" the meeting should maintain a good hold on their sense of humor and be prepared to divert the conversation—without just grabbing for control—if it's heading for the emotional cliffs.

Optimize the environment: Ask everyone to turn off their electronic devices, and make sure that any family members who are not involved with the meeting are occupied and that any young children have appropriate supervision. Hire a sitter, if necessary, and split the cost. A pack of running grandkids can create a grand diversion. Exile them outside or to the basement and let older kids choose their own videos or use the computer while the meeting is ongoing. (Ordering pizza helps.)

Choose a facilitator: Give some careful thought to who will serve as the facilitator for the meeting. The person who initiates the meeting does not necessarily have to be it. In fact, you might consider having an objective third party who doesn't have a stake in the game act in this critical role. The facilitator is the person who will keep the meeting on schedule by managing the agenda and make sure that the ground rules are followed. Depending on the subject matter of your meeting and your family dynamics, using an outside facilitator may be the only way to accomplish a successful meeting. You'll know if you are the family who almost comes to blows over each year's Thanksgiving turkey or can't talk politics without someone storming out in a huff.

Discuss next steps: Before you adjourn the meeting, be sure to discuss next steps and make assignments and set deadlines if appropriate. Maybe your sister can check out local assisted living facilities, or your younger brother can contact transportation companies your Dad could use instead of driving if his sight is failing. Also circulate a brief meeting summary to all participants within a few days of the meeting, noting any follow-up commitments or the date of the next meeting, if you've set one.

Whether you are the Older Adult parent or Adult Child, such end-of-life or care discussions have great potential to be incendiary. Thoughtful preparation can prevent the whole meeting from going up in flames.

3

CAREGIVING AND CARE GETTING

LENNY IS A LONG-DISTANCE caregiver for his mother, Arlene. He does the best he can to make sure that Arlene has the support she needs while maintaining as much independence as possible. Yet the reality is that Lenny is stressed by the responsibilities of his work and being present for his wife and two young adult children, and he feels guilty that he doesn't spend more time with Arlene. At the same time, Arlene feels sad that her only son is so far away, but she doesn't want to be a burden so she omits telling Lenny about her struggles to handle her finances and manage her medications. He has no idea there is trouble until Arlene falls and breaks her hip. The crisis causes him to put his own life on hold, miss his daughter's recital, leave his boss high and dry during an important project, and arrange an emergency trip to evaluate the situation himself and try to arrange for his mother's proper care.

Take Charge, Don't Take Over

Adult Children: Whether you are teaching your young daughter how to knit or helping your aging mother balance her checkbook, how do you take charge without taking over? How many times have you found yourself "showing" your daughter or parent how to do something by doing it for them?

It's human nature.

But while it might make sense to show by doing when you are "teaching" someone younger or less familiar with a particular topic than you are, it usually leads to anger when you do this when you are "assisting" someone with a task that he previously has been perfectly capable of handling himself.

Older Adults: It's enough to make you grit your teeth. All you have asked your Adult Child for is a little help—perhaps figuring out something on the computer or trying to make sense of a particularly complex medical bill—and the next thing you know, your son or daughter is rolling their eyes, grabbing the bill or keyboard, and doing it *for you*.

You recognize the behavior from when they were teenagers, but you are pretty sure you were not that impatient with them when *they* were growing up.

No matter.

What needs to happen here is that new boundaries need to be laid out—adult-to-adult.

Older Adults: You need to express clearly, and without anger, that when you ask for an explanation of the bill or to be shown how to make the computer software do what you want, you wish to *be taught*. Then, of course, you must be willing *to learn,* and that includes asking for further clarification of things you don't understand. It also means that, if a reasonable amount of time passes and you still don't understand, be willing to admit that you need more help—perhaps even asking your Adult Child to handle the project for you.

Adult Children: You must be willing to teach your parents, to the best of your ability, and have the same patience as you would for a child of yours learning a new skill. Treat your parents with dignity, give the instructions slowly, and summon the patience you will need. They aren't dumb and can learn; it would be good to remember they managed to keep you alive to adulthood and have navigated the road of life much longer than you. Realize that acknowledging that they need help with the business of life is really hard for most Older

Adults. If they come to the point where they need your help, they are confronted with their own limitations. And those limitations won't "get better" in most cases. Deep down, your Mom knows that this is the beginning of the end of her independence, as she has come to know it, and that is an uncomfortable, and possibly frightening, thought.

Finding a Happy Balance

So how do the two sides come together? How do you Older Adults get the help you need without becoming totally dependent, and how do you Adult Children give them that help without taking over?

If possible, do the tasks together: Adult Children, work alongside your Mom rather than doing the task for her. While this approach might take longer than doing it yourself, you allow your Mom to retain some self-esteem by letting her fully participate. Older Adults, instead of surrendering all responsibility for your situation, work alongside your Adult Child. You'll stay more involved in your own life, be more mentally active, and won't be plagued by the awful feeling that you are a burden to your Adult Children.

Share responsibility: Adult Children: Let your Dad tell you what aspects of a particular activity he needs your help with, and if possible, try to limit your assistance to just those things, at least for now. Of course, if your Dad doesn't have a realistic picture of what he can do for himself, you will need to gently find a way to help him see your perspective. And Dad, it is okay to acknowledge you don't know how to do something. There is no such thing as an ignorant question. Ask the Adult Child who is acting as your instructor and stand ready to receive information with an open mind.

Mind your manners: For both sides—be respectful. Adult Children, ask permission before you just jump in. For example, when you take your parent to a doctor's appointment, don't just assume that they want you to come into the examining room with them. Instead, ask if they'd like you to be there the whole time, or if perhaps you can just be called in toward the end of the visit to make sure that *your* questions are answered. Older Adults, don't be instantly hostile or resentful that you need help at all. Try to see your own situation clearly and accept what is—not what you would wish it to be. Ask for help, but do make allowances for the fact your Adult Children have lives of their own and might not be able to drop everything the moment you say you need help. Be as courteous and thoughtful of their time as you would if you were asking a neighbor for help. Hold your own temper, too. If their explanations are going over your head, don't get frustrated and angry. Ask for more clarification and be patient with yourself when it comes to learning something new.

Don't work without a net: Set up invisible safety nets. Adult Children, if you come every Sunday and set up your Mom's medications in a weekly medication management system, you can have some expectation that she will take the correct medications at the right time. But it wouldn't hurt to also have a way of checking that system once or twice during the week. This might take the form of a medication management visit by a home care company or trusted friend or perhaps daily medication reminder phone calls from you. For the Older Adult's part, you might make this failsafe system a little better by marking off a daily space on a whiteboard mounted near your medications, noting when you took the medication, so it is easily seen at a glance, and make reading the chart's notations a standard part of your "reporting" during your regularly scheduled call with your Adult Children.

Safety comes first: Make a distinction between safety and everything else. Adult Children: When your Dad's safety is on the line, you might just have to take charge by taking over. On the other hand, if you'd just prefer that something be done a certain way or at a certain time, there might be an opportunity to loosen your grip a bit. Older Adults: Be reasonable. If your infirmities don't allow for you to take your own safety in hand in the way that you should or if your situation has changed (your eyesight has worsened or you can't get up the stairs without falling anymore), it is your responsibility to share this information with your Adult Children. They need to be able to trust you or else they will really have no choice but to launch that coup and overthrow the current system. If your safety is in jeopardy, not only is your health endangered, but the entire situation *vis-à-vis* your Adult Children as caregivers needs to change. Such drastic changes are better addressed before they reach a crisis point; that's only fair to all involved.

Adult Children: Your job as your parent's caregiver is to keep them safe, comfortable, and happy.

Older Adults: Your job as the one receiving the care is to facilitate your own safety and your comfort—as much as your age and health allow—and to make up your mind to be happy.

As long as both parties keep that in perspective, you should have no trouble about who is in charge. You both are—hand-in-hand as partners, not adversaries.

Manage Emotions

Overwhelmed. It is the most common first word that I hear in nearly every telephone call that I receive from a prospective client. It is a loaded word—one filled with raw emotion and urgency.

In these initial conversations prospective clients have with me, the word takes on a negative meaning, as in, "Caring for my ill spouse has left me feeling overwhelmed." But this very same word can also be used in a positive way, as in, "I was overwhelmed by the outpouring of love and support." Or, "I was overwhelmed with joy when I held my son for the first time." Feeling overwhelmed is the catalyst that leads so many to reach out for guidance, assistance, and reassurance, so we know it is a powerful thing. But let's deconstruct the word itself to get at a deeper understanding of the feeling of being overwhelmed.

The dictionary definition of "to overwhelm" is "to bury or drown beneath a huge mass" or "defeat completely" or to "subject to incapacitating emotional or mental stress." Synonyms include "overpower" and "crush." The word is derived from Middle English *over - whelm*. In this context, *over* means "too much" and *whelm* means "submerge or engulf." So it seems that the correct use of the term really is the negative, because after all, is it so terrible to have "too much" joy or to be "submerged or engulfed" by love?

So how do I help my clients get "over" being "whelmed"? Or, to put it another way, how do I help people to feel less submerged by life when it seems waves of problems keep crashing over their heads? Here are some suggestions I share with them:

Acknowledge and name: Start by asking yourself some questions: What are you engulfed by? Why do you feel defeated? What is overpowering you?

Sometimes the answer is relatively clear, as in the case of an Adult Child trying to fill the role of caregiver for her Older Adult, who may say, "I feel guilty that I can't do more for my Mom, but I have my own life."

An Older Adult, who has physically recovered from surgery only to face mountains of medical bills from the hospital stay, may answer, "There are too many bills to pay and forms to be filled out, and I don't know where to start."

Often, the root cause is that my client knows that he can't change an inevitable outcome, such as the Adult Child's inability to reschedule his work hours to care for Mom. Or the Older Adult's need to admit her diminished capacity means she can't handle all the responsibilities she once did and has to relinquish some of her independence. Both realizations can leave people feeling sad and frustrated by their reality. Whatever the cause, the outcome—feeling overwhelmed—typically leads to inertia and profound stress.

Define a successful outcome: I start by asking a powerful question like, "How will you define success?" I encourage my clients to give themselves permission to define success as working within the simplest parameters. For example, perhaps success will be defined working out a flextime option with your employer to come in early two days a week to allow you to spend Tuesday and Thursday afternoons with your mother. Or perhaps, Older Adult, you want to hire someone to help handle your mail and bills. Typically, any given situation will call for multiple definitions of a successful outcome. The simpler the definition, the better it is.

Create a plan: You need a plan to achieve those success milestones. I come to this with a bias, and that is that I see that life has a larger purpose, as something with meaning. I find that clients who share this view find it easier to deal with stress than those who believe that life is random chance. They seem better able to put events into perspective, perhaps because they realize that there may be a larger lesson to incorporate in the scheme of things. Such people believe that problems in life are challenges to aid our growth and development, rather than seeing them simply as causes to feel overwhelmed.

I often need to spend time discovering my client's life's purpose and trying to understand how the immediate challenges fit in as a way to mitigate the stress they feel. What starts as a task-oriented need like, "Help me figure out whether my Dad should go to an assisted living facility and how to pay for it," or "I know I'm not eating right, but I can't seem to manage to cook for myself anymore," often becomes a transformational experience on the journey of life.

Adult Children should know that the role of family caregiver is filled with emotions, both joyful and trying, and Older Adults, you will also be faced with some strong feelings as you adjust to being the one receiving the care.

Yet as anyone who has served in either role—as a caregiver for a family member or as a care receiver—knows, it is the negative emotions that seem to have the biggest impact in the moment. When working with families on the subject of caregiving, I often spend time helping them to work through the negative first, so that I may help them learn to recognize and focus on the positive of this new relationship dynamic.

Let's first discuss how Adult Children, as the family caregivers, feel about the role they have been called upon to play. When I ask such questions, I typically hear things like, "I never feel like I'm on top of everything" or, "If it's not one thing, it's another" or, "I have no time to myself." If I ask these caregivers to label their emotions, they will say things like, "I'm scared that I won't do the right thing or I won't do enough" or, "I'm angry that my siblings have dumped this on me and don't help." Fear, anger, and feeling overwhelmed are the most common caregiving emotions I hear about from Adult Children.

I've developed a method of helping these caregivers through a two-step process. The first step involves the caregiver learning to *stop doing* certain things. The second step requires the caregiver to answer a series of questions that can help him or her to *start doing* things that will make those caregiving emotions more manageable.

Stop doing: The first thing on the "stop doing" list is to stop trying to make *everything* better. Unlike taking care of a young child who will, over time, grow and learn to do things for himself, taking care of an Older Adult means accepting the reality that he or she will probably need *more* help in the future, not less. Things are not necessarily going to get better.

As the caregiver, your role is not to find a solution for every new problem, but rather to make sure that your care recipient is safe and happy, and allowed to remain as independent as possible. Until you, as the caregiver, let go of the expectation that you can make everything the way it once was, you will feel tremendous stress, wondering if you can ever do enough.

The second thing on the "stop doing" list is making assumptions or projecting your needs onto your caregiving recipient. Have you ever caught yourself saying something like, "If it were me, I'd . . ."? Or how about, "I can't believe you would . . ."?

In these situations, you are expecting your care recipient to have the same feelings and preferences as you do. While the care recipient may be your parent who you've known your whole life, by the very nature of your roles now, you do not have the same feelings and preferences. To be blunt, in the current situation, Adult Child, this really isn't about you. It's about your parent. The more you try to understand how they truly feel and what they need, without judgment, the less stressed you will be.

Start doing: The "start doing" side of the equation is based on some introspection on the part of the caregiver. I challenge caregivers to ask themselves the following questions:

- What scares me about my role as a caregiver or my care recipient's needs?

- What is the worst that can happen if my fears are true?

- What if the opposite were true?

- How can I plan ahead or prepare for the situations I fear most?

Taking the time to examine what underlies your caregiving emotions is the first step to managing them.

This is also the time when a caregiver support group can be helpful. Your local community undoubtedly has in-person groups, as well as numerous resources online. You might prefer a group centered on a particular disease or condition or one sponsored by your church, synagogue, or community organization. What brings the group together is less important than the skill of the facilitator and the positive support that is shared. Just to know you are not alone can be a great relief valve.

Sometimes it can also be helpful to work with a caregiver coach who is familiar with the issues faced by caregivers, as well as with the resources available to you and your care recipient. By seeking help and reaching out, it is possible to stop being overwhelmed and begin to feel as though you can handle the situation at hand and any future challenges that arise in a competent and loving way.

For you Older Adults, preparing yourself mentally to be cared for—in a life where you undoubtedly spent much of your time caring for others—is a hard transition, but it needn't be too bitter a pill to swallow.

The most beneficial change you can make to ease this transition, for both yourself and your caregiver, is to adjust your attitude. No one likes to surrender one inch of his or her independence. I understand that and I recommend that you make clear to your caregiver—in a loving and not dictatorial way, even if it is your daughter and you've been bossing her around her whole life—that you want her help in maintaining your ability to live your life as independently as possible.

You may need his help getting in and out of the tub, but prefer to clean your dentures in private. Someone might assist you to walk to the toilet, but the bars you have had installed on either side of the commode will help you once you are in the enclosure. Your Adult Child can wait outside in case you need help. You might wish to do your own laundry and only have the caregiver carry the basket. Maybe you prefer to make your own toast in the morning. Whatever you can still do, you *should* still do, and you should enlist your caregiver's cooperation in helping you do so.

Also, one of the traps of your increasing dependence upon others is to resent them for the fact you need them at all. This twisted piece of logic is common to many of us and is part of the vital internal work you must do within yourself.

If you are angry because your body is failing you in ways it didn't do when you were thirty, learn to come to terms with aging. Don't be angry with the caregiver. Try to learn not to be angry at all, but to accept the changes in your lifestyle with good grace and good humor. Aim for an attitude of gratitude for those who are helping you. I am not advocating a simpering, overly officious, oh-I-am-sorry-to-be-such-a-bother relationship. Keep your dignity, but also try to mind your tongue. It is not their fault you are getting older. It is no one's fault. It is just the way of things.

Don't take abuse, certainly, but don't dish it out, either. Speak your mind, but try to do so with love and balance. The crotchety old lady or cranky old man needn't be your persona. Every day of your life—even those when you are older, less mobile, and more dependent—can be sweet. Stop to smell, no longer the roses of early spring perhaps, but the rich aroma of the falling leaves in the autumn of life. Each has its blessings.

Remember to try to look for those blessings and be grateful for both what you have *had* in your life and what you *have* in your life. One of those blessings is the family caregiver trying to help you live it to the fullest.

You Can't Fix It

Nobody rides for free. When it comes to this life, there is only one way out, and the end comes for every one of us. But, whether you are an Older Adult seeing that "Exit" sign loom ever closer or an Adult Child struggling with the concept that your parents may soon leave the stage, the concept of "fixing it" has to be addressed.

Older Adults: Perhaps you were a captain of industry, used to figuring out ways around obstacles in your company and commanding underlings to fix any problems. Or Adult Children, maybe you are a baby boomer, ever busy, with a cell phone in one hand, Bluetooth set up in your car, and an iPad at the ready in between times. Present you with the problem and it just gets added to your to-do list to figure out, fix, and check off.

Either scenario means you are oriented to getting things done, to figuring out any situation, to fixing things. The trouble is, aging is natural and inevitable and cannot be fixed. No amount of tennis games played can enable you to outrun death, and no checklist, no matter how well you accomplish all the tasks on it, will prevent that day from coming for your parents.

As the Older Adult, you are going through a natural process, and Adult Children, you can't make everything okay for your parents. Everything *is* okay and unfolding as it should. Both of you can make this natural process a little easier, though, by paying attention.

Older Adults: Note your needs and express them.

Adult Children: Ask questions, listen well for the answers, and watch carefully for opportunities to help.

Neither of you will have all the answers. This is not a road that you have yet traveled. You will have many questions and not all of them will be fully answered, making you feel as though you don't have all the information you'd like. Life—even the end of it—isn't perfect, but you can still make good decisions.

Adult Children: The day you stop looking at your caregiver role as Ms. or Mr. Fixit is the first day of the rest of *your* life. The next time you have a caregiving challenge, stop for a moment and think about the situation. What does your parent really need? Have you asked? Have you asked in several ways—without badgering or nagging? Have you tried to see the situation through their eyes? If you're sure about the need, then what are the possible ways to fill it? Is there really only the one way, the way that seems impossible right now and has you (and your Dad) so frustrated? Or might there be another way to skin the cat?

Let's take the situation of Lisa and her Dad, John. Lisa is in her mid-fifties, married, and has one teenager still at home and two in college. Lisa works full time outside the home. Her Dad lives about an hour away from Lisa and her family in a condo he owns. John is in his mid-eighties and was widowed two years ago. Lisa has one sibling, a younger brother who lives across the country. John's in pretty good health, but he has become increasingly frail over the past six months and seems to have lost a lot of weight. Lisa is worried about her Dad, but with her other responsibilities, it's hard for her to get to John's home more than once per week.

Over the past week or two, Lisa has concluded that John is not eating well and that's the cause of his weight loss. Every time she visits, she brings a load of groceries and meals she's cooked at home. Ms. Fixit to the rescue. Yet, on subsequent visits, the food is pretty much right where Lisa left it. She's frustrated because, "No matter what I do, Dad won't eat." When she begs him to eat, John gets angry and tells Lisa that he's just not hungry. The situation escalates and ends with Lisa storming out of John's home in tears.

What if Lisa had stopped for a moment before her Ms. Fixit instincts kicked in? Instead of jumping right in to fix what she saw as a "problem," Lisa might have talked with John about how he was doing. Had she done so, she would have learned that John was very worried about his finances. He was afraid that he was going to outlive his money, and as a result, John had decided that he could get by on less. The last thing that John wanted was to be a burden on Lisa and her brother. So when Lisa starting bringing food to John, he felt guilty because exactly what he feared seemed to be coming true. He felt that if he didn't eat much of the food that Lisa brought, maybe she'd stop bringing it, and, by being less of a burden, he would feel less guilty.

Had Lisa just asked the right questions and really listened to John's answers, she might have come up with another way to solve the problem. In any event, by allowing John to participate in the solution, she would have allowed him to preserve some of his independence and feel more in control of his situation. And Lisa herself likely would have felt less stressed and less frustrated.

Of course, it's possible that John wouldn't have shared his fear with Lisa directly, but Lisa might have included John in identifying the problem and trying to solve it. Even if that approach failed, maybe Lisa could have arranged for some of John's friends to invite him over for dinner so that he would have the social interaction and not feel as though he were imposing on his daughter.

For John's part, he could acknowledge, at first to himself and later to his daughter, just what was actually worrying him. He could have talked the situation over and perhaps asked Lisa to recommend her friend, the daily money manager, to set an appointment and come discuss rearranging his finances to alleviate his worry about outliving his money.

By communicating clearly and honestly with his daughter, he could have saved her stress, helped his own anxiety by voicing his concerns, and spared making his daughter "guess" what his predicament was. The real problem would have been addressed and a lot of good home-cooked food would not have been wasted.

Without question, the road to the end of life has some bumps. As both the caregiver for your Older Adult parent or as the Older Adult parent yourself, you have many choices and decisions to make, and the sheer volume of what needs to be done can be overwhelming.

To the extent that you can remember that it is not your job to fix everything, that you can ask for help and treat each other as partners, either you as the Older Adult or you as the Adult Child will both be better off.

You share the job of making the natural progression of aging easier on you both, but as hard as you try to keep this train from rolling down the tracks, you won't be able to stop it. Once you can acknowledge and accept this reality, it will be easier to keep things in perspective. Your job is to do your best with this ultimate reality and to do it with positive intentions.

Preserve Independence

Older Adults: You spent the first eighteen years (or longer) of your life under your parents' supervision. You then spent years of life answering to teachers, bosses, and perhaps even your spouse, and now, in your later years, you have finally achieved independence and are loath to relinquish one iota of it to anyone. That is perfectly under-standable and, when you were a bit younger, stronger, and healthier, even commendable. But now you need to reassess what independence means to you and how asking for help or turning over some chores to others may be the best independent decision you make.

Adult Children: One of the most difficult aspects of helping your parents as they age is the very delicate balance between preserving their independence and taking charge. If you don't believe the situa-tion is combustible, just organize a coup, take over your parent's busi-ness without their permission, and watch the flames erupt.

It may seem "easier" for you just to take on an activity once handled independently by your parents but, believe me, it is almost always better to find a way to get the job done in a manner that allows your aging parents to remain in control of as much of their affairs as possible.

Here are some examples of how the generations can work together on these possible prickly problems:

You, Mom, may be having difficulty managing your bills and keeping your checkbook balanced. Perhaps it wasn't your strongest suit when you were younger, or your husband handled the finances. Now you feel like a fish out of water, but you don't want your children to do it for you. After all, you are the parent here.

You, the Adult Child, could just take over the situation, have all of Mom's bills delivered to your house, set up automatic payment for them, and grab up her bank statements to balance her checkbook yourself. Though that is a ruthlessly efficient way of getting things done, it takes all control from your Mom and will likely make her feel angry toward you, even if she doesn't say so. A resentment unspoken is resentment nonetheless.

An alternative might be to ask your Mom to put all of the mail in a special place each day, and then for you to come once a week and sit with her while she sorts through the bills and prepares her checks. Sure, this will take you more time, but you will allow Mom to feel as though she is still responsible for herself and allow yourself to rest easy that her bills are being paid and her money managed.

It is true that you, as Adult Children, sometimes have no choice and will have to take charge in order to keep your parent safe. If Dad has cracked up the car and you (or worse, the police) have determined that it is no longer safe for him to drive, you must make sure that he no longer is behind the wheel. How can you preserve Dad's independence in this situation?

One idea might be to arrange for transportation services that he can access when he needs them so he isn't required to ask you for a ride. In some areas, local taxi companies will allow you to set up an account and pay the bill monthly. This way, if Dad wants to meet a friend to play cards, he can do so without the extra stress of arranging to get there and back or having to carry the right amount of cash for the fare.

Or perhaps you are an Older Adult with mobility issues who is finding it hard to go grocery shopping for yourself. Many major supermarket chains now have online delivery service. Ask your Adult Child to set up the account for you (the funds come from your bank account via a debit card) and then, using the electronic checklist, it is the easiest thing in the world to place your order right from your computer. Better still, the system remembers what you have ordered in the past and keeps your favorite brands on file to make ordering even easier. Alternatively, you may be able to arrange for a volunteer to shop for you once a week, and your Adult Child can help you purchase supermarket gift cards to make it easy for the volunteer to pay for your groceries at the store.

For your part, Older Adults, you have to avoid reacting stubbornly to inevitable changes in your life as you age. Wouldn't it be nice to know that all your bills were being paid on time and your checkbook balanced each month with no nasty surprises like insufficient funds notices? You really do want to act the part of responsible adult when it comes to your finances, don't you, Mom?

Dad, do you really need the expense of owning a car, paying insurance premiums (sure to increase as you age), and handling maintenance when the object of the game is just to get where you are going when you want to get there? Isn't it the correct choice to acknowledge your sight and reflexes aren't what they used to be so that you don't endanger other people by sheer stubbornness? As the Older Adult in these situations, you have a responsibility to act the part—that of an adult.

Cooperation and flexibility are the keys toward both generations working together to find solutions and solve problems. Adult Children: Help preserve your parents' independence whenever possible and treat them with dignity and respect. Older Adults: Acknowledge that changing circumstance does not indicate failure or total capitulation of your independence.

You always have choices about how to solve the problems you will encounter. If you make a real effort to overcome challenges together, both sides can have their needs met and preserve their mutual independence, while working together in harmony.

Stay in Touch

For an Adult Child, one of the toughest parts of being a family caregiver, especially a long-distance caregiver, is keeping aloft all the balls you are juggling. The truth is, the more organized you are, the less stressed you will be.

Checklists and calendars are a big help for keeping yourself organized. But family caregivers are often expected to keep others informed, too, and taking the time to make all of those phone calls can sometimes just be too much.

Luckily, many wonderful tools are available that will help you facilitate communication between yourself and your parents, your caregiving resources, friends, and family.

Conference calls can be a terrific way to get far-flung family members involved with important decisions. For example, if you are the primary caregiver but have several siblings who each live in a different city, you can use one of the many free conference call services to set up a number that each of you can dial into at the appointed time. In this way, all of those who should be part of the decision-making process can participate in real time. Similarly, if you are a long-distance caregiver, you might find it helpful to convene a monthly conference call with all of your caregiving resources so that everyone is aware of the others' insights and concerns.

"CarePages" (www.CarePages.com) are a great way to keep your Older Adult's friends, family, and support network up-to-date on his or her condition and activities. Also free of charge, CarePages are essentially personal websites or blogs. They allow you as the caregiver to post entries and photos, and allow visitors to post words of encouragement to you and your Older Adult. You can set up the CarePage with various levels of security so you can control who sees what information. This can be a really convenient way to communicate when you don't have much time. You determine when you post and when you read what others have posted. Many people who have used CarePages find that they develop a wonderful network of others in similar situations, creating, in fact, a virtual support group.

Social networking sites like Facebook can serve a similar function to CarePages, in that you can post updates to the page that interested parties can follow. You can create various levels of security on Facebook, so make sure that you don't expose personal or medical information to the world.

Similarly, many blogging sites are available. You can then post your thoughts or updates, and viewers can post comments on what you've written. Blogs are generally very public, so you might find that a CarePage is a better tool for this purpose.

Finally, webcams allow you to get a look at your Older Adult care recipient if you are a long-distance caregiver. Unlike a phone call where you can only hear their voice, the webcam allows you to both see and hear the person on the other end. Many computers today have built-in web cameras, or inexpensive freestanding ones are available. Once the web camera is set up, most Older Adult care recipients are able to follow simple instructions to use them.

By putting updates in one place and allowing those who wish to do so to access them, you eliminate the need to make multiple phone calls. You are freed from worrying about whether it is too late at night to call your sister who lives three time zones away, since she can read your update when it's convenient for her. Likewise, if all of those involved with the hands-on caregiving report their activities and observations in one place, the information is available to all of the caregivers without the need for long conversations. If you establish a regular schedule for updating the caregiving reports, everyone involved can also be assured that the information posted is timely and up-to-date.

If you are the Older Adult who is the recipient of the care, you, too, can make use of the methods set up above to keep your family informed. Or, if you find it easier, you can add to the information to be shared with your whole family and give it in a timely manner to your local caregiver to post to the rest of the group.

For example, let's say you find yourself in need of some items—like several sets of slip-proof socks or extra mattress protectors. Have your caregiver list what you need online—he or she can even set up an Amazon Wish List for you, where you choose exactly what you need. An online list of those items is collected, sent to everyone on your list, and items are taken off the list when one of your Adult Children buys them. Your long-distance Adult Children will be delighted to know what you need (without guessing) and will probably be happy to provide it. Keep a list updated every month so your needs are met.

Or perhaps you need a bigger item, one not fully covered by your insurance, like a high-end electric wheelchair. By listing the item online, everyone in the family can donate money toward the purchase. Your local caregiver can even set up a PayPal account allowing remote family members to transfer money electronically from their bank accounts to a PayPal account online, where the money is "stored" until retrieved by your local caregiver for the purchase. Such an account may also be used if your Adult Children all want to contribute an amount of money to your general care each month, and it can all be done, conveniently for everyone, online.

When it comes to webcams, have your local caregiver arrange to set aside a specific time for you to make a cameo appearance on a "web broadcast" so that all your Adult Children can "see" and talk to you. Just have the local caregiver bring in a laptop and sit you in front of it. Or ask for time on the family conference call to speak to your Adult Children or to be involved in the whole call. It is your life they are discussing, after all.

Perhaps you would like to write—or even use a software program like Dragon Dictation to dictate what you'd like to write—on a family blog. A blog really is just a way of sharing your thoughts "on paper," though your words will appear on a computer screen as opposed to on paper, and a dictation program allows you to talk into a smartphone and have your words appear onscreen. With such a blog, your thoughts can also then be saved and shared as part of a family archive.

My point is this: Technology can help you stay involved in your own care; help your family understand your wishes; eliminate the miscommunication that happens when your Adult Children are asked to "read your mind" or guess your desires; and can keep you, as a family, closer, despite geographical distance.

Using technology is nothing to fear and, if you are an Older Adult, can be a big help in ensuring you receive the care you need and helping your Adult Children along on the caregiving journey.

Lifesavers for Long-Distance Caregivers

What if you have no siblings, or all of you Adult Children live far away from the Older Adults who need care?

Long-distance caregiving can be a scary proposition. You may feel as though you have no control or are doing a bad job of taking care of the parents who took such good care of you. Put that latter notion out of your mind. You are doing the best you can, and by doing some prep work and staying organized and informed, you can gain the control you need to feel less anxious about the situation.

Caregiving is all about control. If you are the Adult Child, you want to control everything so that "nothing bad" happens to your Older Adults. If you are the Older Adult being cared for, you want to remain in control so that you can continue to feel like a complete person. If everyone concerned can remember that control is at the core of every action and every reaction, it will help all of you to keep things in perspective.

When you become frustrated, ask yourself why you are trying to control the situation, what will happen if you stop, and why you feel out of control. Take a deep breath (or several), write down your concerns, then put the list and the obsessive thoughts away for a while. Go see a movie, take a long walk, pour a cup of tea—then return to the problem with a clearer head. You may want to talk over the situation with a friend—particularly one who has been down this road before—or a professional, like a life transition coach. While it might seem expensive, engaging a professional to help you may be a wise investment. A life transition coach can assist you in putting all of the pieces in place early, ideally even before your loved one's health has deteriorated. This professional can help you select your caregiving team so that you know exactly who to call when the time comes. As a neutral third party, your coach can help navigate the family dynamics that often are heightened during times of transition.

Older Adult, if your Adult Child is trying to manage your caregiving over a long distance, the most important thing you can do for them is to have your affairs in order. As I wrote in the "Creating a

Life Transition Plan" section, you should gather in one place all your health and medication records; contact information for your doctors, lawyers, and financial planners; all information about your bank accounts, including signers, passwords, and safety deposit box keys; power of attorney and health proxy papers; and any end-of-life information (organ donation permissions, funeral wishes, burial plots) that your Adult Child will need to access in the event of your death or incapacity. Let the Adult Child know where that place is located.

The easiest way to think about this information and what it should consist of is this: What questions will your Adult Children have if you go into a coma or die, and who can they ask if they can't call you?

Adult Children: It is critical that you have all of the information that you need to handle your loved one's affairs at your fingertips, and that you have the appropriate permissions in place to tackle issues as they arise. You, too, should reread the section on "Creating a Life Transition Plan" and ensure that a Life Transition Plan gets created so that you are prepared for every eventuality. For your part, the best way to think about this is: What would happen in an emergency? Do you have access to all the documents you'll need to make medical, financial, and end-of-life arrangements if something happens to your parent? Who will be your Older Adult's advocate if Mom falls and has to be taken to the emergency room? How quickly can you or another family member arrive on the scene? If your parent lives in an area with blizzards, hurricanes, brushfires, or earthquakes, what is the emergency plan in place for their evacuation? How will you remain informed? Does your parent know what to do in case of emergency and who to call?

Life isn't all about emergencies, thankfully, but *is* made up of a million little details. As an Older Adult, you may need help with these smaller issues. You, as the Adult Child, want to help ease your parent's day-to-day situation in any way you can, but you can't show up every Saturday to mow their lawn. What to do?

Hire someone.

A reliable local handyman can be engaged for household repairs or to install handrails, stair lighting, and treads to make the Older Adult's upstairs bedroom accessible again. Worried about hiring someone long distance? Ask your parent's neighbors for recommendations or, for a nominal fee, join Angie's List and read the ratings and reviews other users have left. Be sure to ask your Older Adult when such work could be conveniently scheduled and get back to them about when the workmen are expected to show up. About that lawn—maybe a college kid might be willing to earn a few extra dollars landscaping the garden. Check local college bulletin boards or Craigslist. If the Older Adult is having mobility issues, perhaps the local dog groomer also doubles as a pet walker, or maybe a neighborhood middle school student can handle walking the family pet.

All problems have a solution, but first the problems themselves must be identified and shared. Older Adults, help your kids help you and help alleviate some of the worry they feel from having to be far away from you as you age.

The best time to start hammering out solutions to problems is when you are all together—Older Adults and Adult Children both. Parents, talk about what you think you need, and Adult Children, feel free to throw in your two cents about what your parent needs help with. Remember that a dialogue means that *everyone* gets a chance to speak and that you're having a conversation. It isn't necessary to convince Mom right then and there that she has to abandon preparing her garden beds herself as she has each spring for years. There's time enough after your visit to work through details or logistics by telephone or email, after you've had a chance to find alternatives to help that Mom might find acceptable.

Adult Children, when you visit, take home a copy of the local Yellow Pages. This can be very helpful if you need to marshal resources for your parent from a distance. Don't assume that you will find everything that you need on the Internet, because it might not be listed the way you expect it to be and the perfect resource might sneak by the search engine. Get to know a few of your parent's neighbors and make sure to take their phone numbers home with you. Make a list of other important phone numbers, such as your parent's doctors or providers of household repair services. Anything you can do to be prepared for the day-to-day "crises" will help keep your stress down later on.

Older Adults, you can help here, too. Gather such information and give it to your Adult Children to take home.

One of the most important caregiving lessons is to ask for help. And then, ask again. So many wonderful people and resources are available to help you Adult Children who are acting as caregivers. Don't feel like you are less of a caregiver when you accept help. Be specific about what you need. It's much easier for someone to respond to your request to bring Dad dinner one night a week than to respond to the vague request to "keep an eye on Dad."

And speaking of asking for help, remember that you are no good to anyone if you get sick, so take the time to take care of yourself. Eat well, exercise, and get plenty of rest. Ask for help for your own needs if that will make it easier for you to be the best caregiver that you can be.

Look at your care as a team effort—the Older Adult and the Adult Children working together—often in full view of *their* children. Consider it an object lesson for the next generation in how families care about one another. Remember to show them, too, how to enjoy the time you share—every precious minute of it.

The Five Languages of Family Caregiving

You may be familiar with Dr. Gary Chapman's timeless best-seller *The 5 Love Languages,* originally published in 1992 and updated many times since. If not, I recommend you read it to help you form a framework for how you, Adult Children, think about becoming a caregiver or how you, Older Adults, can better understand the family dynamic if you find yourself needing to be on the receiving end of that care.

Dr. Chapman's premise is that people who understand each other's "love language" have a distinct advantage because they are able to effectively communicate with the people with whom they are in relationships—be it a spouse, child, parent, boss, or business partner.

Over the past several years, I have applied Dr. Chapman's approach in my family caregiver coaching and have seen tremendous benefits for my clients. As Adult Children learn to identify their own caregiving language and that of their Older Adult care recipients, they are better able to navigate the inevitable challenges.

One of the most common frustrations I hear from Adult Children acting as caregivers is that they feel taken for granted, not so much by their parent, but by other family members who seem to expect them to just keep managing everything with little help or support.

When I work with these Adult Children caregivers to get underneath the surface of what is really going on, I often find that the caregiver has never explicitly asked his siblings for help, or if he has asked, he has made a vague request like, "I wish you'd help out more with Dad," without discussing the specific need or spelling out what actions they can take to help.

When we dissect what the true problem is, I almost always find the disconnect to be a communication issue. Even if messages have been exchanged, the parties are speaking in two separate languages. Both sides feel misunderstood and frustrated by the lack of opportunity to make one side truly grasp what the other side is trying to say. Communications break down, feelings get hurt, and resentments build up. It is fertile ground for creating family rifts and makes an already stressful time even worse for both the Adult Child and the Older Adult they are caring for.

Since it is very rare that two individuals in any kind of relationship will have exactly the same love language profile, Dr. Chapman counsels that it is very important that you communicate *exactly* what you need to your partner and that you make sure your partner has communicated *exactly* what they need to you. Communication must be two-way, and when it comes to Adult Child/Parent relationships, clarity becomes not only more vital, but somewhat trickier.

Family members assume they know what each other thinks or

will say about most subjects, just from having spoken to each other their whole lives. The problem with this assumption is that family members too often speak "at" each other, not "with" each other, and each has preconceived notions of exactly what the family member will do or think or say in any situation, based on previous experience. But people *do* change. Kids grow up and become Adult Children who have to deal with the reality of their parent's situation in real time—how things are *now*—not how they once were. For their part, Older Adults have to accept that their children are now responsible and fully grown adults capable of making good decisions, even about so delicate a situation as caregiving. All involved need to relearn how to truly *listen* to each other and understand the "language" the other is speaking.

Dr. Chapman identifies five distinct love languages: *Words of Affirmation, Quality Time, Receiving Gifts, Acts of Service,* and *Physical Touch.* I have found that these very same languages can be applied to caregiving relationships.

A caregiver whose language is *Words of Affirmation* is someone who thrives on verbal compliments or hearing encouraging words. If your sister is the one who is the primary caregiver for your Mom, and this is her language, telling her how very much you and the rest of the family appreciate her excellent caregiving may be the boost she needs to keep going through what can be an exhausting time.

If, however, her language were *Quality Time*, your sister would value you stopping by to visit and centering all your attention on *her* for a while, not the parent for whom she is providing care.

Or if your sister's language is *Receiving Gifts,* use more than just words to thank her. A gift card for a facial or the offer to sit in for her one afternoon so she can run errands is the best way to say thank you.

Giving a gift certificate for a massage or just a big hug after a long day with the Older Adult may be the way to show love to someone craving *Physical Touch.*

These same love languages can be used to communicate love to the Older Adult, too.

Offering to give a manicure/pedicure to your bedridden Mom

is a way to share touch and provide an *Act of Service*. *Quality Time* may be employed by offering to spend a scheduled afternoon each week reading to your low-vision parent (and then staying afterward for your own personal little book group to discuss what you've read). Bring a box of diabetic chocolate to the assisted living facility or roses on Mother's Day to a parent who enjoys *Receiving Gifts*, and tell your parent you love them—every day—to please any parent who needs *Words of Affirmation*; and as people age, those words become ever more important.

Older Adults, if you are the receiver of the care, remember to say "thank you" often to those Adult Children helping you. Perhaps even write a note that can be reread during tough times and cherished by your Adult Child when you are gone. For caregivers whose language is *Receiving Gifts*, have a florist deliver tulips, or ask a grandchild to help order football tickets to be sent to your son to thank him for his help. Remember that everyone gets worn out—on both sides of the issue of caregiving—and replenishing people in a language they can understand does much toward keeping everyone going.

I encourage the caregivers with whom I work to identify their own caregiving language and then to effectively communicate that to their care recipients.

One of my clients said, "You know, I can get through even the toughest day taking care of my husband when one of our children comes over and asks me about what's going on with me."

Can you guess which language this caregiver prefers? If you guessed *Quality Time,* you are correct.

This woman doesn't need to be told she's doing a wonderful job or get sent a gift certificate for dinner and a movie. She doesn't even really want you to take her husband to his doctor's appointment or give her a hug. This caregiver might welcome all of those gestures, but the thing she most craves is that you sit and really *listen* to her when she talks. Paying attention to what she is thinking and feeling is the greatest gift she can receive.

If family caregivers knew this important reality from the outset of their caregiving journey, the road would grow smoother for all the travelers.

Learn to speak a new language—the language of love as understood by the person with whom you are trying to communicate—and brand-new relationships can be forged with chains of affection and contentment on both sides of the conversation.

4

HOUSING

HAROLD IS IN HIS EARLY EIGHTIES. He lost his wife of fifty years a decade ago. Ever since, Harold, who lives in Florida far away from his three children, has been trying to decide whether to move "up north" to be closer to them or to stay where the warmer weather is better for his health conditions. If he stays put, his biggest concern is whether to age in place or move to a senior living community. The problem is, Harold has been considering these options for more than five years now. During that time, he has been diagnosed with a neurodegenerative disease that now makes him ineligible for several of the communities he was most interested in.

"I'm Not Ready Yet"

So often, Older Adults intellectually know that their current living situation isn't right for them anymore but seem unable to take the steps necessary to do something about it. Studies consistently show that most people would like to live independently, in their own residence, for as long as possible. While this makes sense in the abstract, many Older Adults do reach the point where this is not practical or possible for one reason or another, unless some changes are made. Whether you are the Older Adult planning for your own future or the Adult Child of a parent and the time has come for those aforementioned changes to be made, the question is the same: "Where to go?"

As you plan for your future or help your parents plan for theirs, think about the options of aging-in-place, sharing a home with your Adult Child or another family member, or moving to a senior living community. Which makes sense for you as an Adult Child, or your Older Adult parents, will often depend on economics and available resources. Be sure to consider not only traditional assets like investment accounts, but also the proceeds from the sale of your parent's home, possible VA benefits, disbursements from long-term-care insurance policies, or the option of a reverse mortgage. As an Adult Child, you might even figure out the costs to add on to your own home to accommodate your parent or explore if it might be a better use of your finances to sell your existing home and use the proceeds to buy another better suited to fit Mom or Dad along with the rest of your family.

Consider your (or your parent's) physical, social, and transportation requirements. Don't focus only on what you or they need today, but also think about what you or they might need in the future. And, don't consider only your *needs* or the *needs* of your parents. *Wants* are important to consider too.

"Aging in place" commonly means staying where you live right now with appropriate modifications that will keep you (or your parents) safe and comfortable as you or they age. For example, if you are an Older Adult who has been diagnosed with a condition that pretty much guarantees that you will have increasing mobility issues, remodeling your bathroom with a roll-in shower, grab bars, and a wheelchair-accessible toilet is necessary.

On the other hand, aging in place might just as easily mean transitioning to another, more suitable private residence. For example, if your parent's current home has a second-floor master bedroom and no elevator, you might discuss with them selling that home and purchasing one that is all on one level. A variation might be sharing a home with an Adult Child or other family member.

Alternatively, if you are thinking about senior living options, your choices include rental, purchase, and life care. Each alternative has pros and cons, and which is best for you or your parents will depend on many factors.

One common objection I hear from Older Adults when the topic of where they will live in their final years comes up is, "I'm not ready yet." You may have many reasons why you are not ready or are reluctant to discuss the subject, but the most common objections tend to fall into three categories: fear, denial, and anger.

Older Adults, getting old stinks, and no one wants to admit that it's happening to them. Whatever the reason, being "ready" means acknowledging that the home you are moving to is likely to be your last home, and that implies confronting your mortality. Plan early, because it is inevitable that each of us will have a "last" home, and most of us would like to be able to choose it for ourselves. The longer you take to get ready and confront this and make some decisions, the more likely you won't get to make the decisions at all.

Adult Children, don't discount a little denial on *your* part. All of us tend to stick our parents in amber, suspended forever, with us seeing them always as the ones in charge, the head of the family, the Matriarch or Patriarch. When you finally get past that compartmentalization and come to the realization that your parents *are* getting older, you too have to face some new realities. You need to acknowledge your parents will need more help, may in fact become more dependent on you, that you may have to assume more responsibility in what may already seem like your overburdened life.

Many emotions can hit you at this time. Anger at your added "burden" or fear that you will be unable to help properly (or are too far away to do so), and the perfectly natural reluctance to face your parent's mortality—that is *your* denial. The sooner you begin to plan the necessary conversation you and your Older Adults must have, the longer you have to face the inevitable changes that aging brings to families and the more time you have to *control* your reaction and instead *craft* your response.

Handling Possessions

Next, understand that the mere thought of downsizing is a tough idea to contemplate. As an Older Adult you have collected a lifetime of possessions and certainly wonder what it is you are to do with all your "stuff." Conversely, as an Adult Child, you may have to temper your initial reaction, which is often to yell, "Just throw the junk out."

Recently, I was working with Mary, who was planning to move from her large home to a one-bedroom independent living apartment. On my first visit to her home, Mary opened the cabinet where she kept her wine glasses and showed me that she had three-dozen *each* of glasses for red and white wine and champagne. I asked her whether she planned to keep any and she told me that she would keep all of them because she still entertained regularly. Upon further questioning, I learned that Mary actually invited a few people over about once a month. A dozen of each type of glass would be more than adequate. Once we talked about it, Mary agreed, and we were able to send the excess to her recently married granddaughter who was planning dinner parties of her own. Sometimes just coming up with a plan for disposing of the extra household possessions is enough to help yourself (or your parents) get ready for the necessary transition.

Adult Children, accepting the job of helping your Older Adult part with their possessions is a delicate thing. What seems like unnecessary trash to you may be treasure to your parent. Allow plenty of time to go through the things with your Older Adult. Each item may have a story associated with it. Pour a cup of tea and take time to listen to that story before gently assisting your parent to part with it. Have a list of places to donate the items; know, for example, that the Salvation Army may send a truck for furniture and the location of the nearest Am Vets clothing donation box. Or find out which of your siblings is interested in those photographs of your great-great-grandparents from Poland, and tell your parents who wants what. Knowing their possessions are going to someone within the family or some worthy cause may help make the parting easier for your Older Adult. If you decide to have a yard sale, volunteer to run the whole thing—from organizing and pricing to final cleanup, and be prepared for your Older Adult to change their mind on some items and "rescue" them from the sale pile at the last minute. Realize, too, that the things are *their* things to part with or keep, and know that anything that gets moved to their new home and doesn't fit can be given away later. That isn't as efficient, perhaps, but it may be less wrenching for your parent.

Finally, thinking about the move itself is overwhelming—for everyone concerned. Getting bids. Coordinating the packing. Supervising on moving day. Unpacking. Furniture layout. Hanging pictures. Everyone hates moving, no matter what his or her age. If you are an Older Adult, it's likely that you don't have the stamina to do this all yourself. Enlist your Adult Child or, if they are too busy or too far away, consider hiring a "senior move manager." You can learn more about these professionals later in this book, or check the resources section for a link to their national organization.

Adult Children, don't make the mistake of thinking that by offering to supervise your parent's move that you've undertaken a small chore and you can get the truck and be packed in a weekend. Leave plenty of time for discussion and planning of the destination and even more for sorting, packing, and disposing of the things your parent will not be taking with them.

One of the biggest mistakes I see is folks who wait too long. By the time they decide what they want to do, their choices are more limited and they feel like they've lost control of the situation. Planning ahead saves much heartache when it comes to choosing where to age.

Where to Age?

Recently, I've found myself working with several client families: Older Adults who are deciding where and how they should live as they age, and Adult Children trying to make this vital decision about one or both of their parents who are unable or unwilling to do so.

While your situation may differ from other families in some important ways, a set of common tools works well in these situations.

If you are thinking about this important question for yourself or are helping a loved one to make the decision, give this approach a try:

The first step is to have an open and honest discussion about the wishes, wants, and needs of each person who will be affected by the decision, and that goes for both the Older Adult and the Adult Child. If you are an Older Adult who doesn't have a spouse, partner, or child to engage in this discussion, then enlist a friend or a trusted advisor. It's important to have someone there who will ask the tough questions and make you think about the answers rather than just validating what you say you want to do just because you said it.

Neither should you, as the Adult Child, just take over the situation, make all the decisions, and ramrod them down the throat of the Older Adult. A clear, honest, and thorough *exchange* of ideas is the key to harmony.

It's important to talk about all kinds of parameters without judging at first. You must get a clear picture of your (or your parent's) current needs and try to envision what will be needed in the future. Write down everything that comes to mind. Focus on *making* the list at this point, not on organizing or editing it. Whether you are the Older Adult tending to your own future or the Adult Child making such an important decision for or with your parents, trying to envision the big picture is very important. The basic options are to "age in place" in your current residence or that of a family member, or to transition to a senior living community of one kind or another.

Questions to Consider

Here are a few questions for you, the Older Adult (or for you, the Adult Child, to pose to your parents) to get you started:

- **How much space do you really need? How much space do you want?** If the two answers differ, explore why. I've observed that many women feel they want a large kitchen with lots of storage, but when the discussion gets specific, they acknowledge that they no longer cook as much as they used to and might rather make reservations to eat out.

- **Do you plan to age in place? Why? Have you thought about the logistics of that decision?** For example, is there a flight of stairs to get to your unit or to the master bedroom? Is there at least one bathroom that can accommodate a wheelchair or could be easily modified to do so? Is there a second bedroom and private bathroom where a caregiver could live if that becomes necessary? How comfortable would you be having a caregiver living in your home with you?

- **Do you have a readily available social support structure nearby?** If you begin to have mobility issues or can no longer drive, will you quickly become isolated, or do you live in an active community with lots going on nearby?

- **How do your personal finances stack up?** Do you own a long-term-care insurance policy? Are you still paying a mortgage and/or equity loan on your residence? What financial resources are available to you to fund possible future care needs? Are you living within your means today? Can you find ways to reduce expenses or increase income?

- **Have you considered sharing a home with a family member?** Would your family member move into your home, or would you move to theirs?

- **What worries you the most about the decision regarding where to live?** Is it running out of money, being a burden on family members, feeling isolated and alone, or losing your independence?

Once you have addressed these sorts of questions, it's time to articulate a couple of scenarios and then analyze them. For example, one of my clients was trying to decide whether to sell his condo and move to a senior living community. We looked at the two scenarios based on the economics of each choice, by running cash flows for each scenario out for five years beyond his statistical life expectancy. This client was more worried about running out of money than anything else and wanted to be sure that he had adequate resources to fund his decision. For another client, the main concern was not becoming a burden to her children, so we evaluated her options by placing the most weight on that parameter.

Also, you should ask yourself, and try to answer honestly, how willing you are, as the Older Adult, to take care of yourself because that answer will weigh heavily on your decision (or the decision being made for you). There are no "right answers" when it comes to this important decision about where to age. Rather, find the answers that are right for you, the Older Adult, given your current and expected future situation or that of the Older Adults in your life. A frank and realistic discussion of the options is the basis for a successful outcome, no matter what the final decision.

Age in Place

The option that most people say they prefer is to age in place in their own home (or that of a family member). This is typically feasible as long as you can manage activities of daily living (ADLs) such as dressing, bathing, toileting, preparing meals, etc., and as long as you are not suffering from cognitive decline that could cause you to be a harm to yourself or others by, for example, leaving the teakettle boiling on the stove and starting a fire. As your abilities decline, you can get help from family, community agencies, or faith communities, or through private individuals or services.

In Case of Emergency

Making a commitment to staying safe is a prerequisite for successfully aging in place. For example, sometimes we forget to take even the most basic steps to protect ourselves in the event of an emergency. I've been surprised many times when I ask clients if they have added ICE to their cell phones, wallets, and glove compartments. Most often, I'm greeted with a questioning look. Of course the "ICE" I'm asking about isn't the kind you find in a cocktail. I'm talking about that most basic of preparations for times of trouble: ICE—In Case of Emergency.

Today, emergency first responders such as police officers, fire-fighters, paramedics, or emergency medical technicians (EMTs) are trained to search a victim's cell phone for an entry labeled "ICE." This is how they know who to call in the event that something has happened to you.

The first thing I advise my clients is to obtain a simple cell phone if they don't have one and then create at least one emergency contact in their cell phone. It is possible to find very simple cell phones made especially for older adults. In addition, I suggest placing a laminated card with the same information in the glove compartment of each of their vehicles and in their wallet. Finally, if you take walks and don't tend to carry your phone or your wallet, I suggest punching a hole in a laminated emergency card and attaching it to your house key. That way, if you collapse on the street during your walk, you will be quickly identified and your emergency contact may be notified.

The first question that usually comes up in this discussion is who should be listed as your emergency contact. I recommend that you list at least two people, one of whom should be the person you have named as your health care surrogate. Ideally, this person will also know other important information about you and your health; don't forget to supply them this information, including who else needs to be contacted and the name of your primary physician.

The next question I'm frequently asked is what information should be listed on the card when you need more room than what can easily be incorporated into an ICE contact in your cell phone. Start with your name. It is easy to be separated from your wallet containing your identification, especially in an emergency.

Older Adults, it is particularly important that you list your medical conditions, major surgeries you've had, prescriptions you take, and your insurance numbers, along with your people/doctors/attorneys to contact. Include these with the cards physicians often provide if you are a heart stent patient (indicating which ventricle the stent is located in) or alerting EMTs that you are taking anticoagulants. Diabetics often opt for a bracelet alerting people to their condition. You may wish to include your blood type and date of birth to store with the other information as well.

As with so many other parts of our lives, technology is available for this purpose as well. If you choose to, you can subscribe to a variety of services that store your emergency information and/or your medical history and will provide it to first responders in the event of an emergency. Such services require that you wear or carry an identification tool such as a bracelet or wallet card that tells emergency workers what number to call and provides your member identification number. You will also have preloaded your personal information into the service's database, usually via a secure website, along with instructions regarding the circumstances under which your personal information can be accessed and by whom. Of course, this type of a system only works the way you intended if you wear or carry the identification at all times and keep your data up-to-date in the service's repository.

If you prefer, special encrypted flash drives are available to hold your complete medical record, including recent test results and your full list of medications and conditions. If you go this route, you must also remember to carry this with you at all times if it is your only form of emergency information because if it isn't with you, then no one will know that it exists.

Adult Children, you should offer to have the cards laminated, the key ring card or flash drive made, and your parent's information entered into their cell phone for easy access. While you are at it, don't forget to take care of your own ICE information. It you are old enough to act as caregiver for your parents, you are old enough to know you are not immortal. It's best to be prepared.

Medical Alert Systems

Older Adults, another way to take care of yourself, and one you should not resist if you are choosing to live alone as long as possible, is using a medical alert system. The TV commercial scenario "I've fallen and I can't get up" is a true one. By agreeing to use such a system, not only will you never be alone in the case of emergency, but your Adult Children can have more peace of mind knowing the proper professionals will be alerted if something were to happen. If you are unfamiliar with the whole idea, here's an explanation of how a medical alert system works and why they are so valuable for independent-minded Older Adults: The basic idea is that if you are ill, injured, lost, or disoriented, you simply have to push the button on a transmitter device that you wear or carry with you at all times. The person receiving the transmission can then call emergency responders, a neighbor, or a family member to come to your assistance.

Many people supplement this system by putting a lockbox on their front door containing a house key. The person receiving the emergency transmission can then provide the lockbox code to the responder, avoiding the need to waste valuable time trying to get to the ill or injured person or having to break a lock or window to gain entry.

Medical alert systems typically consist of a receiver or base station that allows a central monitoring station to communicate with the client and a waterproof transmitter (typically on a wrist band or necklace) that allows the client to communicate with the monitoring station. The central station then maintains a call list indicating who should be called in the event of an emergency and in what order. Such systems are typically available for a monthly or annual rental fee or as a one-time purchase. Another choice is the "no fee" alert system that you can set up to call your friends or family, instead of a monitoring service, thus avoiding the cost of monitoring.

Some of the newest technology even incorporates monitoring sensors that tell the central station whether the client has deviated from his or her normal schedule or has forgotten to take medications that are stored in a special medication management container.

Medical alert systems also differ from each other in the radius from which their signal can be received. Some medical alert systems work only within a set distance from the base station (receiver), which is usually connected to a home's landline telephone. This means that the system will work within the home and sometimes for a short distance outside, such as to the end of a driveway where the mailbox is located. Many newer systems work anywhere in the world through GPS technology and do not require a landline. Some are hybrid or dual systems and work via a base station in your home and via a portable unit that you carry with you when you are out. So, the first decision you need to make is whether to obtain a home-based system or one that works wherever life takes you.

When selecting a medical alert system, be sure that you under-stand both the technology and the terms of the contract or service agreement. Also, be sure to compare the different systems carefully. For example, some systems come with only one transmitter while others provide a second one at no extra cost. Some provide assistance with setting up the system while others expect you to do it yourself. Finally, some providers include back-up batteries for the parts of their system that require electricity to operate, but others do not.

The most frequent objection that I hear from my clients regarding acquiring a medical alert system is, "I carry a cell phone. What do I need a medical alert system for?"

Here's my answer: A cell phone is terrific, until it's not. For example, let's say you are the Older Adult and have fallen. You've hit your head and are knocked out. You won't be able to dial your phone. If you are confused or disoriented you might not remember the pass-word on your phone or what number to dial in an emergency. What if the person you've managed to call doesn't answer? And finally, do you take your cell phone into the shower with you? The biggest advantage of a purposed-medical alert system is that it is designed to be with you all the time, twenty-four hours a day.

That brings me to perhaps the most important point of all: Older Adults, your alert system only works if you remember to have the transmitter on your person all the time. I can't tell you how many times I walk into a client's home and see the neck pendant on the bedside table or the kitchen counter. It won't do you any good at all in those locations. Be cooperative. The system is being provided for your safety, it's true, but it is also for the peace of mind of your Adult Children and other caregivers who can't be with you all the time.

Adult Children, you may find that sometimes the Older Adults in your life get recalcitrant and dig in their heels about not wanting to wear the alert system monitor. It may feel like a kind of leash to them. I have two strong suggestions: Make sure to fully discuss why the monitoring system should be considered—and by "discuss" I mean a two-way conversation where the Older Adult gets to vent their frustration at having reached a stage in life where such monitoring is necessary—and try to overcome the Older Adult's objections and gain their cooperation *before* choosing the monitoring system. Remind the Older Adult they should be wearing the monitoring transmitter device. Sometimes Older Adults will fight wearing the device in passive ways, like simply "forgetting" or frequently losing it. Don't give up the fight. You must convince them to wear the device even if you risk being considered a nag. Not wearing the transmitter is the only "fail" in this vital "fail-safe" system. Explain why wearing the device is a selfless act on the part of your Older Adult and that it means you will gain serenity and peace knowing help for them—and communication with you—is only one button push away. If the Older Adult realizes it's not just about them, but about you, too, you may have won the battle. It is a battle well worth winning.

Combine Households

The author of *How To Set Up A Multi-Generational Household,* Ashlea Ebeling, wrote, "One of the side effects of the [recent] economic contraction is that Americans are about to rediscover the virtues of three-generation households. This is how families used to take care of their oldest members before that newfangled invention, the retirement home, arrived on the scene."

Ebeling goes on to outline an excellent guide on how to "do it right" if you plan to have a multi-generational household, covering zoning laws, space planning, and ownership/estate planning/tax issues. But perhaps most important of all, she also suggests that both sides of the equation, the Adult Children and their Older Adult Parents, have a sit-down talk about everyone's expectations regarding the proposed new living arrangements.

Adult Children, are you planning to rely on Grandma as unpaid childcare? That's called "Gransploitation" in some circles. Older Adult, are you looking forward to leaving your lonely life and assuming your kids will spend every weekend fishing or watching the game with you? Both these scenarios rely on unspoken assumptions, and until such things are brought out in the open and discussed—*prior to anyone moving anywhere*—you all may be setting each other up for disaster.

Money should be discussed also, as it serves as the flashpoint for lots of burning resentments and fires of anger. Older Adult, do you want to pay your fair share of household expenses so as not to be a burden and seem dependent? Adult Children, are you counting on your Older Adult to split the monthly expenses, when in fact your parent may plan on leaving all their money untouched until their death and then leave it all to the grandkids? Who handles the household accounts? Who writes the checks? Can all adults access house accounts? Are the Older Adult's supplemental medical expenses to be paid out of one combined account? For tax purposes, is the Older Adult going to be claimed as a dependent? These and many other questions should be discussed in detail, not only among the two generations, but with any tax advisor, insurance agent, or any other professional who is needed to bring clarity to the situation.

How about the other domestic issues? Will everyone dine together? Do any adjustments have to be made in meal planning to meet dietary guidelines in that instance, or will the Older Adult maintain their own grocery buying/cooking schedule? Will the Older Adult have a key to the house and come and go as he or she pleases, or will some method of checking in with each other be in play? Will the Older Adult get added to the Adult Child's cell phone family plan? How will laundry be handled? Does either generation have a pet that needs to be considered? Small pets can be hazardous to low-vision Older Adults, and longtime pets may be as much a part of an Older Adult's family as the human children are to the Adult Children. Can the household accommodate another pet? Does the house need to be made more universally accessible (more or better lighting, grab bars, stair railings, etc.) to make it safer for an Older Adult? Is one of the grandchildren going to give up their room to accommodate their grandparent? As a member of the family, perhaps that child should also be included in family discussions about the merging of the household.

These and other questions can and should be discussed and a Life Transition Plan crafted once all parties have reached agreement. This is not something to drag into court if things go awry, but rather a document that clearly states what everyone has agreed upon, so all can see what is expected of them and what they can expect. If you encounter trouble crafting such a Life Transition Plan, consider consulting a life transition coach or other trusted professional.

The last thing you want to do is sacrifice quality relationships with your family for what may be short-term economic gains. Family is priceless and, though a rich tapestry can be woven by multi-generations living together, it is not the solution for every family. Only a frank, open, and thorough discussion will let you see if it is the right solution for you.

Transition to Senior Living

So, you are an Older Adult, and the day you've been dreading has finally come. You have concluded that you simply can't live in your home a moment longer. Or you are an Adult Child and you have decided—with or without input from your parent—that the time for the move has arrived. You, Older Adult, need to move from your home or condo for your own safety and/or convenience. But because many Older Adults resist facing this reality (and many Adult Children don't want to bring up what their parent sees as such a disagreeable subject), the question of where to move still looms large. Each choice has different implications with regard to cost and logistics, and what is right for you will depend upon your needs, financial resources, and family dynamics.

An option for some is an **independent living community**. While the details of what is included in an independent living contract will vary by state law and property, they generally provide a maintenance-free lifestyle, some meals, and communal activities. Some communities will also provide transportation to doctor's appointments, local shopping and banking, and entertainment venues. As with living in your own home, you can bring in additional help à la carte as you need it.

At the point that you need more help with activities of daily living (ADLs), you might want to consider an **assisted living community**. While details regarding what is included will again differ by state law, this option will generally provide hands-on and standby assistance with ADLs and all meals, in addition to the things that independent living communities provide. Each state has rules about what physical and cognitive abilities a potential resident must have in order to be admitted to an assisted living community, as well as rules regarding limitations in the services such facilities can provide.

The scenario that most Older Adults dread is the thought of ending their days in a **nursing home**. Most such facilities offer two types of care: rehabilitation and long-term care. The rehab unit typically provides physical and occupational therapy for those who have been discharged from an acute care hospital, allowing them the opportunity to regain their strength so that they can go home again, wherever home may be. The long-term-care (sometimes called custodial care) unit provides care for an indefinite period of time, and in addition to providing custodial care (such as bathing, incontinence care, etc.) can provide skilled care related to wounds, oxygen, and IVs, to name just a few examples. Some states license "adult-care homes" or "convalescent homes," which might be relatively small facilities that provide only custodial care.

Specialized **memory-care facilities** offer secure surroundings for those suffering from dementia or another cognitive decline. Memory-care units come in several different models, ranging from freestanding "cottage-style" communities to secured units within another facility. The objective of these dedicated units is to keep residents safe, while at the same time providing them with a stimulating environment staffed by specially trained personnel. This can be very important for some patients who may have dementia and related complications but who are otherwise physically healthy.

Some parts of the country have integrated offerings called **continuing-care retirement communities** (CCRC) or life-care communities. These are regulated by each state. In general, the concept is that you pay an entry fee and monthly fees that entitle you to certain services and amenities during your lifetime. Depending on the contract, your estate may or may not receive a refund of a portion of the entry fee upon your death. In return, the CCRC promises to provide you with the level of care that you need for the rest of your life. Most CCRCs require prospective residents to pass both financial and medical entry tests and will generally accept you only if they believe that you will be able to live independently for at least three to five years before needing assisted living or nursing home care. Emerging models include "CCRCs without walls," where a similar concept is employed but the care is delivered in your own home.

Choose a Specific Community

I recently had the opportunity to participate in a health fair in a local assisted living community. I was able to engage with several residents, and I noticed some striking differences among them.

The first lady I spoke with was very pleasant but completely out of touch with what was going on around her. She was calm, polite, and immaculately dressed, and if you saw her at the cosmetics counter in Saks Fifth Avenue, you wouldn't have thought that she was anything other than a sweet older lady. That said, after spending just a few minutes chatting with her, it became clear that she was (happily) in her own world.

Along came an older gentleman who, with the exception of a pronounced limp, looked like he belonged on the golf course. He was charming and articulate, and I was wondering to myself why exactly he was living there, since he looked like the picture of health.

A few moments later, a gentleman stopped by in a blue blazer, crisp dress shirt, pressed trousers, and well-shined shoes. He spoke in French for a few moments and gave me the two-minute version of his life story. When he was done speaking, he began again and repeated the story, word for word. When he started in for the third time, the truth of the phrase "looks can be deceiving" became startlingly clear to me.

Finally, a woman came in riding a scooter. She was the self-appointed leader of the book group and was concerned that she couldn't find her "flock." She had a mission, and that was to get her fellow residents to read and discuss great works, and to write their autobiographies as a legacy for their families. She and I spent quite a while talking about her frustration that so many of her peers didn't seem to think that anyone would be interested in their life stories. This lady was clear in her thinking and well spoken—as vibrant as most people half her age. It was her body, not her mind, that caused her to be there.

Remember that each of the people you will encounter is an individual. The same admonition can be applied to you Older Adults who think assisted living facilities are just for "those really old people." Don't assume that everyone's circumstances are the same or that such facilities are just Heaven's Waiting Room. Though some residents' bodies may be failing them, their minds are sharp and their personalities intact. Conversely, don't assume that if someone "looks fine" that they will be able to process everything that you are telling them. You should take each person as they come and realize that each of these individuals is a blessing in their own way. We all, Adult Children and Older Adults, need to stop making snap judgments and see people for who they are and how they can contribute to our lives.

So, after taking all of the above into consideration, it is time to make a choice. From past experience, I know that once you have arrived at a decision, it is important that you move ahead with it quickly. As the saying goes, "time kills all deals," and this situation is no exception. You will always be able to come up with a reason why this *isn't* the right time to move. But the truth is, if you or your parent has reached the point where you have even started visiting communities, you probably know in your heart that this move really is in everyone's best interest. Look at the move not as an ending, but a beginning—of the newest chapter in your life or the life of your Mom or Dad. Making the right decision now will help make that chapter a happy one.

Top Strategies to Determine the Right Choice

Scout ahead of time: Options for senior living are many. If you remember going to look at colleges, you'll know exactly what I mean. It can be overwhelming to figure out what you need and what you want. So start the process sooner rather than later, even if you can't imagine that you'll ever choose to move or if you are an Adult Child who can't envision having the conversation with your parent.

Understand the math: Money *does* matter. Your resources as an Older Adult will determine the range of available options. For example, if you have equity in your home, are a veteran, or own a long-term-care insurance policy, you may be in a very different situation from someone whose only resource is a monthly Social Security check. Crunch the numbers ahead of time to figure out how much you can spend each month and what is included. Most communities provide a worksheet that will help you understand this calculation.

Don't confuse the issue by spending time visiting a place that is beyond your means. Adult Children, you can volunteer to help here. Gather the brochures and price sheets from various places for your Mom or Dad and sort out the choices that must be excluded before presenting the others for consideration. Note your parent's and your own questions and make the calls to get the answers. Write the answers down and add the Q&A to any discussion about the suitability of any destination. Offer to arrange and drive to visits to each locale and take photos to help you and your parents remember each individual place. Have lunch out afterward to quietly discuss the pros and cons of each place while the memory of the visit is still fresh. Listen carefully to what your Older Adult has to say about each place. It is, after all, where they will be living, no matter what *your* preference.

Narrow the choices to no more than three or four using the "Six S" method: Once you have a list of possibilities that are within the budget and preferred geography, it's time to narrow the choices to a few where you think you (or your parent) will be happiest. My "Six S" method considers size, sights, sounds, smells, services, and, most importantly, similarities. Older Adults, with the help of their Adult Child as advisor, should notice these categories and ask themselves these questions:

Size: Will you be more comfortable in a larger community with many residents or a smaller, more intimate setting? Can you still get around reasonably well, or will a large campus become frustrating? Will you take advantage of the facilities that might be available in a larger community, or will these amenities likely go unused? Will the size of the living unit work? To many women, having a full kitchen is very important, even if they will receive two meals each day as part of their living package. On the other hand, many men are sure they need a den or office within their living unit and won't hear of moving into a space without it.

Sights: The classic line I hear from people exploring senior living options is, "Everyone here is old!" Sometimes that's true. Some communities cater to an older crowd with more physical limitations, and you'll see lots of walkers and wheelchairs. Other communities attract younger, more physically active residents, where jackets and ties at dinner are expected. You'll also find distinct differences in the "look and feel" from one residence to the next. Some have a homey feel, while others look like an upscale hotel or even a cruise ship. Still others give a more clinical or medical impression. Ask yourself whether you can see yourself in a particular community. Take the time to notice the details, especially in the public spaces.

Sounds: When you first enter the community, do you hear a hush or a loud television set? Or perhaps you hear ringing phones and beepers, much like you would in a hospital. Do you get the impression that the residents are socializing, gathering, and participating in activities? Is music playing? Are people talking to each other or each in their room watching TV or, worse still, lining the hall, sitting in wheelchairs, looking listless?

Smells: Try to visit about a half an hour before mealtime, and notice the smell. Is it appealing? When you are in the living areas, do they look and smell clean? Does there seem to be a strong air freshener odor everywhere that might be used to mask less than optimal cleaning? Your sense of smell is a fabulous clue to what's really going on.

Services: Some communities offer a continuum of care so that residents can come into an independent-living situation and then move to assisted living, skilled nursing, or a memory unit if needed. This is ideal if you and your spouse need different levels of care or if you suffer from a condition that you know will progress over time. You'll also want to look at the services available to help with activities of daily living, transportation, physical therapy, etc. Take a close look at the social calendar, since interaction with others is one of the huge benefits of community living. Ask to look over meal plans and menus and ask to have a meal in the dining room. That will not only give you a hint of the quality of the food served, but will allow you to see some of the residents.

Similarities: You are looking for a place where the residents are as similar to you as possible in terms of age, activity level, mental acuity, hobbies and interests, and socio-economic factors. Ask about the demographics of the place you visit.

Ask for and check references: Before you decide that a particular community is on the short list, be sure to ask for and check a few references. Ask for permission to talk with the family members of two or three residents, in addition to the residents themselves. When you have these conversations, don't be shy about asking some tough questions. Ask to meet some of the staff as well—and not just the marketing staff, but the servers, aides, nurses, even the director of the place. Make a list of things you want to know and literally interview them.

I would also counsel you not to jump to conclusions, but take time to really observe the residents you might encounter at any senior living community you visit.

The Move

While no two family situations are the same, Older Adults and Adult Children face several common scenarios as the Older Adult parents come to the point where it is no longer possible for them to live in their own home without assistance.

If the family has determined that it is not feasible or desirable for the parent to move in with one of his or her Adult Children or another relative, and in-home assistance isn't possible either, the Older Adult will need to move to another living situation entirely.

You, the Older Adult, have decided that it is time for you to move to a senior living community, or perhaps this decision was reached through discussion between you and your Adult Children. Or, failing that, in the case of incapacity of the Older Adult, you, the Adult Children, might make this decision alone.

But a frequent scenario is when you Adult Children might clearly see that it is time that your parent makes the move to a senior living community, but your Older Adult doesn't see it that way. Conflict can result. So what are the steps you, as the Adult Children, need to take to make that move happen without causing a battle to break out?

First, you must deal with your own guilt, which can prove toxic to the entire situation. Despite your Older Adult's initial objections and the natural tendency we all have for self-doubt, I'm sure you have examined the situation carefully and weighed all the pros and cons. If, after that process, you still believe a move is in the best interests of your Older Adult, you should act. Realize that the longer your parent stays in his or her current living situation, the more likely it is that a crisis such as a fall will occur, making the move ever more urgent. It is always better to transition calmly than to do so in crisis mode.

So, what can you do to help your Older Adult accept that the move is the correct choice for them?

First, talk it over with them calmly. Lay out your case and the facts you used to arrive at the decision that moving to a retirement home is a good move for them. Take your time and be patient. This is a conversation you might need to have more than once. Allow the Older Adult to think things over—after all, they've been making their own decisions all their lives. Be prepared to address their objections; under no circumstances should you lose your temper. Treat your Older Adult with the respect they deserve.

For your part, Older Adults, don't be recalcitrant and dig your heels in. Treat your Adult Child with enough respect to allow them to present the case to you, and try to keep an open mind. Do your part to help fight the notion that Older Adults are inflexible. Consider that your Adult Child's decision is based on love for you and their hope that you stay safe, happy, and healthy.

One of the best ways to see the benefits of a move is for the Older Adult to literally see what they are moving *to*. Many communities will allow short stays for prospective residents. Such a stay can be a great way to introduce the Older Adult to the new environment, while still letting them come home again before making the move permanent. A week or so is a good length of time for a short stay. I've actually heard of Older Adults who decide not to return to their former residence once they've tried out their new community.

Adult Children, you can do the legwork and investigate which places allow such visits and make the arrangements once the Older Adult agrees to the visit. Older Adults: Don't just say "no" arbitrarily. Consent to the visit. Think of it as an adventure or the beginning of a new chapter in your life. Your attitude can determine how positive this new living arrangement can be for everyone involved. Abraham Lincoln was speaking truth when he said, "Most people are as happy as they make up their minds to be."

Another way for Adult Children to help their Older Adults get a little further down the road toward making the beneficial move to a senior living community is by helping choose the household items and personal treasures the Older Adult wants to bring along to their new home. It is true that one of the hardest things for an Older Adult is parting with all of those things he or she has accumulated over a lifetime. Moving to a senior living community usually means downsizing and getting rid of some of those things. Perhaps there is a favorite chair or dresser that will make the new space feel more like home and help you or your Mom or Dad get over having to get rid of the rest. Maybe some special window treatments or new bedding can be made for the new space that will make it feel fresh. Hanging favorite photos or art on the walls and making sure the place is all set up before you or your Older Adult moves in will help to make the whole move less overwhelming. Older Adults, if you can try to look at this as a positive new experience where you get to move to a clean, new, safer place and can enlist the help of your Adult Child to make it your own, the time of preparation for the impending move can be a bonding experience for you both.

Adult Children: If you are good at visualizing an empty room as a home and have the time and energy to set up the new space, then by all means you should take on this project yourself. If not, you might consider engaging a **senior move manager** (SMM) who can coordinate the entire project.

Senior Move Managers

SMMs are professionals who specialize in assisting Older Adults and their Adult Children with the emotional and physical aspects of relocation. They can also be enlisted should you be attempting to age in place and need modifications to the Older Adult's or the Adult Child's home to do so.

The SMM can help you determine the optimal community and unit that will best serve your needs. If you and your Adult Child enlist their aid, your SMM will create a floor plan for your new home, organize and sort through belongings, arrange for the shipment or profitable disposal of unwanted items, locate storage where needed, interview and oversee packers and movers, unpack and set up your new home, and coordinate related services such as cleaning, waste removal, selecting a realtor, or preparing the home you are leaving for sale.

These professionals are part organizer, part psychologist, part coach, and part conductor. They are often very familiar with the layouts of local senior living residences and will know at a glance whether that favorite sofa will fit in the new space. They are also invaluable when it comes to knowledge of local consignment shops, organizations accepting donations, and specialty sellers of collectibles.

Most SMMs will orchestrate the move in all ways—unpacking, hanging pictures, and even stocking refrigerators on the day of the move. In fact, I was so impressed with a senior move manager with whom I regularly work that I engaged her firm's services to help *me* downsize and move. On the day of the move, I thought I had died and gone to heaven when I came home after working all day and found the beds made up with clean sheets and the coffee pot ready for the next morning. The next day I came home to find the pictures hung and the boxes empty. Amazing!

With their expertise in resources and approaches that save money and time, SMMs reduce stress for both the Older Adult and their Adult Children. Imagine how nice it would be to go away for a long weekend and return to your new home with everything unpacked and put away. That sounds like the perfect cure for the exhaustion everyone fears when facing a big relocation, doesn't it?

When picking a SMM, be sure to choose someone who is bonded and insured. Also, make sure the person you choose specializes in working with Older Adults and their families and is not simply a moving company employee.

Household transitions are difficult for everyone, but even more so for Older Adults who have accumulated a lifetime of possessions that often won't fit in their new home. As the Adult Child, you don't want to be the bad guy making Mom or Dad part with their treasures, or perhaps you live far away and logistically can't be in charge of overseeing the move. An expert, affordable, and compassionate SMM can help both you and your parents to navigate this important life transition.

The National Association of Senior Move Managers (see resources) provides more detailed information about these professionals, including where to find one to help make the move a smooth transition.

Billing Errors

You may be an Adult Child handling the bills generated by the senior living community where your parent now lives. Or you may be an Older Adult resident of one of these communities who pays your bills yourself. Either way, you may notice that many senior living communities don't do a bang-up job of bookkeeping.

They are notorious, in fact, for not properly recording payments, causing duplicate bills to be sent or late charges to be applied. Since, as a caregiver, you may be working long distance, or as an Older Adult, you may have problems with mobility, it is not always as simple as walking into the facility to sort things out. Often, the person responsible for generating the bill is at a location far away from the facility.

So how can better communication be implemented with the facility?

I recommend that prior to moving in, the Adult Child who will be responsible for overseeing Mom's care or the Older Adult himself or herself make an appointment and go in to meet with the various department managers at the facility. Whoever is handling paying the bills should meet with the person who generates the bills for the facility—just as whoever will handle medical issues should meet with the director of nursing.

The purpose of these meetings is to establish open channels of communication. This is usually done better in person than over the phone. We are all more likely to respond positively to someone we know than to a frustrated stranger on the other end of the phone, and fitting a face with a name is always a good thing. However, if the correct person works in another location, then a phone call is better than nothing.

Then, keep a close eye on every bill and make sure that the payments are posted properly. If you have a question, take the time to call and ask, and document the date, who you spoke with, and the outcome of the conversation. When necessary, put things in writing. If either of these tasks is too inconvenient for the Older Adult, you Adult Children can step up and offer your help in getting things straightened out. Be sure to help institute and keep up a paper trail of any conversations to avoid misunderstandings. If long-term-care insurance or other third-party payments or reimbursements are involved, the probability for error increases exponentially.

If you find chronic errors, speak with the billing manager and ask if there is a better way for you and her to communicate so that the errors will be reduced, taking less time for both of you.

If you are already well into your relationship with the facility, or you've tried the suggestions above to no avail, then you are in a tougher spot. If you can find someone on the other side that seems willing to help, then make friends with her. Find out when her birthday is and be sure to send a card. Try to catch her doing something right, and then say "thank you" or write a brief thank-you note. You might even write a note of praise or thanks to her boss and send her a copy. The idea is to have someone who will be willing to go the extra step to try to solve problems on your behalf. Develop a personal relationship because it's harder to be rude to someone who has been nice to you in the past.

Another suggestion is to assume the facility is innocent until proven otherwise. That is, instead of calling with a huffy tone of voice about the error you are sure they have made, tell them you are confused by the bill and ask for an explanation. Even if you know that you are correct, if the other person can see the error, he might simply acknowledge it and make the correction, thereby avoiding an argument.

The key lesson is to keep a close eye on things and act on them immediately if you have a concern. The newer the possible error, the easier it will be to solve.

Settle In

For many Older Adults, the move to a senior living residence is emotionally very difficult. True, the move is a smart one if you are no longer able to safely live on your own. But that doesn't make the change any easier. The realization that it is necessary is very sobering, as is the inescapable conclusion that you are another step down the road.

Such a move is wrenching, too, for Adult Children, who tend to think of their parents as living in one place—set there firmly in their imagination—never to be anywhere else. Truth be told, it's a bit like putting your dolls away in a toy chest and expecting them to be right where you left them when you return.

In either case, the scenario of moving into a new place—no matter how nice the new residence is—can be jarring. Adult Children may look at it like a new opportunity. Older Adults, at first, may see it more as an ending.

Simple Ways to Make a Senior Living Residence Feel More Like Home

Resist the assumption that new is better: Be sure to bring along some *familiar items*. If you are an Adult Child, you might be tempted to buy a new bedspread for your Mom, much like you would do for your daughter who is heading off to college. However, Mom might much prefer that familiar old spread that makes the new space feel like *her* bedroom and not a hotel. Older Adult, you will probably be parting with much of your home or condo furniture, but you can always make room for your favorite chair and footstool. Make sure to place lots of family photos around the new space, too. Updated photos of the grandkids are always welcome and, Older Adults, be sure to stash a family photo album on your closet shelf, too. A new place doesn't mean there is no room to reminisce.

Feel free to decorate: Make the room your own new space so it doesn't look or feel institutional or generic. Many senior living communities will allow a new resident to specify a paint color at no charge, or will allow you to have the space painted a non-standard color, as long as you leave a deposit to cover the repainting later. Warm colors on the walls will help make the new space feel cozy. Likewise, be sure to bring any favorite wall art or lamps along, and don't hesitate to have some window treatments made. They go a long way toward customizing a space.

Consider the space limitations: When you are considering what should be moved to the new residence, remember to make sure that you have a place for everything. You don't want too much clutter that will collect dust and get in the way. Maintain the delicate balance between having enough of those familiar items to make it feel like home and trying to stuff too much into what is almost certainly a smaller space than you or your parent is used to.

Get organized: Older Adults, if you didn't do it when your kids left for college or when you downsized to move into the condo, it's time to regroup and reorganize. Adult Children should help with this. Have a "Sorting Saturday" and maybe even a yard sale. Call the Salvation Army or AmVets to pick up larger things, and drop clothes off at a nearby clothing donation bin. Maybe your neighbor's son could use the cookware and dishes for his new apartment, or ask at the local homeless shelter if they need such things. Adult Children, you should be careful, though, that you don't bully your parent into getting rid of some of their most cherished items just because you think (secretly, I hope) that they are junk. And Older Adults, don't cling to things you really never will use again. One perfume bottle is fine. Do you really need your entire collection cluttering up your new bathroom vanity?

Everything has a place: Be sure that there is a simple way to keep everything in its place. You Older Adults will feel much more in control of your environment when it is easy for you to find what you are looking for in your new home. Ask the help of your Adult Child to organize your new closets and label new baskets and bins for storage. For a while, until you are used to things, you may even want your Adult Child to label your new kitchen and clothing drawers until knowing the location of everything becomes rote. Adult Children, *if your parent doesn't mind,* when you visit, take the time to look around and make sure that things are where they should be to help keep order in the smaller space.

Jump into the social swirl: The sooner you get to know your fellow residents, the better. Ask the administration to introduce you to others and speak up (after giving them a chance) if you really can't stand the dinner companions at the table to which you've been assigned. Adult Children can help here. Listen to your parent's complaints. Speak to the staff about them and see what accommodations can be made, understanding that your parent may just be reacting badly to a new situation and that his or her feelings may change with the passage of time.

Another thing to look out for is to help get your parent "matched" to other residents with similar memory and physical levels of mobility. If your Mom has some memory issues but is still physically very active, be sure to request that she not be seated that first night with a group who is all mobility impaired. I promise that if you do, she'll notice and tell you that everyone else is "too old" for her to socialize with.

As with any other transition, it's important that you or your parent immediately finds a few people with whom he or she can relate, who are "their kind of people."

Such care at the beginning will make the move into a senior living residence go much more smoothly for all.

5

HEALTH CARE

MR. HUNTER, A RETIRED career military man, also worked in the aerospace industry for many years. Upon retirement, Mr. Hunter became eligible for Medicare and had supplemental insurance from both his employer and the military. With all of this insurance coverage, Mr. Hunter never expected to receive many medical bills, and he certainly didn't expect to have his accounts with his physicians sent to collection agencies. Over the years, Mr. Hunter's former employer changed insurance carriers, and this created much confusion. In the meantime, Mr. Hunter's health was declining and he was suffering from memory loss. The situation became more and more confused, and eventually Mr. Hunter was receiving nearly daily dunning letters and calls regarding his medical bills. He couldn't understand how, with his three insurances, his bills weren't being paid.

The Importance of an Advocate

Recently I was acting as a life transition coach for Fran, who was undergoing a series of significant life transitions all at once, including divorce, the loss of her job, and troubling physical symptoms, including weight loss and musculoskeletal pain. As overwhelming as all of that sounds, perhaps the biggest challenge was that none of Fran's doctors thought to look for an underlying physical condition to explain her symptoms.

While working together to solve many day-to-day issues, I began to wonder if there wasn't something more going on and suggested Fran get a second opinion from another doctor. As it turned out, Fran had needlessly suffered great physical pain because her varied symptoms had been chalked up to "stress."

While it is true that stress played an important role in Fran's distress, the fact is that she had a medical condition that, when treated, caused her situation to become manageable rather than hopeless. The fact that I, as a third-party advocate, was involved and suggested she consult another physician was the catalyst necessary to make a positive change in her situation.

A patient advocate can often bring a fresh set of eyes to a situation. In this case, I began to research possible causes of the constellation of symptoms that might be causing her discomfort, apart from the generic diagnosis of stress. And while I am no doctor, it immediately became clear to me that it was very possible that at least a portion of the symptoms could be explained by one or more medical conditions or be due to an adverse reaction to prescribed medications.

Such research is sometimes beyond the capabilities of some Older Adults, many of whom grew up in an era where a doctor's word was sacrosanct, and even researching other possibilities related to their own condition meant at least a day in the library and more likely a lot of frustration and resignation.

While I had no illusion that my findings would explain everything, my hope was that a proper diagnosis by a physician—perhaps pointed in the proper direction by some of my research and observations—would allow Fran to get some relief from her many physical complaints, gain strength, and have the energy to focus on the hard work of dealing with the financial issues she faced.

Fran's physicians were skeptical and brushed aside our request for a thorough reexamination. They thought we were playing doctor and didn't welcome a cooperative relationship between my client, me as patient advocate, and themselves. They stuck by their guns that all of my patient's symptoms were perfectly explained by stress. In their eyes, there was no need to look further. Such a paternalistic and righteous attitude proved unhelpful for my client.

As an advocate, I was able to engineer a second opinion involving a thorough workup of her medical condition. That workup revealed a diagnosis for a treatable condition. Fran is now recovering well and is in a much better place to tackle her many challenging life transitions.

In another recent case, I became involved after the fact as a **medical billing advocate.**

In many medical billing cases that require untangling, the simple act of a medical billing advocate sending a letter that begins, "I have been retained as Mr. Bailey's medical billing advocate," changes the dialogue between a patient and a physician's office or hospital. Often the mere mention of a third party's involvement in the situation is enough to start or reopen a conversation that had once seemed stagnant and immovable.

A third-party advocate in this situation also has the benefit of looking at a situation with new and objective eyes. When those around you say no, an advocate can ask why. An advocate has the energy and expertise to push harder than you, the Older Adult (or even the always-busy Adult Child acting as caregiver) might be able to on your own, and the third-party advocate doesn't necessarily even have to be a professional.

Adult Children themselves can act as third-party advocates for their Older Adult parents, with some caveats. While gathering, organizing, comprehending, and explaining medical bills and services to the Older Adult is part of the job of the advocate, the other task is to do some medical detective work. Interview (not grill) your parents about their medical conditions and care. Try to discover what symptoms they are still experiencing or perhaps have never revealed, as well as what medications they are taking and if they are taking them properly. Do some online research about their conditions to see what new findings or treatments are being used in the field, as well as what medications are indicated and if there are any contraindications with any of those they are taking for any of their other conditions. Consult with a pharmacist about their whole medication regimen.

Accompany the Older Adult to their doctors' appointments and listen carefully. If your parent (and the doctor) agree, you might even consider making a recording of the conversation on your smartphone or a handheld recorder. Ask any questions you need to in order to understand what is going on with your parent's condition. Press politely for clear answers and keep asking until you understand the answers. Arrange for a second opinion if you feel it is required.

But bear in mind that often Older Adults feel a great sense of loyalty to their physicians and are very reluctant to see anyone else. It is almost as though they feel they are being disloyal to their original physician by asking for a second opinion. Diplomacy must play a part in your dealings with them then. Don't push or bully, but suggest—repeatedly if necessary—that a second opinion won't hurt anything. Ask if you may share with them what your research revealed. Assure them that second opinions are not only valid and covered under their insurance, but part of taking an active part in managing their own care.

Don't put your foot down too hard unless your parent is endangering themselves or their health. Do watch carefully for overmedication. Physicians too often overprescribe strong drugs—like painkillers or sleeping medication—before comprehensively discovering what other medications your parent may be taking or understanding that your Dad still enjoys that martini before dinner.

Don't be too confrontational with either your parent or their physician. Arguing usually is not the way to handle this new relationship of doctor/patient/advocate. The old maxim, "You catch more flies with honey than vinegar" may apply here, but don't be too meek, either. Some physicians are used to geriatric patients who are often submissive and do as they are told. You are not there to do as you are told, but rather to help discover and arrange the very best care for your parent. Be reasonable, informed, and willing to listen. But, at the end of the day, know for whom you are "working." You are there as an advocate for your Older Adult, and it is their well-being that is paramount.

For your part, Older Adults: You, too, must try to be reasonable. Just because you have always done something one way does not mean that is the only—or the best—way to do things, whether it's treating a medical condition or seeing only the doctor you've had for the last twenty years. Doctors are only human, and the landscape of the medical field changes as quickly as scenery flying by a car window. Not every physician can be expected to keep up with every advance.

Listen to what your advocate or Adult Child has learned through research or thorough question-and-answer sessions with your physician and pharmacist. There may be a better way to help gain control of your medical condition.

When it comes to medical billing, Older Adults, you should welcome the advocate's help in unscrambling the codes, copays, and terminology "word-salad" that comprises today's medical bills. Consider it a gift that your advocate is willing to call, clarify, collate, and, if necessary, *command* the medical billing staff to track down the proper information, work with your insurance company, and ascertain that you are being billed correctly, while keeping a record of it all. Don't consider it a mark of dependence; just graciously accept their help and be glad of it.

Advocates, whether professional or family members, don't carry a magic wand and can't always get you the desired outcome, but they often can make an enormous difference and make the road through doctors, pharmacies, hospitals, and medical billing a smoother one for all concerned.

Home Health Care Services

Older Adults, if you have decided to age in place in your own home or live with a family member, and have overcome your natural objections to having a "stranger" in your home to help you with some chores that, once easily performed, are proving more challenging as you age, good for you! It was a hard, yet practical, decision.

Adult Children, you are glad your parents have arrived at that decision. It is, in one way, a weight off your shoulders. You have been watching your Older Adult struggle with domestic or medical chores and couldn't always be there to provide such help yourself. But, no doubt, you had some trepidation about either choosing or helping your Older Adult choose the right home health care provider. It was an important choice and a big responsibility.

Choosing the Right Home Health Care Aide

If you find yourselves in the situation where a home health care aide would be useful, how best to choose the right one?

Correctly identify the needs: Older Adults, take a long, hard look at your situation and be honest with yourself. What do you need help with? Are you no longer able to drive and need transportation to run errands or make your doctor's appointments? Do you need help grocery shopping or with meal preparation? Perhaps you need help safely bathing or with house cleaning? Maybe you just need companionship—an important item on the list of things to keep yourself mentally and spiritually fit. Loneliness can lead to depression, a dangerous condition. Or maybe yours are more medical needs. Do you need skilled services such as wound care or help managing oxygen or a feeding tube? Make a list of what tasks you feel you need help with and discuss the list with your health care advocate or Adult Child.

Next, you should both understand that several levels of licensure are necessary for caregivers, according to the different services they perform. You should arrange to obtain a professional assessment from a licensed home health provider or a geriatric care manager to help refine your specific needs and the appropriate level of licensure required.

Licensed agency/registry vs. private hire: I have a strong bias toward working with a licensed care organization because it puts a professional in the position of selecting candidates for you and because it creates a backup plan in the event that the caregiver you hire quits, is ill, or doesn't show up one day. While particulars vary by state law, a licensed care organization usually also checks references for those they employ or refer, provides the necessary liability insurance, and ensures that their employees or contractors are licensed themselves, drug tested, and, in some cases, bonded.

If you choose to work with a licensed care organization, be sure that you understand the differences between using an *agency* model as opposed to a *registry* model for the particular provider you are trying to hire. These distinctions vary by state.

Generally speaking, *agencies* employ their caregivers, whereas caregivers working with *registries* are treated as independent contractors. This has implications for insurance, liability, pricing, and supervision. However, that does not mean that you should only work with one or the other, because it is the ownership and management of the entity that determines the quality of the operation.

Start with those who know. As with so many services, it is critical that you obtain recommendations from people you trust to narrow your search down to a few registries or agencies. People who have already worked with the home health care agency or registry are your best bet. Ask them the probing questions. Were the home health care workers reliable, punctual, trustworthy, helpful, and kind? Did they speak English (or the language that is the Older Adult's mother tongue)? Were they safe drivers? Were they good cooks with some informed ideas of healthy nutrition? Did they have any problems discussing their education, licensing, or insurance? Were the clients sent a revolving door of different health care workers, or were the same workers available day after day? What problems did they encounter? Would the reference highly recommend the agency or registry's health care workers? If so, why? If not, why not? Compile a "database" of information you'll need for future dealings with any of the agencies or registries and listen for questions you should be asking.

Meet with the ownership or local management: Get comfortable with how they do business. Don't be afraid to ask lots of questions, such as, "What happens if the caregiver and care recipient aren't a match?" Or, "How are issues that arise over the weekend handled?" Find out about how the company selects, trains, supervises, matches, and disciplines its caregivers and management team. Make sure you understand what will happen if your care needs exceed their license in the future, as well as all contractual obligations such as minimums, cancellation notices, and extras.

Select the caregiver: Once you have settled on a care provider, it's time to match up your needs or the needs of your parent with an individual caregiver. If you have any special requests or concerns, the time to mention them is before a caregiver is matched to you. For example, one of my clients had several exotic pets and we wanted to be sure that this wouldn't become an issue for a caregiver. In another case, the client was quite large and we wanted to be sure that the caregiver would be strong enough to properly assist her. Such requests might be directly related to the ability to provide the care or may simply be personal preferences, but it is always best to disclose and discuss them upfront.

Ask to interview at least two potential caregivers for every shift. In other words, if you will have someone coming in three days each week, make sure that it will generally be the same person each time, and then interview two candidates for that job. If you are looking for a live-in person, try to meet a couple of possibilities before agreeing to a placement.

Once your caregiver is on the job, give everyone a chance to settle in to the arrangement. It will probably take at least a few days or a visit to have an idea about how well the situation is working. It is not unusual to have to tweak things a bit, and using a licensed organization to source your caregiver should facilitate this.

Change is hard for all of us, so give it a chance and don't jump too quickly to make a change unless you feel that the situation is dangerous.

Special Transitions
Adult day care

Adult day care centers usually operate during regular business hours and provide social interaction and a safe place for Older Adults who need supervision. This allows family caregivers to go to work, enjoy some respite, or take care of their own activities. Most adult day care centers offer flexible hours and some have transportation services—picking up clients and then returning them home at the end of the day. Many Adult Children struggle with the idea of entrusting their loved one to the care of these centers, but this is often an excellent way to begin to have the care recipient adapt to a congregate setting. Often, the Older Adult will benefit from the increased socialization and stimulation provided in this setting.

After rehab

Often, Older Adults and Adult Children caregivers are faced with the decision about whether they (or their parent) should move directly from a rehab facility to assisted living, or whether they are better off coming home for a short time in between. As with so many decisions involving Older Adults, it depends. It depends on five considerations: safety, cognitive status, resources, logistics, and psychological needs.

Safety

Considering your safety if you are the Older Adult, or your parent's safety if you are an Adult Child, is the top consideration when deciding which destination is best after rehab. Generally, the purpose of rehab is to help the patient regain strength and skill with balance, walking, and transferring from sitting to standing. In addition, the patient may have been receiving therapy related to day-to-day tasks in the home, such as preparing meals or dressing. Sometimes, despite the best effort of the therapy team, you or your loved one will simply not be able to safely care for herself at home and it is best to face the truth of that situation.

Older Adults, it can be dispiriting to have given your all during your stay at rehab, only to reach the end of your stay not yet able to handle everything on your own, but it is a mark of self-care to admit you need a little more help. It doesn't necessarily mean you will be unable to care for yourself always. It just means you need to be realistic about the situation at present so you can get the further help you need in a safe environment until your situation changes and another decision can be made. Pride truly does go before a fall in this instance. You are doing yourself no favor if you are too proud to admit you still need help and further injure yourself—having to start the rehabilitation process all over again. Adult Children have a right to point this out to you if you appear to be ducking the truth of the issue.

Cognitive status

A second consideration is the cognitive status of the Older Adult, and obviously this speaks more to the Adult Child caregiver of such a parent. If your Older Adult suffers from confusion or dementia, she may be unable to manage her own medication administration. Or, he may be prone to wandering around the neighborhood or getting in the car and driving away. In addition, transitions from one location to another are always difficult for an Older Adult, and this can be exacerbated in the presence of dementia or cognitive impairment. If your Older Adult cannot safely manage at home alone or suffers from cognitive issues, going home might not be a realistic option unless appropriate help can be provided. In this case, a specialized memory-care residence may be the best option.

Resources

If you as an Older Adult have sufficient resources to get yourself the necessary care in your home, or you as the Adult Child can yourself (or with your siblings) marshal the financial resources to hire appropriate caregivers, then having your Older Adult return to their home might be feasible. You'll need to familiarize yourself with the different levels of caregiver licenses and the requirements for providing an appropriate living space for the caregiver. In addition, you will need to determine whether a live-in caregiver is the best option or whether you will require multiple shifts of caregiver to cover your or your Older Adult's needs.

Logistics

If assisted living is the best option, it needs to be determined whether the assisted living residence will be ready at the time of discharge from the rehabilitation facility or whether there is a waiting list. Is the new place fully furnished, or do you have to furnish it? If you need to supply the furnishings, do you plan to buy new items or use things from your or your parent's former home? If the assisted living residence is available for immediate occupancy, it is often possible to make it comfortable on short notice by using a senior move manager, so that shouldn't be a deciding factor. You can always have personal items moved over the ensuing few days or weeks. It doesn't all have to be there on Day One.

Psychological needs

Finally, we must consider what is best for you, the Older Adult, or if you are the Adult Child, what is best for your parent. Many families (and certainly lots of you Older Adults will lobby for this) feel that returning home "one more time" is beneficial. Sometimes it is. This is especially true if you are an Older Adult who is both physically and cognitively strong and an active participant in the decision making about where to move. On the other hand, if you are an Adult Child in the role of caregiver and the Older Adult is an unwilling participant in the move or is really unaware of his or her surroundings, moving home again might be challenging.

As with so many other issues when caring for Older Adults, preserving independence and decision-making authority must be balanced with managing safety and resources. You, as the Older Adult, must strive to be reasonable, and you, as the Adult Child, must be as respectful, patient, and understanding as possible. Only in those ways will the decision about where to go be a balanced one, taking into consideration everyone's feelings and opinions.

Memory care

When an Older Adult suffers from Alzheimer's disease or another form of dementia, it often becomes very difficult to continue caring for them at home. This can be true whether they are living in their own home or a senior-living community's independent or assisted living areas. Sometimes the challenge arises because the Older Adult is an "elopement risk," meaning that he or she is prone to leaving the building and wandering away. At other times, the precipitating problem has to do with aggressive or uncooperative behavior. Finally, the degree of assistance the Older Adult requires with the activities of daily living (ADLs) might exceed the capacity for the family or paid caregivers to manage.

Adult Children, if you find yourself in this situation, you will need to make the decision to transition your Older Adult to a specialized memory-care unit or nursing facility (more on them in the next section). Memory-care units differ in some ways, but all share some general characteristics. Namely, the staff-to-resident ratio is generally higher than in other levels of care, and that staff is usually trained specifically in memory impairment and the special needs of these residents. In addition, memory-care units are typically secure, meaning that a special code is needed to enter or exit, preventing residents from wandering away. Finally, most memory-care units place a heavy emphasis on delivering the highest quality of life possible for their residents by offering an environment and activities that allow them to remain safe but stimulated by appropriate activities.

One popular model for memory-care units is the "cottage" model. In these centers, several smaller, typically single-story, buildings are arranged around outdoor space that is fully secured. Each cottage has bedrooms arranged around a common living/dining/kitchen area. Residents are assisted with bathing, dressing, and other grooming needs and encouraged to be out of their rooms during the day with free access to all indoor and outdoor common areas. The idea is that these smaller living units are less confusing for those suffering from dementia and easier for them to navigate. They also take into account that very often, residents suffering from dementia are otherwise physically quite healthy and able to move around on their own or with limited assistance.

Adult Children commonly tell me that making the decision to transfer their aging parent to a specialized memory-care unit setting was both the most difficult and the best decision they made on their caregiving journey. They report that after the initial settling-in phase, their parent was more social and seemed generally happier and more engaged. At the same time, the caregiver knew that their loved one was safe, and the amount of worry they carried around decreased significantly.

Nursing home care

The care setting that most people fear the most is the nursing home. As was explained earlier, most such facilities have sections providing post–acute rehabilitation services, while other areas of the building are set aside for long-term custodial care. If your Older Adult is bedridden or requires certain medical procedures and interventions, you may have no option other than considering a nursing home.

It seems that horror stories appear daily in the press about nursing home neglect and abuse. Unfortunately, these circumstances really do occur, so it is absolutely critical to be a careful consumer if you must place your loved one in such a care facility. Visit the Medicare website and look for the Nursing Home Compare tool, which allows you to learn about how to select a nursing home, gives details about Medicare- or Medicaid-certified nursing homes in your area, and provides five-star quality ratings of nursing homes. Note that not all nursing homes are certified by Medicare or Medicaid, so you may also want to visit your state's nursing home regulation department's website. These are also listed on the Medicare website (enter "State Survey Agency" in the search bar).

Hospice and palliative care

The National Hospice and Palliative Care Organization (www.nhpco.org) defines hospice care as "expert medical care, pain management, and emotional and spiritual support expressly tailored to people facing a life-limiting illness and their loved ones." In most cases, hospice care is provided in the patient's home but may also be provided in freestanding hospice facilities, hospitals, and nursing homes. The hospice team develops a care plan that meets each patient's individual needs, and this care plan is implemented and delivered by an interdisciplinary team. About one-third of Medicare beneficiaries are found to have availed themselves of hospice care, with the average length of service in 2011 being about nineteen days. Medicare does pay for hospice care for its beneficiaries. Most hospice organizations offer caregiver and bereavement support as well.

Hospice care organizations are located throughout the country. The majority of hospices are independent, freestanding agencies with the remainder being part of a hospital system or other care organization. About one-third of hospices have not-for-profit tax status, and most of the others are for-profit organizations. About 5 percent are government-owned programs.

Treatment that enhances comfort and improves the quality of an individual's life during the last phase of life is called "palliative care." No specific therapy is excluded; the test of whether care is "palliative" is whether the care team believes that the expected outcome is relief from distressing symptoms, the easing of pain, and/or enhancing the quality of life. The decision to intervene with active palliative care is based on these measures rather than the desire to affect the underlying disease.

Many Adult Children tell me that they wish they had learned about the availability of hospice and palliative care much earlier while caring for their parents. They believe that considering involving the hospice team sooner (or at all) would have made an enormous difference for both their Older Adult and themselves as caregivers and then survivors.

Make Sense of Medicare

Medicare is the federal government's health care insurance program for people age sixty-five and older (and younger people who meet very specific criteria). Adult Children: Have you ever walked into your aging parent's home and seen a stack of Medicare papers on the kitchen table? Has the thought crossed your mind that maybe you should have these papers come directly to you since they seem so confusing to your Mom? Older Adults, do you find yourself puzzled over which Medicare Part D drug plan you should select, or whether you should consider a Medicare Advantage program? Have your claims been denied for services that you thought were covered? If any of these situations have happened to you or to your parents, you're not alone. Many Older Adults and their Adult Children find dealing with their medical paperwork overwhelming—the sheer volume can intimidate even the stoutest-hearted among us.

What about if you or your parent simply needs help selecting the right plans? Each year, Medicare-eligible people are allowed to switch between original Medicare and Medicare Advantage and/or select their Part D prescription drug plan during "open enrollment." This process begins on October 15 and ends on December 7 of each year, although these dates are subject to change. The best place to gather information for this decision is to start at the Medicare website at www.medicare.gov. There you can learn about "original Medicare," as well as about "Medicare health plans," "Medigap policies," and "Medicare prescription drug plans." Which offering is right for you or your parent will be determined by a number of factors, including your or your Older Adult's overall health, finances, and the degree of choice desired. You may find that while one approach works well for you and another for your spouse, Mom and Dad might be better off on different plans. It is perfectly fine for you or your parent to select the coverage that works best for him or her as an individual.

How to Read an Explanation of Benefits

One area of continuing confusion for just about everybody is what all the jargon on the medical bills means in the first place. You can't evaluate possible errors without learning this language.

You've received a paper titled "Explanation of Benefits" (or EOB) from Medicare or your insurance company. Typically, just below the title, it reads, "This is not a bill." That said, it has dollar figures all over it. So if this isn't a bill, what exactly is it?

The EOB is exactly what it says it is—an explanation of the benefits provided by Medicare or your insurance plan for a particular service on a particular date. Its purpose is to report to you (the subscriber or your caregiver) and your doctor or hospital (the provider) exactly how the claim was processed. It is critical that you review each and every EOB you receive for accuracy and the need to take action. Not doing so may cause you to become financially responsible for charges that otherwise would have been covered by your plan.

However, most people are intimidated by the EOB and have no idea what to look at or what to do about what they see. This is particularly true for Older Adults who may suffer from some incapacity or simple frustration over the ever-changing format of medical billing. Adult Children, who may have more patience, can be a help here, offering to review the bills, explain them to their Mom or Dad, and even handle any discrepancies or question details that need clear explanation by making phone calls or sending correspondence.

But with all the codes, jargon, and terminology, whether you are the Older Adult dealing with your own bills or the Adult Child stepping in to help translate the bills for your parents, medical bills may seem like a journey through a foreign country—one where you don't know the language.

Guide to Your Explanation of Benefits

While every EOB uses slightly different terms and formats, the key items you need to review are:

Patient name: Is this you or your dependent? If you don't recognize the name, call the insurance company immediately and report the error.

Date of service: Refers to the date that the visit or procedure or other service happened. Is it accurate? If not, report it immediately.

Provider's name: This is the doctor, hospital, or other entity that provided the service. Often, you will know that Dr. Jones was your surgeon, but the provider on the EOB will be Everytown Surgical Associates. This is fine, as long as Dr. Jones is indeed part of that group. If you're not sure, call the surgeon's office and ask. Likewise, sometimes you will receive a bill for a provider you don't recognize at all. If you had surgery, it's very possible that this is an anesthesiologist, radiologist, emergency room physician, or pathologist who participated in your care and who bills separately. When in doubt, ask.

Procedure code or type of service: This is the shorthand where the provider communicates the service for which payment is being requested and is often a five-digit number or an abbreviation. You may see several codes for one date of service as when, for example, you visit the orthopedic surgeon and have an office visit, x-rays, and a cast applied. Likewise, when you have surgery, multiple procedure codes are often reported. One common question occurs when a service is reported as "surgery," but sometimes it's not clear if the procedure you had done was surgery or not—like when you had a skin lesion removed in the office. That's hardly surgery, is it? It probably is. This doesn't mean that your provider is doing anything wrong or trying to get away with something. Rather, it is simply the language of insurer-provider communications.

Total charge or billed amount: This is your provider's standard charge for the service.

Allowed amount: This is the amount your insurance plan will pay under its contract with your provider.

PPO discount: This is the amount that is "adjusted" off the bill due to your insurance plan's contract with the provider.

Not covered amount: This is the amount your plan does not cover. Sometimes, this refers to any charge that is above the allowed amount or the "reasonable and customary" charge, and other times this refers to services that are not covered under your plan.

Copay, coinsurance, deductible: These are the amounts that are the subscriber's responsibility under the terms of your insurance plan.

Patient/subscriber responsibility: This is the total dollar amount that you may be billed directly for the date and services reviewed on the EOB and may include amounts that you have already paid at the time of service. Typically, you will pay this directly to the provider.

Remarks/remark code/message code: This is the method by which the insurance company communicates with both you and your provider to explain how the claim was processed. Most often, the codes will be several letters or numbers next to the particular service. Elsewhere on the EOB you will find the "key" to these codes, which might read something like "Duplicate charge," or "Not covered on the same date of service as the related charge," or "Not covered due to lack of timely filing." There are many, many codes and they vary by insurance company, but this is where you will learn what you or your provider might need to do to have the claim processed and paid correctly. You must review this and take the appropriate action in a timely fashion.

Payment assigned to provider: This means that whatever payment is being made by the insurance plan is going directly to the provider. He or she is a participating provider in your plan, and you signed an authorization with the physician to submit the claim on your behalf and receive direct payment. Where this is not the case (as when you use an out-of-network provider), the check may come directly to you, and you are responsible for paying the provider.

If you are confused or overwhelmed by your or your Older Adult's medical paperwork (and who could blame you?), there's no shame in calling in help. As I mentioned earlier, you might consider a medical billing advocate. These professionals are well versed in the ins-and-outs of medical billing and can help you get problems with your claims resolved quickly and efficiently. Calling in the cavalry may save you not only hours of confusion and frustration, but lots of money.

Untangle Medical Billing

Once the health insurance coverage is in place, everyone involved—whether that is you and your spouse and/or Adult Children helping in this arena—should be thoroughly familiar with all the details of your coverage.

Adult Children, if you are acting as caregiver for an Older Adult, it is very useful for you to also understand exactly what is covered under your care recipient's policy. Take time to familiarize yourself with Medicare and any recent changes to the program by visiting www.medicare.gov, and ask for a copy of the Older Adult's supplemental policy and go over that. If possible, schedule a meeting with your parent or Older Adult to make sure they understand what is covered under their policy, too. If you find that you also don't understand exactly what is covered, make an appointment with the agent who sold the supplemental policy and ask any questions you or your Older Adult may have. Keep asking until you get the crystal clear answers you need. Keep any notes you make with a copy of the policy in your papers relating to your Older Adult. They will come in handy if you ever find yourself in a dispute with the insurance company.

For example, if the Medicare plan you've selected has both *in-network* and *out-of-network* benefits, you need to understand the difference. When you make an appointment with a new provider, be sure to ask if they are in your network, and then check this out yourself on your insurance plan's website or by calling their customer service number.

Likewise, some Medicare plans require a referral and/or pre-certification for certain visits to specialists or for specific procedures. *Don't assume that your doctor's office has checked this out for you.* If they say that they will take care of it for you, call your insurance plan yourself anyway and find out if the provider did indeed call and whether the service will be covered and at what level.

Horror stories abound, even when an Older Adult is covered both by Medicare and a supplemental policy. One recent client learned after the fact that neither Medicare nor her supplemental policy would cover her procedure because it was considered to be experimental. In this case, the patient assumed that her doctor would not recommend something that wasn't covered by Medicare because he clearly knew that was her insurance. She was wrong. The experimental procedure was *not* covered and she had even signed an "Advance Beneficiary Notice" indicating that if Medicare refused coverage, she would accept responsibility for payment. Since Medicare didn't provide coverage, neither did her supplemental plan because they generally pay only the coinsurance and deductibles for *covered* services.

Figuring out exactly what you are covered for *prior to any services* is the key to being an informed medical consumer. Ask questions up front—lots of them, particularly about the endless details covered (and not covered) by your policy, like your deductibles and coinsurance responsibility.

If you are an Older Adult and all of this all seems overwhelming to you, be sure to ask for help. Reach out and perhaps ask your Adult Child to help clarify all the details. If the task is beyond them, hire a medical billing advocate. Either way, getting your facts straight will save you endless trouble in the long-run.

Let's say you are long on patience or short on funds and want to have a go at straightening out your own or your parent's medical bills yourself. I applaud your intrepid spirit, but don't go into the fray unarmed.

Mistakes in Handling Medical Billing

Here are some mistakes people commonly make when dealing with medical billing. Avoid these and you will be ahead of the game.

Ignoring the mail: Have you received mail from a medical provider, Medicare, or insurance company and put it in the "I'll get to it later" pile on the kitchen counter, often unopened? From my work with hundreds of clients, I know the reasons for this avoidance are most often:

The paperwork intimidates me.

I don't understand what I'm looking at.

I have insurance, so I don't need to review this stuff.

I can't pay it anyway, so why open it and stress out about it?

While I can certainly understand each of these reasons for avoiding the medical bill mail, the reality is that taking this approach is very likely to come back to haunt you in the form of your account being sent to collections.

If you don't understand the bills or explanations of benefits (EOBs) you receive following a medical service, ask someone to explain them to you. You can call the patient-billing specialist at your provider, or try the customer service representative for your insurance plan.

Everyone needs to review their medical bills and how the claims were processed, even if you believe that you have "good" insurance or Medicare and a supplement. Billing mistakes can and do happen, and the patient is often responsible for paying for them. While you have the right to appeal, you must do so within the time frame required by your plan. By ignoring the mail, you risk missing this important appeal deadline.

If you're worried that you can't pay what you owe, you're always better off negotiating a payment plan and possibly a reduced charge than simply ignoring the demands for payment and ending up damaging your credit.

Not asking for (or reviewing) itemized statements: The best way to avoid medical bill problems is to make sure that the charges are correct in the first place. While no one expects you to be an expert in medical terminology, by requesting and reviewing a detailed itemized statement following every episode of care, you can often avoid some of the obvious problems.

For example, I recently saw a man's bill for his annual physical. The charges included a line for a pap smear, which even most laypeople know is a test that is only performed on women. Had he reviewed the bill right there at the checkout window, that charge would have been removed before the claim was ever sent in to the insurance company.

I also recently saw a hospital bill that itemized seventy-seven of the same item at $198 each. That's more than $15,000 of charges! This item (a urinalysis) was something that no one could have done seventy-seven times in the space of a three-day hospital admission. Not only was the charge itself very high, but the number of tests just didn't make any sense. If this patient had requested and reviewed the bill, she would have picked up on the repetitive charge.

Always take the time to ask for and look at an itemized bill, and if you see something amiss, try to get it resolved immediately. If you feel you are being charged for services you did not receive, ask for a copy of your medical record. If you find discrepancies, these may be used to negotiate with your provider.

Not asking for what you need: Medicare and many insurance plans limit the amount of services you are eligible for under your plan. For example, physical therapy visits are often limited to a certain number within a period of time. While this works out in many instances, sometimes more sessions might be needed in order to optimize your recovery. When that happens, ask your physical therapist and/or physician to write a "letter of medical necessity" *in advance* of the provision of services. Don't wait until you've run out of visits before you ask your providers to help advocate for you. It's your responsibility to be aware of the limits on your policy and not to just assume that your providers are on top of it.

In other situations, doctors will prescribe a certain drug, not realizing that a particular patient's plan only covers a less expensive alternative. There is no way that a physician can keep track of the frequently changing approved drug lists for each of her patients, so if you go to fill the prescription and find out that the drug your doctor prescribed is *not* covered, let your doctor know and find out whether something that *is* approved can be used as a less expensive alternative. If your doctor feels very strongly that you need that original specific drug, request that the doctor's office make a phone call or prepare a letter of medical necessity. The doctor may not agree, but if you don't ask, you definitely won't get covered for the intended medication.

Not reading before you sign: You *know* that you should never sign something you haven't read and fully understood. When the clipboard is shoved in your face, it's tempting to just acquiesce and sign on the dotted line. However, by doing so, you are making yourself responsible for a bill that is not your own.

Another hidden danger is signing for someone else. If you are the Adult Child and acting as caregiver for an Older Adult who cannot sign medical paperwork him or herself, it is very important that your name is not the only signature on the document. If you alone sign, you are accepting financial responsibility for your parent. Instead, if you hold power of attorney, it's better to sign their name and then your own name alongside it with "as power of attorney" noted. If you don't hold power of attorney, it's better if you don't sign at all. If the provider insists on a signature prior to rendering treatment, make sure you sign your Older Adult's name and then your own name and add the phrase "as representative." *Whatever you do, don't accept financial responsibility for another adult, even your spouse.*

Not understanding the coverage: The most common mistake I see is that Older Adults or their caregivers may have no idea how Medicare or their supplemental insurance works and are shocked and confused when they discover they owe money for medical services. It is critically important that you, as the consumer, take responsibility for understanding how your health care is paid, what is covered, the types of services that require referrals or pre-authorization, and so on. As painful as it can be to take the time to slog through this material at the start of each plan year, the more informed you are, the more benefit you will receive from the coverage that you have.

If you, the Adult Child, or you, the Older Adult, don't understand something about your policy or are embroiled in a confusing billing situation, realize there is no such thing as a stupid question. Even experts in the field sometimes are confused. Some would argue that insurers encourage such confusion, as a lot of money is made from less-than-vigilant consumers.

Fight Medical Billing Errors

You Older Adults (or you Adult Children helping them) may have successfully navigated through the treacherous waters of medical billing only to run up against the most frequent problem of all: human error. What do you do if some person along the chain just screwed up and the mistake is now something you have to deal with?

Medical bill errors, including those on hospital bills, can quickly become a nightmare for both you Older Adults and you Adult Children if you don't keep on top of them. The longer an error goes uncorrected, the less likely it is that you will be able to successfully fix it. Hospitals, physicians, and other providers are likely to send your account to collections if it is not paid within five to six months. While each entity follows its own guidelines with regard to how quickly it considers an account to be delinquent, most expect your bill to be paid in full unless other arrangements have been agreed to within ninety days of the date of service or forty-five days of when Medicare or your insurance plan has processed the claim. Failing to pay your medical bills is very likely to affect your credit, and unpaid hospital bills are a major reason why people file personal bankruptcy.

It is particularly critical that you stay on top of billing errors. This is because there is something known as "timely filing" in the insurance business. The regulations for Medicare and the plan documents of your supplemental insurance must indicate how long you or your provider has to submit claims. Once that time has passed, it is permissible for Medicare or the insurance company to deny your claim because it wasn't submitted within the required time period. At this point, the entire bill becomes *your* responsibility.

Similarly, if you don't agree with how your claim has been processed, you have a finite period of time to appeal the decision and escalate it through Medicare or the insurance plan's dispute resolution process. If you miss the appeal deadlines, you're usually out of luck.

Many different kinds of medical bill errors are possible, so you must have an eagle eye when you review your bills. Perhaps the simplest error for a layperson to find is a charge for a service that was never provided. For example, if you were billed for a test that you never took, make sure to dispute it. The fact that the clinician ordered the test and marked it on the "superbill" at the time of the visit is irrelevant if the lab never performed the test and recorded the results. Your medical record is the governing document when it comes to these disputes. If it's not in the records, it shouldn't be billed.

If you find yourself in this situation, request a complete copy of your medical records and a detailed itemized statement for the dates of service in question. Then, take the time to compare what's in the records with the statement and dispute any discrepancy.

Another common situation is duplicate charges where the provider has billed you for the same service more than once on the same day. While this makes sense sometimes, such as when you have an x-ray of both your right foot and your left foot, the provider needs to use a special code called a *modifier* to explain this to Medicare or the insurance company.

Also, keep watch for charges for things that the hospital or doctor isn't supposed to bill for separately. For example, if you have had surgery, the follow-up care should be included in the "global fee" for that service. For major procedures, that means that you shouldn't be charged for a follow-up visit within ninety days of the date of the surgery. You can, however, be charged for additional services other than the office visit itself, such as an x-ray or cast. Similarly, if you are hospitalized, the hospital shouldn't charge separately for sheets for your bed or your hospital gown, both of which are included in the room-and-board charge.

Handling More Difficult Billing Issues
But, even when you do everything suggested above, there will be times when you don't agree with a provider's bill or how Medicare or your insurance plan has processed the claim. What to do in that event? Here are some vital tips:

Keep detailed written records: Keep a log of every contact you have with the provider, Medicare, or insurance company— dates, times, who you spoke with, what they said, next steps, etc. If you mail something, keep a copy. You may wish to send all correspondence with proof of delivery, so both you and the recipients know you have a receipt and that they got your correspondence. If you fax something, keep a copy of both the item you sent and the fax receipt. If you email something, keep a copy—and don't just enter a running email dialogue back and forth only hitting "Reply" each time. All the "subject lines" will end up the same and make searching for individual ones later troublesome. Start a new email with each new exchange; your email provider will automatically sort them by date.

If the customer service person makes you a promise, get it in writing. So if the hospital says they will adjust or write off a charge, ask for written confirmation, preferably by email. If the claims adjuster says that they will investigate your issue, ask for them to write you a note indicating this, along with a projected time frame for their response. If your account has wrongly been sent to collections, demand that the provider immediately correct this and provide you with a written explanation that you can send to the credit reporting agencies.

Request detailed bills from your providers and review them carefully: If you don't understand a charge, ask for an explanation. If the explanation doesn't make sense to you, ask to speak to a supervisor. If you believe that a charge is inappropriate (either an error or outright fraud), don't hesitate to challenge it, preferably in writing. If you believe fraud is involved, report it to your state's insurance department and/or federal agencies, in the case of Medicare, for example. If something doesn't make sense to you on a bill or explanation of benefits, question it *right away*. Grievance or appeal procedures are common, but these must be done within the time frames stated in your policy documents. If you are told not to pay a bill while it is being researched or revised, ask whoever told you that to put it in writing. If you agree to a payment plan or a partial payment as "payment in full," get that in writing also.

Get help: If you don't have the time (or the tolerance) to handle your medical bills and related insurance claims yourself, professionals are available to assist you. Medical bill advocates are there to take care of these issues for you. You can choose to have such an advocate review all of your medical bills, or engage one only to assist with sorting out a difficult issue. Many states offer free assistance via the SHINE (Serving Health Insurance Needs of Elders) program. Check with the bureau that handles elder affairs for your state.

By understanding your or your parent's coverage, tracking, and organizing the reams of paperwork in a *timely* manner, and paying strict attention, the Gordian knot of medical billing paperwork can be untangled.

Need I say again that a medical billing advocate can be a sanity-saver in this situation?

Medical Billing Advocacy

Terminology and complexity are the rules of today's health care system. Most consumers are not even aware that there may be hidden problems with their bills. Whether you are a busy Adult Child, a slightly confused Older Adult, or are simply not feeling well, you may not feel up to the work necessary to get the corrections made. Or worse still, you might not even realize that you are being overcharged.

As I wrote in the last section, all kinds of errors are found on medical bills. I've seen many examples of billing more than once for the same service, billing for services or supplies not received, using the wrong diagnosis and procedure codes, unwarranted denials by the insurance company, and plain old human error. All of these causes can add up to you, the patient, paying more than you should be for your health care services.

Medical billing advocates not only help individuals review medical bills for errors and act like medical bill analysts, they also make sure what you are being asked to pay is something that you actually owe, that you are not being overbilled, and that Medicare or your insurance company is paying the amount it is obligated to pay. They also go over your bills and your coverage with a fine-tooth comb and make sure you get the benefits for which you are paying and to which you are entitled.

According to the Medical Billing Advocates of America, *up to 90 percent of hospital bills have errors, and those errors are not in your favor.* Most people do not ask for and do not receive an itemized statement showing what they are being charged for. If you went to the grocery store and they handed you a receipt that said, "Produce $40, meat $100, and canned goods $50, total $190," you probably wouldn't accept it. You shouldn't accept bills lacking in detail from medical providers, either.

So, having established the efficacy of hiring a medical billing advocate, where do you find one? As with most professional services, the best way is through word-of-mouth. Patients who have had a positive experience are happy to share their story. You may also visit www.billadvocates.com, the website for the Medical Billing Advocates of America, for a list of medical billing advocates. Since most medical billing advocates' work is done by telephone and email, it isn't necessary to hire someone who lives near you. It's best to hire someone who has a background in health care, insurance, or related fields.

Medical billing advocates are usually paid in one of two ways: hourly for the time actually spent on your case, or a percentage of the money the advocate saves you off your medical bill. In this latter case, if an advocate *can't* secure you a reduction in the medical bill you owe, you should be required to pay only the advocate's retainer (if any) and the costs of obtaining copies of your medical records. Discuss with the medical billing advocate which of these payment methods he or she employs, and then get, in writing, the terms and conditions of their contract with you. Also, as with every service provider, check out the advocate's references before hiring them.

6

MONEY

AT ONE TIME GINNY lived comfortably in a condo she owned outright, and she had a late-model car as well as a sizable monthly annuity payment and money in the bank. By the time her daughter and son became aware of her progressing dementia, the condo was in foreclosure and she could no longer drive the vehicle. On top of that, she had cashed in the annuity and spent the proceeds, leaving her with only her Social Security income and no assets. Ginny had managed to hide her financial difficulties from her children until it was too late, leaving her (and them) with few options.

I'm Afraid I'll Outlive My Money

When I talk with Older Adults, they tell me that the number one thing they lose sleep over is the fear of running out of money. In particular, they worry about the cost of health care, including paying for help with managing activities of daily living (ADLs) and potential custodial care. They worry for good reason, and the situation will get worse as the baby boomers age. Fewer Older Adults have (or will begin to receive) payments from pensions than in the past. This, coupled with economic volatility, the very low rate of retirement savings, and longer life expectancies is a recipe for disaster. Recent studies indicate that fewer than two-thirds of those approaching retirement age have any retirement savings at all, and the vast majority of those who do have saved less than $10,000.

Plans for coordinating and paying for future care needs should be initiated early on, ideally by people when they are in their forties and fifties. Why so soon? Because, as with so many other aspects of planning, the sooner you plan, the more time you have to implement your plans and the more options that are available to you. For example, the cost of long-term-care insurance premiums are lower the younger you are, assuming your health is good. As time goes on, it is more likely that premiums will be higher due to your age or health conditions, or you might even be uninsurable. Similarly, if you are interested in the idea of a continuing-care retirement community (CCRC) lifestyle, most communities require that you pass both a financial and health standard or you will not be eligible to buy into the community. For some families, the issue may be about planning to protect assets for use by the "well spouse" in the event that one spouse requires long-term care. Since Medicaid has a five-year look back period, it is important to do such planning well before the care is actually needed.

Consider this reality: You are sixty-five years old and newly eligible for Medicare. Based on actuarial statistics, you can expect to live for at least another twenty years. I advise my clients to plan for another twenty-five or thirty years. What does this mean in terms of dollars and cents? For one thing, you will need to plan to pay for your Medicare Part B premiums, your supplemental insurance premiums (if you carry this insurance) and/or any deductibles and coinsurance, your Part D prescription drug plan and your coinsurance, and services not covered by Medicare (such as hearing aids, vision services, etc.). On top of that, you need to plan for care. What does all this add up to? In today's dollars, you will spend:

- Approximately $1,200 per year on Medicare Part B premiums.

- Approximately $2,400 per year for a Plan F Supplemental Insurance premium (and possibly more, depending on your age at enrollment and the part of the country you live in).

- Approximately $500 per year for a Part D prescription drug plan premium.

- A typical $2,500 per year on uncovered services, deductibles, coinsurance, and copays.

This adds up to about $6,600 per person per year. On top of this, as we learned earlier in this book, long-term care on the average will cost in the neighborhood of $125,000 in today's dollars. And, it could be much more if you require extensive home care or need to move to assisted living or a nursing home. Total this up, and you are looking at $6,600 times thirty years, or well over $300,000 per person in today's dollars. That means a typical couple needs to have set aside at least $600,000 in an investment that will keep up with the rate of health care inflation by the time they reach Medicare age. This is, of course, on top of the funds that will be required for all other living expenses. I hope you can see why beginning to plan early makes sense!

Depending on your family's situation, purchasing private long-term-care insurance might make a lot of sense. In some families, one or more Adult Children will agree to purchase and pay the premium for a long-term-care policy for their parents as a gift. Whether long-term-care insurance is right for you must be considered in the context of available resources from other sources and an understanding of the available public benefits. We will cover each of these briefly.

Long-term-care Insurance

This is private insurance offered through insurance companies. Beneficiaries pay a premium, and in return the company agrees to provide certain benefits if and when certain conditions are met. Long-term-care policy offerings have many variations, so it is important to work with an insurance broker who specializes in this area. Some considerations include:

- **How you qualify to go "on claim":** This is typically tied to requiring assistance with two or more activities of daily living (ADLs) such as bathing, toileting, dressing, etc., *or* suffering from cognitive impairment. Some policies require you to need help with three or more ADLs. Some require you to need "hands-on" assistance, while others allow for only "standby" assistance (as in "Mrs. Jones, are you ready to come out of the shower now?").

- **Elimination period:** How long you need to be receiving paid services from a licensed provider before the coverage under the policy kicks in.

- **Site of care:** Some policies are "nursing home only," while others cover care in your home.

- **Inflation protection:** Some policies offer an annual adjustment to the benefit amount (such as 5 percent simple adjustment or 5 percent compounded).

Long-term-care policies have many other nuances, so it is critical that you understand what you are evaluating and purchasing.

Medicaid and VA Benefits

Medicaid is a joint federal and state program of health care services for the indigent. Details vary by state, and it is imperative that you consult with experts in your state. Medicaid is often referred to as a safety net program or program of last resort. Medicaid will pay for a shared room in a nursing home when it is medically necessary, when the beneficiary's income and assets fall below certain threshold amounts, and when there is a bed available. Not all nursing homes accept Medicaid patients, and there is often a very long waiting list at those that do, so planning ahead is critical. Some states offer limited community-based benefits for people who can be served where they live, and pilot programs are being tested around the nation. The specifics of what is available where you live may change often.

Veteran's Administration benefits may be available to service members and their spouses. As with Medicaid, certain income and asset tests must be met, and some VA benefits are tied to whether or not the service member was active during a declared wartime. This area is another with many technical nuances, so consulting with those with specialized knowledge is key. In general, however, those who qualify may get help with prescription drugs or funds to help pay for home care or assisted living care.

Manage a Fixed Income

Living on a fixed income is hard for many Older Adults. Imagine, Adult Children, if you had made all the money you were ever going to make in this life and yet had no idea how much longer your life would be!

Opportunities to spend at every turn are everywhere—birthdays, christenings, bar mitzvahs—and there is the constant temptation to give gifts to one's kids or grandkids. If you are an Older Adult, you may find yourself tempted to send overly generous checks to your grandchildren or buy too many gifts for your favorite caregivers. Perhaps you simply eat out more now that you cook less or can't resist those theater tickets or opera subscriptions. The hardest temptation for you Older Adults may be the pressure to spend more than you should over the holidays.

Adult Children, it may not even cross your mind that your parents feel pressured to overspend at holiday time. Maybe you are unaware of how "fixed" their fixed income is—how lacking in disposable income they actually are. Or it might not occur to you that your parents want to recreate memories of holidays past where the space under the tree overflowed with presents or where the Chanukah *gelt* was real money, and overspend in the attempt. Maybe your parents are embarrassed to admit they don't have the resources to join in your lavish holiday plans. Maybe you are too embarrassed to inquire about their finances.

Given the financial minefield the holidays can be, it's not unusual for those on fixed incomes to wake up in January not knowing how they will manage their bills for the next few months, given previous overspending.

If you are an Older Adult and find yourself in this situation, it's time to do some serious planning. First, you need to take a careful look at your cash flow and determine if you can do without some items for the next few months while you pay off those credit card bills.

It would also be a great time to dust off your budget and make a plan for putting some money aside each month into a "holiday fund" so that you don't wind up in the same boat next year. If you have never operated with a budget, maybe this is the year to start.

Adult Children, you could offer to help set up a budget for your Older Adult. Be sure you don't sound scolding or negative in your offer to help.

Whether you are helping to set up your parent's budget or are the Older Adult who charged those holiday purchases on your credit cards, be sure to pay at least the minimum amount due each month to avoid late fees. In addition, you will want to be strategic about paying off the accounts with the highest interest rates first.

Besides digging you out of post-holiday debt (or helping your Mom or Dad), the new year is a wonderful time to evaluate spending priorities and come up with a plan to stay on track.

If you're not sure how to begin, you might want to consider finding a daily money manager (DMM) to help. DMMs are those professionals I mention often who specialize in assisting with the day-to-day business of life. They can help create a budget—one you or your parent can actually stick to. They can help analyze which bills to pay off first. They can even handle the Older Adult's mail and arrange for payment of the bills.

As an Adult Child, though you may generously offer help, you may find that tackling your parent's finances is a little beyond your capabilities. Suggesting the use of a daily money manager is one big way you can help your parent.

You might also want to consider how to scale down your family's holiday plans so your Older Adult doesn't feel the financial strain. Host the party at your house, with everyone bringing a dish, instead of at an expensive restaurant; insist Mom make her famous pie as the price of admission. Institute a gift exchange where each family member draws a name and only buys a gift for that one person. Or set a limit on the amount each gift can cost—and no cheating. If your parents need to travel to your home for the holidays, send them a ticket using your frequent flier miles, or do the research online at discount travel sites to make sure your parent is getting the best deal.

At the holidays and every day, help your parent stretch his or her fixed income dollar by signing them up for a AAA membership if they still drive, or talk them into replacing owning their car (and hefty insurance fees) with a membership to ZipCar or another car-sharing service if they live in an urban area. Such a service allows one to pick up a car at various neighborhood locations, use it for a day, and pay very little. Or sign Mom up for Freebies for Seniors, where free samples of many nationally known products are sent to her. Or, if you live nearby, sign your family up at a local farm co-op and share the mountain of fresh produce you'll receive with your Mom or Dad. Put your Older Adult's name on your family cell phone plan and help them save a bundle. Look around for other creative ways to help your Older Adults stretch their limited resources.

Those who are trying to make sure they don't outlive their resources and who try to live within their fixed income need all the help they can get. Whether you are the Older Adult in need of help or the Adult Child trying to be sensitive to your parent's needs, carefully managing finances is the best way to accomplish this, and plenty of help is out there. Be sure to make use of it.

Help My Kids; Don't Jeopardize My Retirement

Older Adults often worry about other money issues like how to be generous to those they love without depriving themselves of a safe and comfortable retirement.

A question posed in an email from one of my clients is one I get asked often:

I am retired and live on a fixed income that should last me through my final years. I see my kids struggling and want to help them, but I don't want to give up my financial security. What can I do to help without hurting myself?

This is a very common dilemma. Older Adults hate to see their children struggle, even when the children are Adult Children with families of their own. It's only natural to want to help your kids. However, as this reader wisely asks, how can this be done without creating a tricky situation for you, the Older Adult?

First, take a realistic and close look at your budget and determine if you have any discretionary spending that can be redirected to helping your Adult Child, at least for a period of time. If you do, it is relatively easy to redeploy these funds. For example, let's say you have a satellite television subscription and you hardly ever watch the extra channels for which you've been paying. If these extras cost you $50 per month, you can cancel the services and instead send your son $50 each month. Alternatively, perhaps your daughter can do something that you currently pay someone else to do, like house cleaning. You might decide to pay her to do it for you instead of paying the third party.

If neither of these options is practical, then perhaps you have items you no longer use that you can sell, using the proceeds to help your child. Or, if you are physically up to it, maybe you can help ease the strain on your Adult Child's finances by providing services like cooking, cleaning, babysitting, or dog walking. Another option might be to pool your resources with your Adult Child, perhaps living under one roof to save expenses for both of you.

If you own your own home and have equity in it, you might consider taking a home equity loan or getting a mortgage (either forward or reverse), but this is rarely a good idea if it is your only source of funds. You never know if you might need this to pay for your own needs at some point, and if you take the funds now, then this last resort won't be available in the future.

Yet another possibility, if you are in a position to do so, would be to offer your Adult Child a loan. Ideally, your son or daughter would be able to pay you a fair rate of interest each month, providing you with some cash coming in. *However, don't do this if you can't afford to lose the principal.* While your Adult Child might have every intention of paying you back, that might never happen. Will you have enough money to take care of your own needs under that scenario?

The most important thing to realize is that money you give away, encumber, or spend on behalf of your children today is money that very likely won't be available to you in the future if you need it. Be sure that your desire to help doesn't set you up for an uncertain future later.

For your part, Adult Children, though times are tough and financial strain can cause panicky thinking, try to take a step back and realize that you don't want to overburden your parents and literally kill "the golden goose." Older Adults have no option to make more money in the future—that's why it's called a "fixed income"—and depleting their resources now will only mean trouble for you all down the road.

Try all other alternatives before asking such a sacrifice of your parent and, if your Older Adult *does* give you the money you need, make a clear plan—discussed and agreed upon—to pay it back. The last thing either of you need is to create an indigent Older Adult. This is truly a case of "penny-wise, pound-foolish."

Your parents are well trained over a lifetime of sacrificing for you kids. Such sacrifice is practically encoded in their DNA. They will give until it hurts and likely suffer in silence. Don't let them sacrifice more than they can afford.

And if your parent can bring himself or herself to say, "No, I can't afford to help you," accept their decision gracefully and without resentment. Know they would help you if they could and are really doing you a favor by taking care of themselves like the responsible Older Adults that they are. In its own way, that, too, is a loving act.

Get (and Stay) Organized

Perhaps you are an Older Adult who would rather get (and keep) a handle on your own finances, or maybe you are an intrepid Adult Child who has taken on the project of helping straighten out your parent's financial situation yourself. Bravo. But, as every Older Adult knows, the longer the life, the more possessions one accumulates.

So whether you are an Older Adult who's just been possessed by an urge to clear up the clutter, are downsizing to a smaller home or condo, or are that dutiful Adult Child who has decided to help your Older Adults get rid of the excess paperwork, knowing what to keep and what to throw away is tough. Allow me to share the advice a daily money manager would share with you—so that you keep the treasure and throw out only the trash.

The first general rule is: When in doubt, don't throw it out! Unless you are certain you can obtain the records electronically—say from your bank (and they often charge a hefty fee for old records) or insurance company, better hang on to the originals in either electronic or paper form.

Items to Hold Onto

Tax returns and supporting documents: In general, anything to do with your taxes should be kept for at least seven years. The IRS has three years from your filing date to audit your return if it suspects good-faith errors, and you have the same amount of time to file an amended return if you find a mistake. However, the IRS has six years to challenge your return if it thinks you underreported your income by 25 percent or more. If you fail to file a return or filed a fraudulent return, there is no limit on when the IRS can come after you. Specific items you should keep, in addition to your tax returns themselves, include documentation of income, alimony, charitable contributions, mortgage interest, retirement plan contributions, and any other deductions taken.

IRA contributions: If you made an after-tax contribution to an IRA, you will need to keep your records indefinitely to prove that you already paid tax on the money when it is time to make a withdrawal.

Retirement plan statements: Keep the quarterly statements until you receive the annual summary, and if everything matches up, you can shred or delete the quarterly statements. Keep the annual summaries until you close the account.

Bank records: Keep any checks or statements related to your taxes, business expenses, home improvements, or mortgage payments.

Brokerage statements: You must keep these until you sell the securities covered by them to prove whether you have capital gains or losses for your tax return. If you hold stocks or bonds for many years, you will need to keep the statements. The exception is if the cost basis and date of acquisition is listed on the statements. In this case, you only need to keep the year-end statements to support your tax return.

Bills: Keep bills until you receive the cancelled check or credit card statement showing that your payment was received. Be sure to keep bills for big purchases like jewelry, furniture, art, appliances, cars, computers, etc., so that you can prove the value of these items to your insurance company in the event they are lost, stolen, or destroyed in a covered disaster such as a fire.

Credit card receipts and statements: Keep original receipts until your statements come and then match them up. You can then discard the receipts. Keep the statements for seven years if they document tax-related expenses.

Paycheck stubs or proof of independent contractor income: Keep these until you receive your annual W-2 form or 1099s from your employer(s) and make sure the information matches. If it doesn't match, request a corrected W-2 or 1099 from your employer(s).

House/condo records: Keep all records documenting the purchase price and the cost of all improvements, as well as records of expenses incurred in selling and buying the property for seven years after you sell it. It's also a good idea to keep prior-year homeowner's insurance policy documents in the event of a covered loss that is discovered after the plan year has ended.

Medical bills and records: Keep all medical bills and supporting documentation such as cancelled checks or credit card statements until you are sure that the bill has been acknowledged as having been paid in full by you and/or your insurance company. If you are deducting unreimbursed medical expenses on your tax return, keep all supporting documentation as discussed above. Remember to keep all health-related bills, including dental, eyeglasses or contact lenses, hearing aids, and over-the-counter medications.

Using the above guide, you should be able to clear out the bulk of the saved paperwork and then establish a system for keeping up with things over time. Remember, documents can be scanned and archived electronically; just be sure to back up your computer system regularly.

Personal property: One other bit of archiving may prove vital, and it proves the truth of the old saying, "A picture is worth a thousand words." It is called **the household inventory**.

Imagine that it's the morning after a hurricane has hit your area. You venture out at first light and find that while your house is mostly intact, a tree has fallen into the roof and your master bedroom is open to the sky with two feet of standing water covering the floor. You immediately call your insurance agent, who begins the process of filing a claim with your carrier.

As part of the claim, you'll have to list all of the items that were lost or damaged, in addition to the structural damage to the house itself. That's a Herculean task at a time where just putting one foot in front of another feels like all you can manage due to shock. Eventually, an adjuster will appear to inspect the damage, and you will ultimately receive an offer from the company to settle your claim—an offer that has to cover replacing all your furniture, carpets, kitchenware, china, and even all your clothes.

It's bad enough when your home is damaged or destroyed by fire, flood, earthquake, or hurricane. But it adds insult to injury when all of the proof of what you had was destroyed, too.

This is a completely preventable scenario if you create and maintain a household inventory. The idea behind your household inventory is to document the items you have in your (or your parent's) home so that in the event of a loss, you can quickly move through the claims process with your insurance carrier and be on your way to repairing or replacing the items. This can also be helpful in creating an inventory of personal property when it's time to settle an estate.

The best way to build your household inventory is to go room by room and take still photos or a video, preferably with a visible date stamp. Be sure to open closets and cupboards to show what's inside, and for particularly valuable or rare items, it's worth taking the time to take a close-up. As you build your household inventory, don't forget to document what you have in your garage, basement, or attic. If you do nothing else, this at least provides proof of what you had in your home as of the day you took the photos.

If possible, go one step further and gather all of the receipts for the more costly items and scan them into electronic format. If you have appraisals for any items, scan them, too. Keep the electronic medium, such as a disk or flash drive, in a safe place outside of your home, like in your safe deposit box. Another option is to give your insurance agent a copy, and it is very useful if your Adult Children have copies as well; make sure they have copies of your insurance policy, too. This way, not only do you have visual proof of your possessions, but you also have proof of what you paid for them and when you bought them. Doing so will not only help you prove your loss, but it might also show you whether you are over- or underinsured. (You should meet at least annually with your insurance agent to go over your insurance needs.)

So now that you've done the big job and built your initial household inventory, it's important to maintain it. As you acquire new items, be sure to scan the receipts for major purchases and put the original receipts in a safe place. If you dispose of items, it's a good idea to make a note of that, too. Many people find it helpful to have a spiral notebook in their kitchen junk drawer or on their desk where they can write down the "stuff" they add or delete, the date, and the price they paid for the item. This makes it much quicker when it's time to make a formal update to the inventory. Then, at least annually, make the changes in the master inventory, take new photographs if necessary, and store the results in a safe place outside your home.

Adult Children, your generation is more comfortable with technology than the Older Adult's generation, and this is where your expertise can be very helpful to your parent. Offer to do the videotaping of your parent's house and store the video online in cloud storage. Take the receipts and scan them for your parent and keep an online record available at a moment's notice. Store any still photos you take in software on your desktop, ready to be faxed or emailed instantly from your computer to the insurance company. Create a spreadsheet of the inventory items and their value, and add or subtract from it as necessary. You might even go one step further and offer to scan all your parent's old photos and create an online archive that can't be lost or damaged in the event of a natural disaster. Take their old reel-to-reel or VHS tapes and have them converted to DVD and store those discs for them, too.

Digital belongings: Once you have taken care of cataloguing your physical property, don't forget to turn your attention to your *digital belongings*. If you are an Older Adult, technology may be a brave new world for you, and perhaps one you have resisted exploring. Even you Adult Children may find yourself surprised by the wide reach of your personal digital fingerprints. The Internet tends to give an illusion of privacy, but it is simply that—an illusion.

If you have an email address, you own a digital belonging. If you author a blog or save photographs to an online site, you own more digital belongings. If you do any shopping online or have a Facebook account, you're in the game.

Today, it's pretty hard not to participate in the digital world. But what doesn't occur to most of us is what happens to these things when we die. Dealing with such digital belongings is an emerging and rapidly evolving area of the law.

In his book *The World Is Flat*, Thomas Friedman tells the story of Justin Ellsworth, a United States Marine killed in Iraq. Justin's parents wanted access to his email account to enable them to learn more about his life. After the email provider refused, Justin's parents had to go to court to gain access to his personal email account.

More and more, attorneys who are advising clients about estate planning are recommending consideration of wishes for distribution or destruction of digital belongings along with planning for tangible property. In fact, some people are now naming "digital executors" in addition to standard "executors" or personal representatives. Your digital executor need not be the same person as the one you name to handle the other matters associated with settling your estate.

So what is a digital belonging? And when is that belonging a potential asset to you and your estate? The easiest way to think about this is to make a distinction between digital belongings and digital assets. With tangible property, there is "stuff" and then there is "valuable stuff." In your estate plan, you have probably given some thought to the disposition of the "valuable stuff" and lump the rest together as "my other personal property." The valuables may have monetary or sentimental value, or both.

The same is true for your digital belongings. For example, if you have written a travel blog for the past five years, that might be something that can be packaged and published electronically or in print and sold to a willing buyer. Or if you have created a famous website or a high-demand domain name, it is likely that someone would acquire it from your estate. Alternatively, all the digital photos you took of Grandma Elizabeth might have only sentimental value. However, if Grandma was a famous actress, those photos might have monetary value as well.

In short, your digital property is an asset when it has value to someone else, whether that value is monetary or sentimental.

In addition to the obvious digital belongings like email accounts, blogs, and photos or writings stored online, don't forget about other digital assets such as social media accounts; your financial records; audio, video, or e-reader libraries; and so on. And then there are your frequent flyer accounts, memberships, and anywhere else that you log in to or store personal information.

An emerging industry is seeking to help you organize your digital life. When evaluating such services, pay close attention to their approach to security and privacy, as well as the history of any breach the company has suffered. Whether you are considering a service to help you store your digital assets "in the cloud"—meaning that data doesn't "live" on your computer's hard drive but rather is stored on a company's secure remote server, available to you by signing in and downloading the data to your computer—or one that simply helps you catalog your login and password information, do be a careful consumer.

Adult Children, you can be a help here. Do the research about what type of cloud system your parents should consider using to store their valuable information. Consider longevity and the security credentials of the various companies. Read the fine print of the contract; don't just click "Agree" to the statement you need to okay before accessing the service. Also, both teach your Older Adults how to back up their home computer systems and/or create an automatic backup for both their hard drive and any cloud service they use. Tell your parents to make a *dated* list of their various user names and passwords, and teach them how to store such information on a flash drive (and find out the location of that flash drive) in case they become incapacitated or suffer memory loss. Help the Older Adults guard their digital belongings as they do their physical ones.

Remember also, while there is something appealing to having an online repository of your important information, passwords, and login credentials, the system has obvious risks. You might also want to consider capturing and including your (or your Older Adult's) digital life in an off-line (paper) format such as your Life Transition Plan. In this way, the information is available to your digital executor, but you also greatly reduce the risk of losing this valuable information. Such pre-planning can help you or your parents survive a crisis in the best shape possible.

Older Adults, if these tasks seem overwhelming and your Adult Children can't help, remember you might want to consider the help of a daily money manager, professional organizer, or senior move manager. They can come in and do these projects for you quickly and efficiently. They will use special software and/or storage media like password-protected flash drives or cloud-based storage that safely and securely store all of the information electronically, where it can be accessed from any computer with an Internet connection.

Adult Children, your help may be useful when it comes to sorting papers. If time is an issue, you're unable to make heads or tails of your parent's records, or you aren't handy with a video camera or software storage, remember it is all right to ask for help from such professionals, even if just to set up the initial system that you can then maintain.

Tips for Tax Time

By the end of January you will be inundated with envelopes in the mail that scream "Important Tax Document." Many of you will open them and review them as they arrive. Still others will throw them in a shopping bag and avoid looking at them until April 14. A few of you will let them pile up on the kitchen counter, in the car, and on the washing machine, and you may or may not be able to locate them all when it's time to sit down to do your taxes. If you are in the latter categories, there is a better way.

I suggest to my clients that each January they establish one place to throw any paper that *might* be helpful for preparing their income taxes. This can be a bag, a basket, or a box. The container doesn't matter. The important thing is that you are meticulous about getting every last item to that one place.

Once the flow of tax-related mail seems to have ended—by late February for most people—it's time to sit down and organize the mess. Open everything and sort by the type of document. For example, clip all of the 1099-INT documents together. These are the forms that financial institutions have used to tell the IRS how much interest you were paid last year. Repeat this for each document type.

Once you have sorted through everything, it's time to see if you are missing anything. The easiest way to do this is to start by pulling out the prior year's tax return and looking for the schedules that show interest, dividends, mortgage interest paid, etc. Match each entry on the prior year's return to a document in your stash. If you don't have a document, then it is time to figure out why not. It may be that you closed an account and no longer receive interest from the institution. Or maybe you refinanced your mortgage and have a different lender.

It is also helpful to look through statements for all accounts that you currently have open and make sure that you have documents for each of these if you had income, gains, or losses from them. The idea is to cross-check to see that you have what you need.

Many tax preparers will provide you with a tax guide or tax organizer. Sometimes these are preprinted with your information from last year. If you receive one of these, it is very important to take the time to review it, complete it—especially as related to any changes in your family or situation, and make sure you have the documents you will need to support your return. Here again: If this all seems overwhelming, you might want to enlist the help of a daily money manager. The cost will be minor compared with the potential of forgetting significant deductions.

Adult Children, you might gently remind your Older Adults that tax time is coming up and even offer to organize the paperwork your parents have (hopefully) faithfully gathered all year. You can assemble it all for the accountant or tax preparer and take it to their office. You can make sure that your parents sign the return—and mail it for them by the deadline—or that the tax preparer arranges to file electronically. Make and keep a copy somewhere findable for next year's taxes. Tell your Older Adult what refund they are getting and arrange to have the money direct deposited into their account.

Then start the process all over again—maybe with a new basket or bag labeled with the next tax year, and place it somewhere your Older Adult can find and use it without moving it; hung from a doorknob in the office or wherever mail is opened is helpful. While you are at it, Adult Child, create just such a catch-all for your own tax-preparation papers. Good habits will last you a lifetime; and *your* children will someday thank *you*.

Are Finances Off Track?

What if you aren't the Older Adult who has followed all this good financial organizational advice? Or if you are the Adult Child and *assume* your parents have kept on top of things but are wrong in that assumption?

Perhaps you are an Older Adult and your bills have simply gotten the best of you. Now you are besieged by envelope after envelope of multiple copies of those same bills coming in the mail every day. Maybe you can't answer your phone without creditors dunning you for payment. Possibly a registered letter demanding payment has arrived. You feel under attack and don't know how to get your finances back on track. You are embarrassed and maybe even too ashamed to ask for help or don't know who to ask.

Or you may be an Adult Child who has begun to feel a niggling worry about your parent's financial situation. You might notice your parent seems anxious when money is mentioned or maybe find a couple of unopened bills on the kitchen table when you visit. You don't like to pry, but you are getting concerned and want to know if the situation is becoming serious.

Whether you are evading your own mismanagement or are worried your parents need help, how do you know if your finances (or those of your loved one) are off track?

Signs that Finances Have Slipped Off Track

Piled-up mail: The first sign of trouble is very often an Older Adult overwhelmed by the volume of mail. Once the mail pile gets too big, many people find that it is easier not to open it. And once the mail isn't opened, the situation is on the slippery slope to trouble. If this describes you or your Older Adult, do yourself a favor and get help right away. It is much easier to get back on track before the situation gets too uncontrollable.

Unpaid bills: This problem often (but not always) results from the piled-up mail. Sometimes I meet with people who have a very organized system for handling the incoming bills but then slip up with remembering to actually pay them. A relatively easy fix for many of these bills is available. Assuming that your cash flow permits this, set up automatic payments from your bank account or charged to a credit card. Adult Children, your comfort with technology can be a great help here. Explain how the system works to your parents and then offer to set up such automatic payments for them. Keep track of the passwords for them as well.

Late fees: Unpaid bills usually lead to late fees, and interest charges are typically piled on as well. So if you notice that more and more of your accounts have either of these added on, it is time to get back some control of the situation. Even worse are bouncing checks or excessive overdraft fees. Both of these are signs that you are not managing your cash flow well at all. Older Adults, consider sharing your troubles with your Adult Children. Ask their help in going through and organizing the latest copy of each bill, point out the interest you are being charged, and perhaps even call your debtors to negotiate a lower interest payment or set up a repayment plan.

Mounting credit card debt: This can be a sign that you are living beyond your means and need to rein things in. If you are paying only your minimum balance every month and especially if you are late making that minimum payment, then you are digging yourself deeper and deeper into a hole. Consider paying off all but one card—the one with the lowest interest rate—and keep that one only for emergencies. Adult Children can help here, too. Offer to call the credit card companies for your Older Adult and see if you can get them to lower the interest rate, then monitor future bills to see if the credit card company has honored their agreement.

More charitable donations: Sometimes a sign of finances being off track, particularly for you Older Adults, is finding that you have a new habit of making frequent small charitable donations. Many charities have a strategy of mailing to older people very frequently and asking for small donations, hoping that they will get in the habit of writing those checks every few weeks. I had one client who was making thirty donations of $5 each every month to various organizations. He had no idea that he was spending $1,800 every year on this hobby! If this was part of his philanthropic plan and he was doing this with intent, then I'd have no issue with it (assuming that he could afford it), but in this case he could not afford it and didn't realize the impact these seemingly small donations had on his finances.

Adult Children, you can offer to bring in the mail. Track what charity sends what request and include only one solicitation letter a year from that organization. Throw away the rest. Discuss with your Older Adult which charities they want to support and how much they want to contribute, and get the charities to send e-receipts to *your* email address for each contribution your parent makes. You'll have an accurate record of what donations your Older Adults made that year and you'll end up with a complete record for their taxes as well. A note here: Older Adults, discuss with your Adult Children whether you would like to keep a small contingency fund for charitable emergencies—such as the New Orleans flood, the Japanese earthquake, or the Hurricane Sandy disaster. Set an amount, based on what you can afford, to send to the International Red Cross or charity of your choice if you want to help in the event of such a crisis.

Buying lottery tickets or participating in sweepstakes: Do you find yourself buying more lottery tickets or entering more contests for cash prizes than you used to? A dollar at the grocery every week may be no big deal (though you will be $52 poorer by year's end), but an escalating habit may be indicative of a bigger problem. Are you sure, Older Adult, you aren't hoping to hit it big to pay off old debts or leave money to your kids? Gambling is never the best investment strategy.

Adult Children, if you get to see your parent's mail, notice if the amount of junk mail is going up. Once your parent enters one contest or sweepstakes, other solicitors will be on them like bees on pollen. Some shady companies even unscrupulously target Older Adults.

Again, throw away the junk mail. Ask your parent if you can set up spam filters on their email accounts to cut down on invitations to such contests (and scams), and enter your parent's phone number in the national "Do Not Call" registry at www.donotcall.gov/ to keep unsolicited calls from getting to them.

Explain to your Older Adults why sharing their cell or home phone number, email address, or any private information with anyone (even in the form of filling out a contest entry) is a bad idea. If your Older Adult surfs the Internet, point out that if the address at the top of the page they are visiting starts with "http," it means any information they share on that page can be retrieved by hackers. If they add an "s" to the "http," making it "https," the page is more secure.

Calls from creditors: This is an obvious sign that your finances or your Older Adult's finances are in trouble. If you are the one in trouble, do your best not to get to this point by getting some help early, and if you are the caregiver, pay attention to the situation and resolve to say something to the Older Adult at the earliest opportunity.

Daily Money Management

A woman recently wrote to me to share that her husband had died. He had handled all the family finances, including establishing the household budget and paying all the bills.

"I don't even know where to begin to get everything in order," she wrote. "Is there someone who can help me with this?"

She signed herself "Intimidated Irene."

I couldn't blame her for feeling intimidated. Facing a pile of paperwork, particularly when it's associated with money, can scare even those of us well-versed in financial matters, much less a novice like Irene.

Her situation isn't that unusual for Older Adults. Couples in her generation often had such a division of labor, with one spouse handling the family finances. Convenient in some ways, this arrangement left the other spouse at a real disadvantage when the situation changed—especially if it was a sudden and unexpected change. As a new widow, Irene had enough on her plate without having to instantly learn how to deal with the finances of her new situation.

Adult Children, you are often called in to help your surviving parent when a situation like Irene's arises in your own family, but you may find yourself almost as much in the dark as Irene. Figuring out someone else's system or tangled finances isn't easy, particularly when you may not have all the information you need and the one who had the answers is no longer around to ask.

Whether you are the Older Adult trying to go it alone or the Adult Child trying to figure things out, you may need a hand to help your parent navigate through the unknown waters of their finances. If so, you are not alone.

According to the American Association of Daily Money Managers (AADMM), Adult Children, especially the baby boomers born between 1946 and 1961, face a huge struggle in trying to balance caregiving responsibilities for their Older Adults with other family responsibilities—so much so that they are known as the "Sandwich Generation," stuck between their parents and their own kids and trying to meet the needs of both.

A research study, cited by the AADMM and conducted by the Brookdale Center for Healthy Aging and Longevity of Hunter College, states: "For vulnerable Older Adults, management of daily financial obligations can become an overwhelming burden, quickly spiraling into adverse behaviors and at-risk situations such as unpaid bills, undeposited checks, and the terrifying consequences of cut-off utilities, bank foreclosures, evictions, and financial exploitation."

Hiring a Daily Money Manager

Many Adult Children (or capable Older Adults themselves) are taking some of the stress off of their overburdened shoulders by engaging a daily money manager (DMM).

A DMM brings clarity and order to an individual's daily management of personal bills, budgets, and recordkeeping, assisting clients with activities such as bill paying, day-to-day banking, budgeting, insurance paperwork, and organizing records and receipts in preparation for income tax filing.

An experienced DMM can provide day-to-day personal financial services for elderly parents, giving peace of mind to Adult Children that their parent's financial affairs are being taken care of properly and professionally. Hiring a DMM may allow some seniors with health challenges to avoid guardianship and a complete loss of independence.

In addition to bill paying, day-to-day banking, budgeting, and records organization, many DMMs are experienced with handling Medicare and other insurance paperwork, offering seniors and their families increased peace of mind. Also, many DMMs are very knowledgeable about social support services for seniors—from Medicare home health benefits to Meals on Wheels. They aren't financial planners or advisors and are seldom accountants or attorneys, but they can help smooth the path for Older Adults and relieve some of the anxiety of Adult Children.

And to put your mind at ease on another point about DMMs, they do *not* have to gain control of the Older Adult's money. If the client prefers, the control of the funds stays with the Older Adult (or their designated Adult Child), and the DMM simply helps organize, plan, and distribute funds on a day-to-day level.

Some DMMs offer a free initial consultation, and after that they charge on an hourly basis or a monthly package rate. They may also charge for travel time and expenses like postage. Most bill monthly, but arrangements may be able to be made to better suit your own situation. In some locales, reduced-fee or free DMM services are available for low-income clients. Though DMMs may come recommended by an attorney or financial advisor, it is good to check their references or to contact their association to put your mind at ease as to their competence and honesty. AADMM members are expected to adhere to a strict code of ethics and standards of practice. AADMM promotes excellence in services through a voluntary certification program that emphasizes both experience in the field and continuing education. Certified DMMs, called Professional Daily Money Managers (PDMM), must also submit to criminal background checks.

Questions to Ask Before Hiring a DMM

Here are some questions suggested by the Association of American Daily Money Managers to ask of any DMM you are considering hiring:

- What types of services do you provide? Do you only do book-keeping, or are there other ways that you can be of assistance?

- How long have you been working as a DMM?

- What kinds of professional insurance do you have?

- Are there industry standards and a code of ethics to which you adhere?

- Are you willing to work with other advisors, for example, my financial advisor, tax accountant, or attorney?

- What are the costs of your services, and what are the common billing methods?

- How often do you usually visit your clients, and what do you charge for travel, if anything?

- Would it be possible for you to assist me remotely, if necessary?

- Do you require and/or provide a contract?

- What about confidentiality?

- Can you provide a reference list?

Take the time to call the references on the list, asking them whether the DMM is respectful, dependable, efficient, empathetic, and professional in manner. Ask if there have been any conflicts, and if so, how they were resolved. Find out if asking for explanations of things not understood has been a comfortable situation for the questioner.

You can find a DMM in your area by visiting www.aadmm.com and clicking on "Find a DMM," which allows you to search by state, city, or ZIP code. Complete contact information for the AADMM is available in the resources section of this book.

Budget for Caregiving

Whether you are an Older Adult planning for your own care or an Adult Child who finds yourself the principal player in helping to arrange care for your parent, one of the more stressful parts of caregiving is the worry about how to pay for it. Creating a realistic caregiving budget is an important first step in helping to alleviate the anxiety.

But creating a budget is not just a matter of tracking dollars and cents. Think through the "what ifs" and create a few scenarios for how your caregiving journey might unfold, whether you are the one receiving the care or are the caregiver.

It's helpful to construct best-case, worst-case, and most likely-case scenarios. Considering such alternate views of what might happen in the future can help you make decisions about what to do now and help eliminate some nasty shocks and surprises the future may hold. Rose-colored glasses have no place in this planning. "Expect the best, but prepare for the worst" should be your catch phrase.

I advise caregivers to assume that the resources available at any moment will be lower than what you expect, and the needs of you or your care recipient will be higher. If you think about things this way, you are more likely to be pleasantly surprised that you have more than enough resources, rather than the opposite.

A budget is made up of inflows, outflows, and the assets and other resources available. Inflows include your—the Adult Child's—contributions and/or your parent's income, Social Security payments, pension benefits, IRA, 401(k) or annuity distributions, veteran's benefits, and long-term-care insurance proceeds. Outflows include the Older Adult's expenses, not just those associated with the care itself. For example, Older Adults, you should include all your expenses—including food, prescriptions, and supplemental insurance payments.

Or Adult Children, if Mom lives in her own apartment, you have to include her rent and utilities, not just the cost of the home health aide.

Always include a contingency, or "cushion," when you are fashioning a caregiving expense budget. Be sure to consider all of the assets or other resources that are available or could become available. These include savings, value of the home or car, gifts from others, loans, credit card limits, and life insurance policies. Research the availability of these resources, along with how to access or monetize them. For example, Older Adults, if a payment won't be available for ninety days, note that. Adult Children, if all you know is that Dad has a life insurance policy, but not with whom or where to find the policy or whether it allows you to withdraw funds to pay for care, the asset isn't truly available to you for use in your caregiving plans.

Once you have crafted the budget, you will immediately see whether the inflows are sufficient to cover the outflows. If they are, you have a surplus, and that's a good thing. When you have a caregiving surplus, *put it away for immediate access in the future.* If the outflow exceeds the inflow, a budget deficit occurs and must be funded. That's where assets and other resources come in. If the deficit is short term, as when extra help is required for respite, it might be feasible to fund it from savings or a credit card or maybe a one-time loan from you, the Adult Child, or one of your siblings. Alternatively, if the deficit is ongoing, it's time to determine if the available resources are sufficient to cover it and for how long. It may be time to consider making changes to the caregiving budget so things are more in balance.

A budget is just like a roadmap—it gives you an idea of where you're headed. When you're on vacation, it's sometimes fun to toss the map and take the scenic route that might lead to an adventure or a great little restaurant, but a budget detour is less likely to be fun. Therefore, whether you are arranging for your own care or have assumed the mantle of caregiver, periodically take a look at your direction and make sure you are heading where you planned to go.

Whether you do this course evaluation weekly, monthly, quarterly, or less often will depend on how tight your caregiving budget is and the stability of the caregiving needs. For example, if yours is a deficit budget and the caregiving needs suddenly and permanently go up, it is critical to keep a very close eye on the budget. On the other hand, if you have a surplus budget and things are stable, it is likely to be fine to check your budget less frequently.

When you review your caregiving budget, you are looking for *variances*. A variance occurs when the actual amount spent differs from what you planned when you created your budget. A variance can be positive or negative. For example, if inflows are greater than planned, that is a positive variance. Similarly, if expenses are lower than planned, that's also a positive variance. On the other hand, if inflows are lagging or expenses are higher than planned, you have a negative variance.

The idea is to explain the variance and determine whether it is likely to recur, not to blame yourself or anyone else for the fact that the variance happened. For example, if the electricity bill is high in August relative to your budget for August, you're unlikely to be alarmed if you assumed that the bill for the year is divided evenly by month. One way to help interpret a variance is to look at both this period (e.g., this month or quarter) and to also look at year-to-date. In this way, you can see if a variance seems to be a one-time matter or a trend. If you see trends, you're likely to be facing a new reality, and it's probably time to revise the budget.

Facing the future squarely is the best way to be prepared for what may be coming your way—whether the planned care is for yourself or your parents. Knowing where you stand always means you will find yourself standing in a better place.

7

FACING THE FINISH

A Caregiver's Last Expense

Coming to the end of what has hopefully been a long and (on the whole) satisfying life is like bringing the curtain down on the run of a great Broadway musical. A lot of great memories were created, people have left the theater singing the score, and the performances will be fondly talked about for years. But it is hard to face the finish, and planning can take some of the sting out of the show's closing.

One area that needs to be discussed is funeral expenses, especially if this "final act" on behalf of their parents is one that is being performed by the Adult Children. While it is always best for the Older Adult to make their final wishes known to their Adult Children and other loved ones, we all know that this doesn't always happen.

The advisability of prepaid arrangements is debatable. AARP and the Funeral Consumer's Alliance both advise against such plans and suggest alternatives like a "payable on death" bank account, making funds available once there's a death certificate to reimburse funeral expenses.

However, I've often heard that the exact opposite proved true in many situations. People actually found that prepaying for funeral arrangements *was* a good idea.

But the executive director of the Funeral Consumer's Alliance says that each state has different laws and protections for consumers, and in some cases, when funeral homes or cemeteries were sold, the prepaid plans were not honored. However, he does acknowledge that a prepaid funeral might make sense in the case of a family trying to "spend down" an Older Adult's limited assets to qualify for Medicaid nursing home care.

No matter what your circumstance, I think it is worth considering the difference between "pre-planning" and "pre-paying." While it might or might not make sense for you (or your parent) to prepay your funeral arrangements, I can't think of a reason why pre-planning would ever be a bad idea. With pre-planning, you or your parent gets to decide exactly what you want, and that decision is documented by the funeral home of choice for later reference.

Adult Children should welcome such arrangements. Trying to establish what your parents or Older Adults might want for their final arrangements is more difficult the closer to the end of life they get. Hospitals and nursing homes are not the best place to hold a private conversation and, at times of stress and crisis, the best decisions are seldom reached. Worse still, having those vital conversations with funeral directors after the fact of the Older Adult's death is putting a lot of pressure on you—at a time you yourself will be grieving. Also, having to make all the arrangements while literally guessing at your parent's wishes can open a pathway to discord with other family members who might have their own opinion about what Mom or Dad might have wanted, and grief sometimes makes people act in strange ways.

Better to encourage your parents to make their final arrangements known, and if those arrangements can be paid for in advance, so much the better. If concerns about prepayment are worrying your parents, they might wish to consider the "payable on death" bank account referenced above or consider a specially designated "burial account" at their bank. Name a trusted person as co-owner of the account so that funds can be accessed immediately upon death to avoid any lag time before funeral expenses are reimbursed.

Such planning allows you and the rest of your family to concentrate on what's truly important at the passing of a loved one—the pulling together of the family for mutual comfort and to celebrate the life of the one who died.

Create an Ethical Will

The end of life isn't all about money and arranging for physical care. As an Older Adult, no doubt a great deal of time and attention has gone into creating "end of life documents" such as your will, health care directive, or durable power of attorney. However, you should consider creating a non-legal document to add to your "end of life" portfolio—an ethical will.

The ethical will is an ancient tradition, the purpose of which was to transmit wisdom to future generations. It can still be employed for such a purpose.

An ethical will, unlike a formal legal will, is not designed to transfer your property to your heirs. Rather, an ethical will's purpose is to allow you to share your thoughts, feelings, and hopes for the future with those you care about most.

There is no right or wrong way to construct your ethical will, and no topics that you must, or must not, include. Some people focus on spiritual matters; others on hopes and dreams for future generations. Still others use their ethical will as a vehicle to forgive others, or to ask for forgiveness.

Writing an ethical will allows you to leave a highly personal legacy for your loved ones, and in the process, you just might learn something about yourself. The process of writing an ethical will may allow you to reflect on your life and to find meaning where perhaps you didn't see it before. It might help you articulate what you really stand for, what's really important to you.

If the idea of creating an ethical will appeals to you, you might be wondering how to get started. There are as many approaches to the process as there are people, and you have to find one that works well for you. Some people prefer to start with an outline or prompts of topics to include. If you fall into this camp, you might want to visit www.ethicalwill.com or one of the numerous other online resources where you can see examples and structures of ethical wills. On the other hand, you may prefer to start writing and see where it takes you. This approach works well, too. You might also find a workshop where you can work with others who are also interested in writing an ethical will.

The process of creating an ethical will might actually help you to make other types of estate planning and end-of life decisions. For example, the process of thinking about things you wish to say in your ethical will might help you to clarify how you want to distribute your worldly possessions. Or, it might help you to conclude what type of funeral or celebration of your life you do (or don't) want.

Most people find that their ethical will takes shape over time, and rarely is it completed in one sitting. And, there's nothing wrong with making changes or additions over time. (Be sure to date each revised ethical will to avoid confusion.) Your ethical will is a living document as long as you are alive.

Adult Children, you may tell your parents how very much an ethical will would be treasured by you—having their wisdom shared with you even after they depart. You may be able to help the process along by agreeing to or even initiating conversations on topics more philosophical and less mundane in nature than just discussions of day-to-day details of your lives. We often get too wrapped up in talk of prescriptions or family gossip and what the grandkids are up to and never find time to discuss anything deeper. Perhaps you could ask to interview your parents about past events or favorite family stories, or just get their view of the world (as they prepare to leave it) looking back over a lifetime of experiences. Or bring out the family photo albums and start them talking. Maybe doing this will help jog their memories and create new ones. Perhaps the most important thing to impart to your parents is that their views are important to you—now and later—and that you would welcome their final words of wisdom to cherish as you cherished the author during his or her lifetime.

An ethical will could be used as a final pontification—a way to truly get the last word in, or press one last dictatorial argument, but it needn't be that type of document. It can be one last talk—a verbal valentine—to those you love.

After the Loss of a Spouse

During our first meeting, a recent client of mine shared her story:

My husband of fifty-nine years died recently, and I'm feeling overwhelmed by day-to-day decisions. I expected to feel the emotions associated with grief, but I never expected to feel helpless. My husband took care of our financial life and I'm really at a loss. I don't want my children to know how much this confuses me, and I certainly don't want their help if that means they take over. I should be perfectly capable of handling my own affairs. How can I get on top of things so that I can manage on my own?

Her emotional challenge is common to Older Adults who recently lost their lifelong mate, and the difficulties may be exacerbated by how the division of labor was handled between the partners during their marriage. Such a division of labor, for example, may have meant one spouse took care of the finances and the other took care of all the shopping and cooking. That was fine as long as both spouses were willing and able to do their jobs. However, if because of illness, attitude, incapacity, or death, one of them can no longer hold up his or her end of the bargain, trouble is brewing.

The best way to avoid this is through "cross training." In this way, one partner teaches the other his or her system for accomplishing their job. If that's not an option, then at least each should document the process and the facts of how they handle their tasks for the other. Each partner should be aware of where financial documents are kept, how to access the funds, and what bills need paying. Both should have copies of supermarket/Costco or Sam's Club cards and debit cards, know the nutritional needs and food allergies of the other, and have the contact information of the housekeeper, home aide, and other service providers.

However, what do you do if such cross training or documentation never happened?

The short answer is that it's never too late to learn if you want to and don't suffer from physical or cognitive complaints that make such learning too difficult. If you don't want to or can't learn, then you can hire someone to take over the tasks on your behalf.

There's a middle ground, too. Maybe it is too overwhelming to step in and figure out how to do something you've never had to do before, but you're not ready to completely outsource it either. In this case, you can bring in a professional who can set up a system for you, teach you how to use it, and then check in with you periodically to make sure that you're on track and to answer any questions that might come up.

That's exactly what my client did. She had me figure out her late husband's financial system, bring it up-to-date, and then modify it until it made sense to her. Once we got to that point, it was easy for her to take over and maintain the process. At first we had a check-in meeting every other week, and then every month. At that point, I felt that she was ready for a quarterly meetings, but she liked the idea that I was looking over her shoulder, "just in case," so we met more frequently.

As the months passed, new issues came up. For example, while the bill paying was well under control, when it came time to deal with the annual income tax return, my client became overwhelmed again. Then her car lease came to an end and she was having a tough time making a decision about whether to lease a new car, buy out her current car, or purchase a new one. We did the analysis together and I helped her negotiate her new arrangement.

Adult Children are often unaware that Mom or Dad may be struggling, as their parent often suffers in silence, as my client was doing. The Adult Child may be emotionally supportive and even smothering when it comes to making sure Mom is allowed or encouraged to cry, offering a shoulder on which to do that weeping, and hanging around for several days after the funeral to make sure Mom is "all right."

Noble impulses all, but what your parent might truly need might not become apparent until weeks later. The Older Adult may be "prepared" for the funeral and even the grief (death is an expected part of life, after all), but two or three weeks later, you should make an appointment with your parent—don't just drop by; respect their privacy—and have an in-depth conversation with your parent and offer *specific* help.

Offer to set up online banking for your parent and explain how it works. Install personal financial software, such as Quicken, on his or her computer and explain (and then explain again) how to use it. Tell your Mom or Dad that you will run the year-end tax return statements for their accountant. Take Mom car shopping after offering to do the initial market research. Find Dad's favorite recipes from the index cards your late Mom used and create ingredient-shopping lists. Then set up online grocery shopping and delivery for him and offer to come help recreate those meals.

The object of your thoughtful offering is not to take over but to empower your parent. That is showing them true support in this hard time.

Losing a life partner is tough in so many ways. It adds insult to injury to feel as though you can't take care of yourself because of your loss. There's help available, whether from family, friends, or qualified professionals. Don't be afraid to ask for help. Encourage your surviving parent to ask for help. It is not a mark of weakness, but one of strength.

Talk about the End of Life

Caregivers, especially Adult Children, often struggle with how much to talk with their parents about the end of life. Their parents, you Older Adults, struggle too, not wanting to cause pain to your kids and perhaps not even wanting to face the fact that your life is coming to a close. In a way, talks about the end of life seem easier to have when the subject is treated in the abstract, long before it seems like an impending reality.

As it turns out, doctors struggle with whether or not to have *the talk*, too, but recent evidence suggests that quality of life for patients and their caregivers is better when doctors level with their terminal patients.

In her *New York Times* article, "Doctor and Patient: Talking Frankly at the End of Life," Dr. Pauline Chen speaks both as a physician and as a family member about the importance of having those "difficult discussions" at and about the end of life. She writes about the conversations that doctors and nurses had with her dying mother-in-law, and also about the important opportunities her husband and the rest of the family were afforded to share final thoughts and sentiments with their Mom/Grandmother/Great-grandmother because the truth was on the table.

Dr. Chen quotes a close friend of hers who said, "One of the scariest things in the world is to look someone in the eye and tell them they are dying." But Dr. Chen goes on to say that, in her practice, she does try to tell patients they are dying because she believes that it is worse when clinicians don't.

Yet, she also points out that every doctor comes to these conversations with some anxiety "because it is hard not to feel as if you have failed your patients and their families, to wonder if taking out an inch more of bowel when removing the colon cancer, starting with a different antibiotic, or ordering a different diagnostic test might have somehow changed the course of events."

She goes on to talk about the conversation itself. As Dr. Chen puts it, "death" and "dying" are "words that can echo in a room long after they are said. Hopes can be shattered in an instant. Patients and families may feel abandoned. It is hard as a doctor not to wonder: Am I doing more harm than good?"

Dr. Chen cited a study, published in the *Journal of the American*

Medical Association, that examined how end-of-life care discussions with terminal patients affected their quality of life and that of their caregivers. The study found that patients who had discussed end-of-life issues with their doctors were more likely to have better quality of life at the end of their lives, with less aggressive care. The study also found that their caregivers also fared better than those caregivers whose loved ones had received more aggressive care. The truth had indeed set them free—free of some of the shock, pain, unnecessary treatment, and, perhaps even more importantly, from the regret of things left unsaid by families who thought they had more time. Hospice and palliative care prove their worth here, allowing families to turn their attentions from charts and medications to sharing true quality time with their loved ones before such vital—and irretrievable—moments together pass away as life ebbs.

It seems that for many people, open and honest conversations about death and dying are desirable. It is a topic that should be broached by you Older Adults, first with your doctor, whose cooperation you require in order to be told the truth about your condition, and then with your Adult Children. Hopefully the first time you address this topic with your Adult Children won't be when you disclose that you are terminally ill. Before you are forced to have the conversation out of necessity, you should discuss with your kids the fact that, should you find yourself in this situation, you will ask your doctor to be straight with you about any of your medical conditions. You should further promise that you will be honest with your Adult Children as well and that you expect them to level with you if they come by any knowledge about your medical condition that you may not have. Honesty all around should be agreed to by all parties.

Adult Children, this, by necessity, means you have to take any news shared with you about your parent's condition as calmly as possible. Tears help wash away the pain, but what is called for at the moment of revelation is caring support and compassion or, if that is beyond you, respectful silence and a willingness to listen until you feel more able to express your feelings calmly. What your parent and the rest of your family members don't need at that moment is to have to channel everything they are feeling themselves into taking care of you. Though the death of your parent will affect you deeply, the situation is not about you—but about your parent and the family unit. Muster up all the maturity you can and then you can all face what needs facing together.

AFTERWORD

IN THE JUDEO-CHRISTIAN tradition we are offered a perspective on relationships between Adult Children and their Older Adult parents that urges respectful, attentive care on the one hand, and on the other, recognizes and supports accepting limits of what Adult Children can do.

In the Fifth Commandment, we're told, "Honor your Father and your Mother that you may long endure on the land that the Eternal, your God, is assigning to you."

This is the only one of the Ten Commandments that promises a reward. Why? Commentators suggest that perhaps this is because fulfilling this obligation is so difficult. Others posit that the reward itself, long life, is the point. We care for our parents in the hope that we will, in turn, be blessed to live to a ripe old age and that we will be cared for by *our* children in a society in which Older Adults are respected.

Much later in the Bible (in Leviticus), we are taught, "You shall each revere your Mother and your Father." Why are we commanded this time to *revere*, whereas before we were commanded to *honor*?

Over the years, this has been interpreted in many ways. The commentary that resonates with me is that reverence is about preserving the dignity of Older Adults. It implies an attitude of respect in that we must not take over their position and we must not make decisions that don't respect their wishes. Honor, on the other hand, involves providing for our parents' material needs. It is our responsibility to make sure that they are well cared for. It is interesting to note, however, that the sources do not require that we provide this care with our own hands.

We are taught to respect and preserve the dignity and sanctity of human life—to do no harm and to make the decisions that ensure that the other person's wishes are honored and respected, even if they contradict our own wishes as caregivers. Put another way, the "right" decision isn't always the "best" decision.

Remember Deborah and her father Saul, the client whose story I relayed in the introduction? In Deborah's case, "right" might be for her and her brothers to place their father in an assisted living facility due to their safety concerns about him living alone at home, even though this was against his will. But "best" might mean finding a way to allow Saul to remain at home because this is what will give him joy.

Complicating matters, there's guilt.

A man calls his mother in Florida.

"Mom, how are you?"

"Not too good," answers his mother. "I've been very weak."

The son asks, "Why are you so weak?"

Mom replies, "Because I haven't eaten in thirty-eight days."

The son says, "That's terrible! Why haven't you eaten in thirty-eight days?"

Mom answers, "Because I didn't want my mouth to be filled with food if you should call."

Sure, the son should have called his mother. But let's face it; the mother was loading on the guilt.

The dictionary defines guilt as "a feeling of regret or remorse for having committed some improper act; a recognition of one's own responsibility for doing something wrong."

In other words, we take on guilt. That means we can refuse it, too. We often create guilt by having unrealistic expectations of ourselves. We say, "I should be able to do this." Or, "I didn't do enough." The truth is, you can't reverse fate. We can't prevent death. With every change in an Older Adult's functional ability, the Adult Child mourns, because grief isn't only about death. It's also about losing capacity. Adult Children: When it comes to caring for our parents, our best *is* good enough. There is no way to give more than that.

I was working with a client's family recently—two sisters in a dispute about how to care for their ninety-year-old mother whose health was quickly deteriorating. When meeting with them individually, I asked each what regrets she would have about the care she had given her Mom if today was Mom's last day. Both answered immediately, "I would have no regrets." The sisters' agreement on this point made my work easy. We changed the focus of the conversation to creating positive memories during these last weeks with Mom, rather than arguing about the daily minutia. Each sister was able to give in, just a little, to reach an agreement by keeping the focus on creating those memories and preserving their relationship with each other.

Mitch Albom, in *Tuesdays with Morrie,* writes, "As long as we can love each other, and remember the feeling of love we had, we can die without ever really going away. All the love you created is still there. All the memories are still there. You live on—in the hearts of everyone you have touched and nurtured while you were here . . . Death ends a life, not a relationship."

Serving as caregivers for our parents allows us not only to fulfill the blessing to honor and revere our parents, but also to create the memories that will sustain that relationship for the rest of our days.

ACKNOWLEDGMENTS

Many thanks to Kitt Walsh, editor and writing coach extraordinaire, who helped make this book happen and who made it fun in the process. Thanks as well to the entire team at Bascom Hill–you all were instrumental in keeping the publication process moving in a most professional way. Finally, thanks to Sue Frederick, who pushed and pushed me to find my purpose and answer the call to service.

APPENDIX

ELEMENTS OF A LIFE TRANSITION PLAN

"In Case of Emergency" information

Biographical information: Names, dates of birth, death, marriage, and military service, etc., for all of the important people in your life: yourself, parents and stepparents, siblings, spouse and any previous spouse, and children.

Minor children and other dependents: Names and contact information of guardians and caregivers for your minor children. Names and contact information of anyone else who depends on you for care and support, along with the names and contact information of anyone else who provides care or support for these individuals.

Pets: Name, species, age, and coloring of any pets or livestock you own. Basic information regarding their care, vet's name and contact information, microchip number, pet insurance information, etc.

Employment: Current and former employers—including contact information, title or last position held, start and end dates, ownership interest, and current benefits.

Business interests: Information about any other owners and key employees, location of ownership documents, and plans for disposition of your share of the business if you become incapacitated or upon your death. Information about the location of business tax records and a list of significant assets or liabilities and information on any prior business interests.

Insurance: All insurance policies owned by you or owned by others that cover your life or your property. Include company name, policy number, contact information, beneficiary designation, etc., for each policy.

Bank and brokerage accounts: Name of institution, contact information, account number and description, debit card and online access information, beneficiary information, location of checkbook, check stock, and statements for each account.

Retirement plans and pensions: Contact information, account number, description, beneficiary designation, etc., for each account/plan.

Credit cards and debts: Credit card numbers, contact information, and PINs. Details regarding any bills or other payments that are automatically paid from your bank accounts or charged to your credit cards. Creditor name and contact information for all other debts.

Government benefits: Social Security information (if currently collecting for retirement, disability, or SSI), along with information on any other government benefits, such as VA benefits.

Memberships: Organizations, clubs, groups, etc., to which you belong, including contact information, membership number (if applicable), and so on.

Service providers: Contact information for physicians, household help, service contracts, lawn care, pool care, or anyone who takes care of you, your dependents, your pets, or your property.

Real estate: Information for property you own or lease such as mortgage/lease details, caretakers, term of rental or lease, landlord's contact information, etc.

Vehicles: Make, model, year, and VIN for all vehicles you own or lease. If you have a loan or lease for a vehicle, include account numbers, contact information, and terms. Name and contact information for service/repair providers, AAA or other auto club, etc.

Other income and personal property: Sources of income and important items of personal property that you haven't covered in any other section; include warranty documents and maintenance guides. Include other property you expect to receive in the future.

Taxes: Name and contact information for tax preparer, location of current year tax documents, and prior year returns.

Secured places and passwords: A list of all online accounts with login information and passwords; location of all locks, safes, safe deposit boxes, and keys, including spare keys; combinations for any locks, secret locations.

Legal matters: Documents such as health care directives, durable power of attorney, wills or trusts, along with the name and contact information of the professional who helped you prepare them, if any.

Organ or body donation: Documents related to donation of your remains, and if you have made any prior arrangements, include those documents.

Burial or cremation: Your wishes and any arrangements you have already made for burial or cremation of your remains upon your death. If you have made prior arrangements, have those documents available.

Funeral and memorial services: Your wishes regarding any service or ceremonies after your death.

Obituary: If you wish to prepare an obituary, include it.

Instructions: Identify where your survivors would find a list of friends and relatives who should know about your incapacity or death. Identify where you keep your calendar with upcoming appointments that might need to be cancelled in the event of your incapacity or death. If this is kept electronically, provide any login or password information.

Letter to loved ones/ethical will: If you choose, include a letter to your loved ones and/or an ethical will to be opened upon your death.

Other information: Any information or materials that have not been covered and that you would like to include.

RESOURCES

AARP
www.aarp.org

AgingCare.com
www.AgingCare.com

Alliance of Professional Health Advocates
www.aphadvocates.org
www.advoconnection.com

AmVets
www.amvets.org

Angie's List
www.angieslist.com

American Association of Daily Money Managers
www.aadmm.com

AttackMedicalBills.com
www.AttackMedicalBills.com

Benefits Checkup
www.benefitscheckup.org

Caregiver Action Network
www.caregiveraction.org

Caregiving.com
www.caregiving.com

CarePages.com
www.carepages.com

Craigslist (by location)
www.craigslist.org

"Do Not Call" Registry
www.donotcall.gov

ElderCare.com
www.eldercare.com

Ethical Wills
www.ethicalwill.com

Freebies for Seniors
www.free4seniors.com/senior-freebies

LifeBridge Solutions, LLC
www.LifeBridgeSolutions.com

Meals On Wheels
www.mowaa.org

Medical Billing Advocates of America
www.billadvocates.com9.docx

Medicare/Medicaid
www.medicare.gov

MetLife Mature Market Institute
www.maturemarketinstitute.com

National Academy of Elder Law Attorneys (NAELA)
www.naela.org

National Alliance for Caregiving
www.caregiving.org

National Association of Professional Geriatric Care Managers
www.caremanager.org

National Association of Professional Organizers
www.napo.org

National Association of Senior Move Managers
www.nasmm.com

National Clearinghouse for Long-Term Care Information
www.longtermcare.gov

National Guardianship Association
www.guardianship.org

National Hospice and Palliative Care Organization
www.nhpco.org

Salvation Army
www.salvationarmyusa.org

SHINE (Serving Health Insurance Needs of Elders)
www.floridashine.org
This is the organization in Florida. Check to see if your state has a SHINE program.

Social Security Administration
www.ssa.gov

Zipcar
www.zipcar.com

INDEX

ABOUT THE AUTHOR

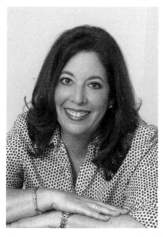 Sheri Samotin is the founder of LifeBridge Solutions, LLC. She has worked with hundreds of families, helping Older Adults and their Adult Children deal with the challenges of aging. Sheri is a life transition coach, National Certified Guardian, and certified Professional Daily Money Manager. She earned a degree in economics from Wesleyan University and went on to gain a master of business administration (MBA) from the Amos Tuck School of Business at Dartmouth College. Sheri is a prolific writer and sought-after speaker on topics related to navigating life's transitions.

NO
HIGH
GROUND

All armies prefer high ground to low,
and sunny places to dark.

—SUN TZU WU, *The Art of War* (500 B.C.)

NO
HIGH
GROUND

by Fletcher Knebel
and Charles W. Bailey II

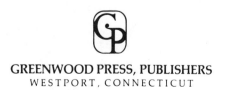

GREENWOOD PRESS, PUBLISHERS
WESTPORT, CONNECTICUT

Library of Congress Cataloging in Publication Data

Knebel, Fletcher.
  No high ground.

    Reprint. Originally published: New York : Harper
& Row, 1960.
    Bibliography: p.
    Includes index.
    1. Hiroshima-shi (Japan)--Bombardment, 1945.
2. Atomic bomb--History. 3. World War, 1939-1945--
Japan. 4. Japan--History--1912-1945. I. Bailey,
Charles W. (Charles Waldo) II. Title.
D767.25.H6K55 1983   940.54'26   83-16384
ISBN 0-313-24221-6 (lib. bdg.)

Reprinted in 1983 by Greenwood Press
A division of Congressional Information Service, Inc.
88 Post Road West, Westport, Connecticut 06881

Printed in the United States of America

10 9 8 7 6 5 4 3 2 1

Contents

Acknowledgments

THIS EFFORT to tell, in a single volume, the full and controversial story of the first atomic bomb has been greatly aided by the interested co-operation of many who played large and small parts in that story. Fortunately, most of those involved are still alive, and almost all of those whose assistance we sought furnished it willingly.

For extensive and excellent research in Japan, credit is due to Mitsugu Nakamura, an old friend on the staff of the *Asahi Shimbun* in Tokyo, and the two colleagues he recruited for us, Miss Reiko Sugibuchi and Masahiro Sasagawa. We are grateful also to Robert A. Hatch, Tiburon, Calif., and Jack G. Knebel, New Haven, Conn., for undertaking specific research jobs.

Special thanks are reserved for several busy people who not only helped our search for facts but also took time to read and comment on parts of the finished manuscript. These are: Major General Thomas F. Farrell, Tullahoma, Tenn.; Col. Paul W. Tibbets, Jr., Tampa, Fla.; Dr. Luis W. Alvarez, Berkeley, Calif.; and Dr. Ralph Lapp, Arlington, Va. Responsibility for facts and conclusions, of course, remains ours.

Among the most helpful of the others whose aid or advice we asked were Dr. Norman F. Ramsey, Cambridge, Mass.; Rear Admiral Frederick L. Ashworth, Washington, D.C.; the crew of the *Enola Gay*; Lieutenant General Leslie R. Groves, Norwalk, Conn.; Nat S. Finney,

Acknowledgments

Charles E. Bohlen and Allen W. Dulles, all of Washington, D.C.; and two former officers of the U.S.S. *Augusta,* Capt. C. L. Freeman, Santa Monica, Calif., and Capt. J. R. Wible, Pensacola, Fla. To the scores of others, in the Manhattan project, the military services and private life, who responded to our requests for interviews and information, we can only offer a collective "thank you."

Officials of the armed forces and of various government archives in Washington were most co-operative. We would especially thank Maj. James F. Sunderman and his staff in the U.S. Air Force Book Program; D. C. Allard of the Office of Naval History, and W. J. Nigh of the World War II records division of the National Archives.

The authors are grateful to the Air Force and Navy for giving us access, without delay or dispute, to all the secret documents we sought from World War II files. The Department of State was kind enough to let us read, in page-proof form, its comprehensive volume of papers relating to the Potsdam conference of 1945.

We also thank the Army for making available, on our insistent request, a few specific papers from the files of the Manhattan project. But we cannot accept without protest the Army's refusal, in the name of "national security," to open the rest of these papers to responsible historical research. It is perfectly clear to the authors that personal and policy considerations, not security, dictated the withholding of these fifteen-year-old papers. During the years since 1945, Russia has developed atomic and hydrogen bombs and has left our pioneer efforts far behind her. It is official government policy, as expressed in a Presidential Executive Order, to make classified wartime documents available for historians unless there are overriding security considerations. The authors of this book were able, in fact, to obtain many of the key Manhattan documents from the files of other federal agencies. Yet the Army still stands on a letter written by General Dwight D. Eisenhower, when he was Chief of Staff, putting the Manhattan papers in the personal custody of General Groves and requesting future Chiefs of Staff to continue this arrangement. Thus to all intents and purposes the records of the Manhattan project remain totally inaccessible until General Groves chooses to allow them to be inspected. Such a policy not only frustrates legitimate research on a vital subject but also flies in the face of a basic principle: that in a democracy the public has an inherent right to inspect the records of the public's business.

Finally we must thank our wives, whose initial skepticism about the entire project soon gave way to warm and helpful support. For their willingness to read the manuscript in each of its draft stages, for the many improvements that resulted from their suggestions, and for their almost uncomplaining acceptance of our antisocial work regime, we can only suggest that they will receive their reward in heaven.

F. K.
C. W. B.

Washington, D.C.
February 1, 1960

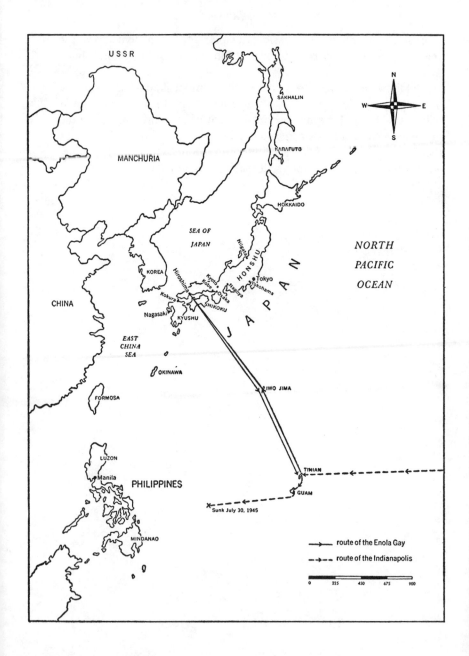

NO
HIGH
GROUND

```
PD TO WA AND OWI
P31148 H30752 JAPANESE HOME SERVICE KON 630 KCS) AT 6:00 AM TUESDAY 8/7
    (TEXT) A SMALL NUMBER OF B-TWENTY-NINES PENETRATED INTO HIROSHIMA
CITY A LITTLE AFTER EIGHT AM YESTERDAY MORNING AND DROPPED A SMALL
NUMBER OF BOMBS.  AS A RESULT A CONSIDERABLE NUMBER OF HOMES
WERE REDUCED TO ASHES AND FIRES BROKE OUT IN VARIOUS PARTS OF THE
CITY.
    TO THIS NEW TYPE OF BOMB ARE ATTACHED PARACHUTES, AND IT APPEARS
AS IF THESE NEW BOMBS EXPLODED IN THE AIR.  INVESTIGATIONS ARE NOW
BEING MADE WITH REGARD TO THE EFFECTIVENESS OF THIS BOMB, WHICH
SHOULD NOT BE REGARDED AS SLIGHT.
    THE ENEMY HAS EXPOSED HIS COLD BLOODEDNESS AND ATROCIOUS NATURE MORE
AND MORE IN KILLING INNOCENT PEOPLE BY THE USE OF THIS NEW-TYPE BOMB.
IT IS BELIEVED THAT THE ENEMY, BEING FACED WITH DIFFICULT CONDITIONS,
IS FEELING RUSHED TO TURN THE WAR INTO ONE OF SHORT DURATION. HENCE
HE HAS BEGUN TO USE THIS TYPE OF BOMB.
    THE USE OF THIS NEW TYPE OF BOMB BY THE ENEMY IN THE FUTURE CAN
BE EXPECTED.  AS FOR MEASURES TO COPE WITH THIS BOMB, IT IS ANTICI-
PATED THAT THEY WILL BE DISCLOSED AS SOON AS POSSIBLE.  UNTIL THESE
MEASURES ARE DISCLOSED BY THE GOVERNMENT AUTHORITIES, IT IS NECESSARY
FOR THE GENERAL PUBLIC TO STRENGTHEN THE PRESENT AIR DEFENSE SYSTE.
    AS FREQUENTLY POINTED OUT IN THE PAST, THE PEOPLE MUST WATCH
THEMSELVES AGAINST UNDERRATING THE ENEMY SIMPLY BECAUSE HE HAS CARRIED
OUT RAIDS WITH A SMALL NUMBER OF PLANES.  THE ENEMY HAS BEEN CARRYING
OUT LARGE-ACALE PROPAGANDA ON THE EFFECTIVENESS OF THIS NEW-TYPE BOMB
SINCE USING THESE BOMBS, BUT AS LONG AS WE FORMULATE STRONG STEEL-LKIE
MEASURES TO COPE WITH THIS TYPE OF BOMB, IT WILL BE POSSIBLE TO KEEP THE
DAMAGE AT A MINIMUM.
    WE MUST BE CAREFUL AT ALL TIMES SO THAT WE WILL NOT FALL VICTIM
TO THE ENEMY'S MACHINATIONS.  (JER-TB)
MRB 8/7-- 1134 EWT
```

The transcript of a Japanese broadcast describing the atomic attack on Hiroshima. At this point the Japanese government was still keeping the true nature of the attack from its people. Picked up by an Office of War Information Pacific monitor station, it was translated by the monitors and transmitted to Washington the day after the attack.

CHAPTER ONE

Another Day of War

THE U.S.S. *Augusta* hurried westward across the Atlantic. It was near midnight and it was wartime—the date was August 5, 1945—but with Germany defeated the war was half a world away and the heavy cruiser, her portholes open to catch the brisk breeze, sparkled with unmasked lights.

Most of them marked duty stations where the night watch kept its vigil. But the officers sitting over a pot of coffee in the wardroom were not held there by duty. They had just been given a glimpse of the future, an advance look at history still to be made, and it had touched them all with excitement and wonder.

That evening they had entertained the President of the United States, Harry S. Truman, who was traveling home with them from the lengthy conference with his British and Russian allies at Potsdam, Germany. Over the dessert and coffee, the talk had turned to that meeting. The *Augusta*'s officers, many of whom had visited the conference while they waited to bring the President home, were especially curious about the Russians and about Truman's impressions of them.

Lieutenant Commander Walter Berberich, the ship's doctor, raised a question they had all been wondering about.

"What did you think of old Joe Stalin, sir?"

Truman thought for a moment, the overhead lights reflected off his thick glasses. Then, looking at Berberich, he replied deliberately:

"I thought he was an S.O.B."

The men at the President's table were silent, their natural urge to laugh quashed by the realization that one does not snicker when the President of the United States makes a statement like that about anyone, let alone the chief of state of a powerful ally.

"But, of course," Harry Truman added with a quick grin, "I guess he thinks I'm one too."

Now the officers around the table could laugh, as Truman's remark broke the momentary tension and restored the pleasant mood that had enveloped the gathering during the meal.

For the President's visit, arranged in accordance with the Navy custom that a distinguished passenger is entertained by each of the messes aboard ship, the officers had provided some almost forgotten peacetime touches: a detachment from the ship's band furnished dinner music, the wardroom was brightly lit and the commissary performed minor miracles to provide a menu that ranged from soup through roast ham to baked alaska.

Truman's joking tagline to his remark about Stalin encouraged Berberich to ask another question about the Soviets. Had there been any commitments at Potsdam, he wondered, in an effort to bring Russia into the Pacific war and thus hasten Japan's fall?

The President again responded with a crisp, clear statement— and one that his listeners would never forget.

No, he said, there had been no such deal made. And if the Russians had been somewhat difficult at Potsdam, it did not matter so far as the war against Japan was concerned, because the United States now had developed an entirely new weapon of such force and nature that we did not need the Russians—or any other nation.

"It is so powerful," he said, "that one weapon is equal to twenty thousand tons of TNT exploded on a single target at one time."

Truman did not wait for the *Augusta's* officers to calculate how many rounds from their eight-inch main batteries would be required to produce such a blast. He plunged on, speaking rapidly, to tell them more: that the new weapon had been developed in total secrecy; that it had been financed entirely by executive order, using a presidential emergency fund so that Congress knew nothing of it; that it had been tested already, and that reports of the tests indicated it could end the war.

When he ended, the table was silent. Truman thanked his hosts and rose to leave. As he stepped away, the President turned back for a moment.

"It is the biggest gamble in history," he said. "Two billion dollars have been spent on it. We will have the final answer on its effectiveness within a very short time."

The officers sat talking for a long time after their guest had retired to his cabin. It was well after midnight before they finally ended their arguments and speculations and turned in, still astonished and still without the vaguest idea of the nature of the new weapon. Harry S. Truman had, for a moment, given a half-dozen relatively junior officers an awesome glimpse of the authority and responsibility of their commander in chief. The authority, in many matters, was absolute; the responsibility, in an

3

equal number, was crushingly final.

Later, Truman was to say of his office, "The buck stops here." There would never be a time when that still-unspoken sentiment would have more exact an application than it did on this August 5.

While President Truman ate Sunday dinner in the *Augusta*'s wardroom on the Atlantic, it was already early the next morning in the Marianas Islands in the western Pacific. The day made little difference to the U.S. Navy Seabees who had been working since 3 A.M. They had been doing the same thing every morning, seven days a week, for over a month. They were the last link in a supply chain that was frantically trying to satisfy the appetite of the U.S. Twentieth Air Force for high explosive and incendiary bombs. Cigar-chewing Major General Curtis E. LeMay had used his B-29 bombers to unload 40,000 tons of bombs on Japanese cities in July; on the preceding Thursday, August 2, his pilots had celebrated the anniversary of the Army Air Force by dropping a single-day record total of 6,632 tons. LeMay was driving his aircrews as fliers had never been driven before. They were logging 120 hours a month in the air, and a recent letup had been due solely to the fact that they were temporarily out of incendiaries after burning mile upon mile of urban Japan in massed, low-level fire raids. Even so, almost 600 Superforts had flown over Japan Sunday night.

West of the Marianas, Karl T. Compton, an eminent physicist and one of the handful of top civilian advisors who had directed the massive mobilization of American science for the war, was in Manila that Sunday night. Compton had flown in earlier that day to open a new laboratory, a sort of front-line scientific first-aid station to give close support to the last big push

4

against Japan. Until a few weeks ago, Compton had been very busy indeed at home on a highly secret project. With his part in that now out of the way, he was off on a new assignment. He would have his plans on the desk of General MacArthur's chief of staff before 9 A.M. Monday.

Some seven hundred miles east of Manila, near the midpoint of Code Route Peddie, the "main line" across the Pacific from Guam to the Philippines, the destroyer escort U.S.S. *Cecil J. Doyle* was steaming a night search course across an empty sea. Sunday was the first night in almost a week that the *Doyle*'s skipper, Lieutenant Commander W. Graham Claytor, Jr., had been able to set a routine night watch and turn in for a few hours. Since midnight Thursday he had been almost constantly on the bridge as his crew hauled from the water the half-dead survivors of the cruiser U.S.S. *Indianapolis,* torpedoed and sunk by an enemy submarine four days after delivering a small secret cargo to Tinian Island in the Marianas. Now, with his load of survivors in the hospital at Peleliu, Claytor was back in the sinking area, ordered to make a final search and to perform the unpleasant duty of recovering and burying remaining bodies. This work, however, required daylight; and after securing ship at twilight, Claytor had time to think ahead. In his safe, unknown to others in the *Doyle*'s crew, were orders for the next operation. With the other five vessels in its escort division, his ship would handle radar picket duties in the next amphibious landing. It didn't take much guessing to figure the next operation as the first landing on the Japanese mainland. It required only a reading of the Okinawa action reports to know that the current life expectancy of a small radar picket ship in such an operation was down to about twelve hours, thanks to the Japanese *kamikaze* planes. The *Doyle*'s only direct contact with the enemy since her commissioning in 1944 had been the rescue of a lone Japanese floating on a raft. It seemed likely that this situation would change drastically before long. To put it mildly, the prospect was not particularly cheering to Lieutenant Commander Claytor.

That same Sunday, August 5, *New York Times* reporter William L. Laurence climbed off a plane at Tinian. He was not sure why he had been sent there (although he could make a well-informed guess), for his orders were sealed. He was sure that he was about to come closer to the enemy, for he carried a brand-new identification card conferring on him the "assumed" rank of colonel—and the card was valid only in case of his capture by the Japanese.

Another reporter for the same newspaper and with almost the same name, William L. Lawrence, was on nearby Guam when his colleague landed at Tinian. The Guam Lawrence was a full-time war correspondent who the previous week had cabled his paper in this fashion:

. . . There are a surprising number of people here . . . who think the Japanese may be forced into unconditional surrender without the necessity of even a token invasion. The existence of that sentiment here is the more important because lots of the people who talk that way wear stars and may therefore be presumed to be in a position to know what they are talking about.

Lawrence confessed in the next paragraph of his dispatch that he did not share this view. He said he had bet "a one-star officer" ten dollars that the war would not be over in three months. Correspondent Lawrence could regret, a month later, that he had not checked with "Colonel" Laurence before putting up his ten-spot.

There was no such wagering going on among the men of the 13th U.S. Marines, one of the regiments of the 5th Marine Division. Pulled out of Iwo Jima in March after fighting in that bloody engagement, the division had been resting, repairing its equipment, training its many replacements and getting ready for the next job: the assault landing on Kyushu, southernmost of the Japanese home islands. The prospect was one that prevented the men of the 13th from fully enjoying the open-armed hospitality of the ranchers on the western slopes of Hawaii, where the division was encamped. For Major William Miller, commanding the 3rd Battalion, the whoop-it-up evenings at the ranch home of Mr. and Mrs. Scott Pratt, who had more or less "adopted" the regiment's officers, were only brief interludes in planning for an invasion in which over-all initial casualties of 100,000 seemed to him a conservative estimate. Miller, who had fought the Japanese at Guadalcanal and Cape Gloucester as well as on Iwo, didn't hear much peace talk at battalion level. What he did hear didn't sound convincing in the light of his previous contacts with a fanatic enemy.

Another military unit whose men were not betting on a quick surrender was the 1st Squadron of the 7th Cavalry Regiment. Two weeks before, Major Houck Spencer had brought his command back to the U.S. lines in the Philippines after a fortnight of bushwhacking behind the enemy front. He had been sent out to find and kill Japanese in the rugged, unmapped ridges and valleys of eastern Luzon. The strategic significance of the foray was nil, but the squadron had found plenty of Japanese. It surprised and killed a lot of them, and then the enemy realized the Americans were there and began to react. When Spencer's squadron came out, it was down to 250 men. The healthier supported the wounded and carried the dead—all their dead—out of the forest.

7

Nothing in either the character of the Japanese opposition or the thinking of the U.S. high command, at least as it had affected their own duties, led these tired troopers to expect an easy end to the war. Their division, the old 1st Cavalry, had spearheaded the Leyte landing and had climbed over its own dead to retake Manila. Now it was preparing for a D-day landing in Japan.

The orders and training assignments which occupied the *Doyle,* the 13th Marines and the 7th Cavalry all had a common source. Men in Pearl Harbor, Guam and Manila were putting the final touches on a plan called OLYMPIC. This was to be the first assault on Japan, and was intended to capture the southern portion of Kyushu so that its airfields and harbors could be used to support a final thrust at Tokyo a few months later.

OLYMPIC was on its way, approved by the President and the Joint Chiefs of Staff in Washington. The details were set down in fine print on over four hundred single-spaced pages of Top Secret Operations Plan A-11-45, issued by Headquarters, Amphibious Forces, Pacific Fleet.

Forty-two aircraft carriers would take part to provide air support. Twenty-four battleships would be there for bombardment. Two hundred and twelve destroyers and 183 destroyer escorts, including the *Doyle,* would screen the fleet and provide close fire support for the assault troops. Six divisions of infantry would go ashore on D-day, with three more following on D plus 2. Four more divisions would be in reserve. In all, three quarters of a million men would be involved.

Houck Spencer's foot cavalry squadron would wade ashore on the east coast south of Shibushi on D-day. Bill Miller's Marine battalion would go in on D plus 2 onto a crescent-shaped beachhead on the west shore, where the 5th Marine Division had drawn a follow-up assignment behind the initial assault by the 2nd and 3rd Marine divisions. The landing beaches had code names chosen from the roster of American automobiles: Buick, Cadillac, Dusenberg, Essex, Ford, Zephyr, Stutz, Studebaker, Reo and others. Each beach was neatly divided, on the meticulous planning maps, into four color zones. Each zone was subdivided into two parts. Thus there would be Buick Green One and Stutz Yellow Two—as there had been, the year before on the French coast, Omaha Easy Red and Utah Fox Green.

The plan would not only get men onto the beaches but also provide for taking them off. The Navy was to furnish ships for evacuating thirty thousand wounded in the first thirty days. Hospitals in the Philippines, the Marianas and Okinawa were to have fifty-four thousand beds ready. Twelve hospital ships would be offshore when the first wave landed. At each beachhead, there would be an LST loaded with whole blood.

The intelligence annex to A-11-45 was only a preliminary one that would be revised as D-day neared. But there was information enough in this first estimate:

Present information of enemy beach defenses on southern Kyushu is meager, but it is known that top priority has been given to preparations for the defense. . . . Recent intelligence indicates considerable activity in the construction of heavy artillery positions. . . . It is probable that fixed defenses cover all of the proposed landing beaches, and minefields have been laid. . . .

The plains surrounding the landing beaches are backed by rugged hills which are being heavily fortified by the enemy. . . . Well developed cave defenses and tactics of the type encountered in Okinawa will very likely be met throughout the area. . . .

One out of every three American soldiers engaged in the fight for Okinawa was now dead, wounded or missing.

9

Not all the members of the U.S. Armed Forces were thinking of the perils that lay before them. In New Mexico, at a place called Los Alamos, an Army non-com named David Greenglass worked in a shop which fabricated bits of machinery sketched by some of the world's most brilliant theoretical scientists. Greenglass was thinking of many things, including his forthcoming furlough in New York City. On his last trip east, he had told his brother-in-law quite a lot about his job, something he had been forbidden to discuss with anyone. Since that time, he had been visited in New Mexico by an associate of the brother-in-law, and had told him more about his shop and what was made there. Now Greenglass had additional information about the project on which he was working. By the time he left for New York, this carefully collected knowledge would cover twelve handwritten pages and include a couple of sketches, all of which he was to turn over to his brother-in-law, whose name was Julius Rosenberg.

While President Truman worked on his Potsdam conference papers during Sunday afternoon, thousands of his constituents were diverting themselves by watching that unique mutation of professional athletics known as wartime major-league baseball. Some measure of the degree by which the times were out of joint could be found in the day's results. The Washington Senators, winning a pair from Boston (5-4, 5-1), moved within a half game of first place in the American League as the leaders, Detroit, lost two games to Chicago. In the National League, the race was about settled. The Chicago Cubs, winning two games this Sunday, stood six games ahead of the pack.

In New York City, August 5 was a bright summer day, with a high temperature of 81 degrees—the first such perfect Sunday, in fact, since early July. The city's millions took full advantage of it. Early editions of the morning papers carried the statistics: 1,500,000 persons were on the beach at Coney Island during the day. Eighteen of them had to be hauled from the water by lifeguards. Ninety-two children were lost, and then found, in the crowds.

The ninety-two sets of parents who got their children back after mix-ups at Coney were not the only families reunited that day. Down the harbor on Staten Island in the early morning, the troopship *Santa Margarita* tied up and unloaded 302 soldiers, veterans of the European war with high scores in the new G.I. game of discharge points. This was a small, off-day installment in the flood of westbound troops. A few days earlier, New York harbor had welcomed the Cunarder *Queen Mary*, carrying 15,000 men, the equivalent of a full division, back to the States.

The flow of men home from Europe was running strong, but not strong enough for some. Senator Ed Johnson of Colorado, for example, called the Army's decision to hold onto many of the men who had served in Europe "blind, stupid, and criminal." Interior Secretary Harold Ickes, worried about the coming winter's demands for coal, wanted Secretary of War Henry L. Stimson to let miners in khaki go home. To these and many other similar pleas and complaints, stiff old soldier-statesman Stimson turned a deaf ear. He pointed out that as far as he was concerned, General MacArthur's requirements were more important than those of the coal fields. He declined to dignify Senator Johnson's attack with a comment. Since Stimson was the Army's boss, that was that, despite the political pressures.

Some American parents that weekend were no longer wondering when or whether their boys would be home: they already knew. Such was the case of Technical Sergeant Kurt J. Hermann II, of Babylon, Long Island. A veteran of seventy-five bombing missions in Europe, including the first raid on Rome in 1943 and the first R.A.F. night raid on Berlin, the twenty-six-year-old gunner had wangled an assignment to Pacific combat when his European tour was up. On his thirty-third B-29 trip over Japan—it was his 108th mission of the war, a record for bomber crewmen—his plane was shot down over Kochi. On this Sunday, August 5, the Air Force announced that he was presumed dead.

Another New York boy who carried his grandfather's name—a name which, in this case, was known in the world's richest counting rooms—was Thomas W. Lamont II, grandson of the chairman of the board of J. P. Morgan and Company. Like Technical Sergeant Hermann, twenty-year-old Tommy Lamont had gone to war with zest. Only a few months after he delivered a moving oration to his graduating class at Phillips Exeter Academy, he enlisted in the Navy. He volunteered for submarine school, was accepted and joined the crew of the U.S.S. *Snook* in the Pacific. On Saturday, August 4, 1945, the Navy had announced that the *Snook* was overdue from its last patrol and presumed lost with all its crew.

There were some young men in America that Sunday who had not yet run the gantlet. To many of them, the surrender of Germany had meant primarily that they now had only one chance to taste the bittersweet brew of war. Such, for example, was Edward Bushnell, a soldier from Williamstown, Massachusetts. Drafted in 1944, Ed Bushnell had believed all along that he was destined for Pacific duty. When he was assigned to an outfit bound for Europe after V-E Day, he wangled a last-minute transfer, the new orders coming through just as the trucks were pulling out for the port of embarkation. Now, with orders assigning him to a

Pacific coast P.O.E., he was home for a few days in the Berkshires, thanks to a delay-en-route furlough. Whatever the apprehensions of his family, eighteen-year-old Ed Bushnell, with the impatience of his years, was anxious to get going.

There was considerably less eager anticipation among a group of war workers in Ambler, Pennsylvania, a Philadelphia suburb. Forty-seven employees of the Keasby and Mathson Company who had taken part in a recent strike were still at home this Sunday, but the next morning they were due at their induction stations for selective-service physical exams, thanks to the action of the Fourth Naval District's labor relations officer and their local draft boards, which had stripped them of their essential-job deferments and put them in class 1-A.

In other places on August 5, other people were looking forward to quite different events. The producers of *Oklahoma!*, for example, could anticipate a small celebration Monday night, when their touring road company, then playing Philadelphia, would take in its millionth dollar at the box office. In Stamford, Connecticut, Clare Boothe Luce, a member of Congress on holiday from Washington, was preparing for the final dress rehearsal of a straw-hat production of Bernard Shaw's *Candida*. The playwright-politician was to open a week's run Monday in the title role, her first starring stage part, at Stamford's Strand Theatre.

Americans who sought escape from the war found it in many ways that August weekend. Some went to the movies: the big new shows were *Anchors Aweigh, Incendiary Blonde* with Betty Hutton, *Wonder Man* with Danny Kaye. Some went to Broadway plays: *Life with Father* had passed another milestone a week earlier with its 2,400th performance. On the radios and juke boxes, there was a bumper crop of first-rate pop tunes, music to dance to with a girl in a short dress and a long bob: "Don't Fence Me In," "The Trolley Song," "Till the End of Time," "Sentimental Journey," "Bell-Bottomed Trousers," "June Is Bustin' Out All Over." If you insisted on merely reading, there was always *Forever Amber,* still a best seller more than a year after publication.

East of the *Augusta,* the time was later. Dinnertime on the ship was mid-evening in England. At a country estate named "Farm Hall" near Cambridge, ten scientists had whiled away a lazy afternoon. Some walked for exercise—a somewhat repetitious pastime, since they were not allowed outside the high garden walls. Others read—for some of them this enforced country sojourn was the first chance in years to read for pure pleasure, and they were taking full advantage of Farm Hall's excellent library. Others talked—of many things, but especially of science. They all knew what they were talking about, and they all spoke in German.

One thing these Germans did not know, however, was why they were here. They had been plucked out of homes and hideaway laboratories by a team of American soldiers—many of them scientists themselves, and some old friends of their captives —and hustled off to England without so much as a by-your-leave, let alone an explanation. The Germans had been at Farm Hall since spring.

The man who had sent them there was himself still in Germany. He was Samuel A. Goudsmit, a Dutch-born physicist whose first stop in liberated Europe had been a visit to his parents' home, empty since they had been shipped off to the gas chambers of a Nazi concentration camp. On this Sunday night, Goudsmit was in Berlin, preparing to spend the next day sifting through the wreckage that used to be Heinrich Himmler's SS headquarters. Goudsmit could have told the German scientists why they were shut up in England. So could Harry S. Truman.

Another who could have cast some light on the scientists' situation was Winston S. Churchill. This Sunday, Churchill was trying to accustom himself to a new role as leader of His Majesty's Loyal Opposition instead of Prime Minister of His Majesty's Government. Ten days earlier he had come home from Potsdam to be present when the results of the British election were announced. He never returned to the conference table, for the war-weary electorate, in a stunning shift of sentiment, swept Churchill's coalition out of office and installed a Labour government. Churchill's moving statement of resignation could have held a hint for the men at Farm Hall:

The decision of the British people has been recorded in the votes counted today. I have therefore laid down the charge which was placed upon me in darker times. I regret that I have not been allowed to finish the work against Japan. For this however all plans and preparations have been made, and the results may come much quicker than we have hitherto been entitled to expect. . . .

In a radish field outside Tokyo, a crew of expert radiomen from the Japanese Navy kept a round-the-clock watch over a room jammed with 181 powerful radio receivers. Members of the "Yamatoda Signal Corps," they were assigned to detect and record all radio signals emanating from U.S. transmitters. Whenever a transmission was monitored, the signalmen not only recorded it and passed it on to the decoding office in Tokyo but also tried to pinpoint the location of the transmitter.

Now, early on the morning of August 6, the men working the

overnight shift picked up a call sign they had first heard almost three weeks earlier. The monitors had located it on Tinian Island, and as it was heard daily during late July they had tagged it "New Task Company" for quick reference. The cryptographers in Tokyo had been unable to break the cipher, but the Japanese monitors had come to recognize it instantly, as trained radio-men will, by the individual touch of the American operator's hand on his Morse key.

Now the signal came out of the air again. To the Japanese, it was merely one more item to be logged and reported. They did not know what the "New Task Company" was. They did not particularly care, either, as they dozed through the last hour of their shift while the new day brightened outside.

Three hundred miles to the east, one of the most powerful striking forces ever assembled steamed into the morning sun. Twenty-four hours earlier, the U.S. Navy's Third Fleet had been lunging toward prearranged targets in southern Japan. Now it had been ordered to turn around and run out to sea—and its admirals were baffled and angry.

Rear Admiral C. A. F. Sprague, commanding Carrier Division Two, summoned his combat intelligence officers to the flag cabin on the U.S.S. *Ticonderoga*.

"Ziggy" Sprague waved an order at his aides. "This is a hell of a way to run a war. What's it all about? What do I have an intelligence staff for, anyway?"

The order, from Pacific Fleet headquarters, read:

It is imperative that there be noninterference with operations of the 509th bomb group. Although their objective has been indicated it may be changed. It is accordingly directed that you send no planes over Kyushu or western Honshu until specifically authorized by me.

Sprague's officers had no answer for their chief. The discussion ended with all hands putting a dollar bill and a sealed guess, to be opened later, into a pool. Lt. Edwin P. Stevens of New York recalled a cocktail-party conversation in 1941 with a physicist friend who had told him how some scientists were seeking to release enormous amounts of energy by breaking the nucleus of atoms. Now Stevens scribbled something about "nuclear energy" on his slip of paper.

Another of the officers, Lt. James H. Rowe, Jr., had been an aide to F.D.R. in the White House before the war. His entry was a suggestion that some attempt to end the war by negotiation might be afoot and that the planned strike had been postponed for that reason.

Both Rowe and Stevens had, in a way, guessed right. But Rowe didn't win the pool. His timing was off. There had been attempts at negotiation, but on August 6, 1945, time had run out on them.

CHAPTER TWO

The Clock Is Running

PER JACOBSSON was not particularly happy to be driving back to Basel on such a beautiful afternoon. He had hoped to spend another day or two at Wiesbaden with his old friend Allen Dulles, enjoying the countryside and the warm hospitality of the American, who had only recently moved north from Switzerland. But Dulles wanted him to report back as soon as possible to the two Japanese whose proposals had sent him hurrying to Wiesbaden in the first place; and Jacobsson, though loath to give up the holiday he had promised himself, had to agree that the job wouldn't wait. It was an exciting job, and a daring gamble: an effort to end World War II.

A big, burly, amiable bear of a man with wide-flaring ears, Jacobsson had looked out through his heavy spectacles at a great deal of history in the making since he had first come to Switzerland from his native Sweden in the early twenties to work for the League of Nations. He had been in Switzerland in the fall of 1941, as economic adviser to the Bank for International Settlements, when two Japanese officials of the bank,

Kojiro Kitamura and Tsuyoshi Yoshimura, confided to him their fear that war was coming in the Pacific—and their unhappy conviction that such a war would be disastrous for Japan. Jacobsson had not forgotten this gloomy conversation, and was thus convinced of their good faith when Kitamura and Yoshimura again approached him in June, 1945. This time, they wanted to talk about ending the war. Specifically, they wanted him to go see Dulles to find out whether the United States might be willing to offer some conditions that would make possible a Japanese surrender.

The two bankers had their eye on Allen W. Dulles for several reasons. Although nominally attached to the U.S. Legation in Bern, the true nature of his work was an ill-kept secret. In the espionage-conscious community of wartime Switzerland, his role as European director of the Office of Strategic Services, the American intelligence agency, was at least widely suspected if not openly acknowledged. He was rumored, moreover, to be a special presidential appointee with great power and direct access to the White House in Washington. Stories of his part in arranging the separate surrender of German forces in northern Italy before V-E Day had leaked out. Some reports had it that Dulles was a personal ambassador of some sort, sent to Switzerland originally by Franklin D. Roosevelt. In any event, he seemed to the worried Japanese like a man who could speak with authority.

As a matter of fact, other Japanese had already contacted Dulles' organization with the same end in mind. In April, as Germany collapsed in its final agonies, the Naval attaché at Bern, a lieutenant commander, had opened conversations with the Dulles group through an American banker and an anti-Nazi German. This approach, however, had failed. The Japanese Navy and Foreign Ministry in Tokyo were irritated by this junior officer who seemed to be trying to act for the entire government. They ignored his urgently worded cables for some weeks, then warned him to be cautious and finally ordered him to stop. But Kitamura, who knew a little about the attaché's efforts, thought he and Yoshimura might fare better. For one thing, they had more standing with the top diplomats and the military at home. They had taken Shunichi Kase, the Japanese minister to Switzerland, into their councils, and he had agreed to support and assist them. They also had a ranking military officer enlisted in their cause. Lieutenant General Seigo Okamoto, former military attaché in Berlin, agreed with their aim and thought he could convince the Army General Staff in Tokyo of the necessity for surrender. They invited Jacobsson to Yoshimura's home in Basel one evening and laid their ideas before him.

What they proposed was that the "unconditional surrender" demand of the Allies, proclaimed at the Roosevelt-Churchill-Chiang meeting in Cairo in 1943, be softened by allowing several conditions. These would include preservation of the Emperor of Japan; no insistence on changes in the Japanese constitution; internationalization of Manchuria; and continuation of Japanese control over Formosa and Korea. The Emperor question, they emphasized, was the critical one. Jacobsson listened, then went home and wrote a letter to his wife in Stockholm telling her that a very important piece of business had come up that would prevent him from getting home to Sweden for his daughter's wedding.

Dulles had moved from Switzerland to Wiesbaden by this time to supervise OSS operations in conquered Germany. The intelligence outfit had its headquarters in a champagne factory that had once produced wine for the table of Heinrich Himmler. The Americans thoughtfully allowed the plant to continue in

Truman ate lunch with the crew on August 5, 1945, as he awaited the news that the first atomic bomb had been dropped on Japan. As Commander in Chief he had made the lonely, final decision to use the bomb. He described it as "the biggest gamble in history."

(Official U. S. Navy Photo)

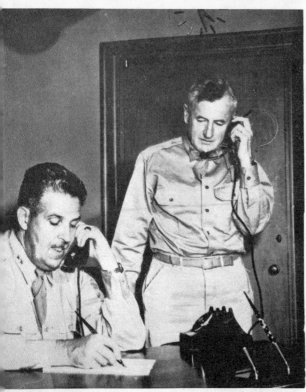

Major General Leslie R. Gro[ves]
(standing), commander of [the]
Manhattan Engineer Distr[ict,]
which made the atomic bo[mb,]
with Brigadier General T. [F.]
Farrell, his deputy for CENT[ER]
BOARD, the operation of deliv[er]-
ing the bomb on Japan.

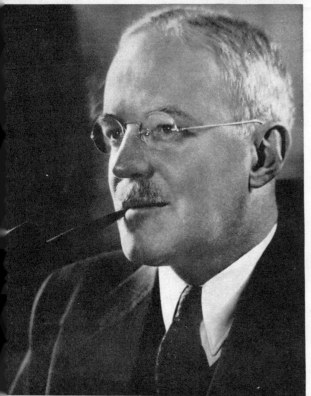

Allen W. Dulles, in Wiesba[den]
as supervisor of OSS operati[ons]
in conquered Germany, was [ap]-
proached through an interm[edi]-
ary with a Japanese surren[der]
proposal. By June of 1945 m[any]
leading Japanese were urge[ntly]
attempting to end the war be[fore]
their country suffered fur[ther]
devastation.

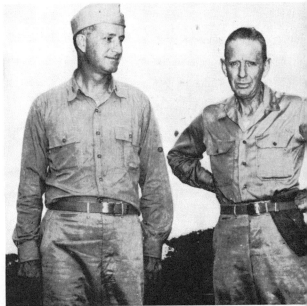

eft to right, Captain W. S. Parsons, USN, head of the technical rew from Site Y, and Rear Admiral W. R. Purnell, Navy co-ordinator, on Tinian Island. arsons performed the final assembly of the bomb aboard the *nola Gay* on the flight to Hiroima.

(U. S. Army Photo)

Crew of the *Enola Gay*. Left to right, standing: Lt. Col. John Porter, ground maintenance officer; Capt. Theodore J. Van Kirk, navigator; Maj. Thomas W. Ferebee, bombardier; Col. Paul W. Tibbets, commanding officer, 509th Group, pilot; Capt. Robert A. Lewis, co-pilot; 2nd. Lt. Jacob Beser, radar countermeasures officer. Kneeling, left to right: Sgt. Joe Stiborik, radar operator; S/Sgt. George R. Caron, tail gunner; Cpl. Richard H. Nelson, radio operator; Sgt. Robert H. Shumard, assistant flight engineer; and T/Sgt. Wyatt E. Duzenbury, flight engineer.

(USAF Photo)

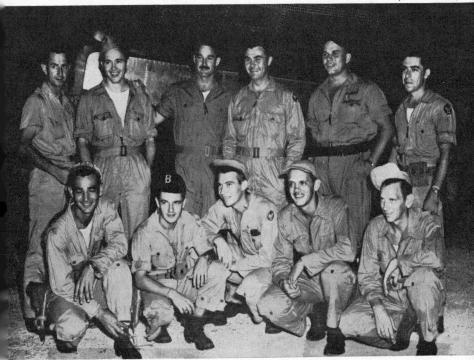

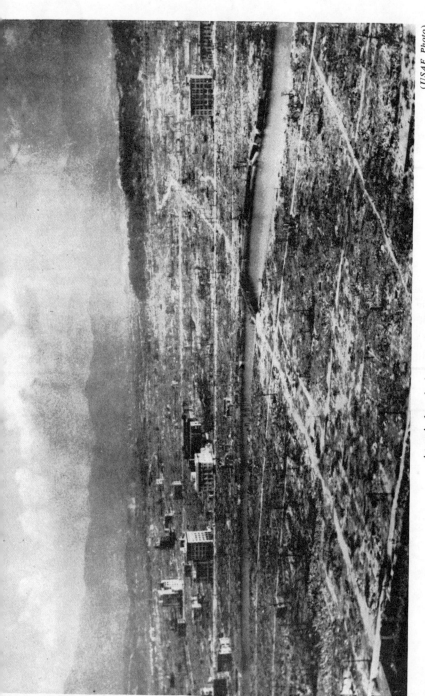

Atomic bomb damage in Hiroshima.

operation, although they soon discovered that the product was so bad it was fit to drink only when heavily laced with brandy. On rainy days, the new occupants found, the place smelled "terrible." Director Dulles was quartered in a big, well-furnished house on a hill near the northern edge of town. The OSS requisitioning officer had managed to find his boss a comfortable billet, a two-story stucco house typical of the region, with an untypically leak-proof roof. It also had such pleasant fringe benefits as a balcony with view and an exceptional rose garden.

When Dulles got word from Jacobsson of this second Japanese overture, he sent a car down from Wiesbaden at once to fetch the Swede. The two men talked far into the night of July 14 in Dulles' house on the hill. Jacobsson urged that the American government go as far as it could in providing whatever reasonable assurances were required to induce an early Japanese surrender. Dulles, aware that he had no formal authority whatever to speak for his government and sensitive to the possible domestic repercussions of a softening of the "unconditional surrender" doctrine, was cautious and skeptical. Jacobsson angrily pressed his views. Finally they went to bed without resolving their differences.

The next morning was bright and beautiful. Jacobsson, despite the shortness of his sleep, was refreshed and determined to keep at the question. At breakfast they plunged into the discussion again. This time, in the clear light of a new morning, their talk ran more smoothly. Dulles left the room for a while to think by himself. When he came back, he had worked out a suggested reply to the Japanese in Basel. His counterproposal reflected his precise lawyer's mind: it drew a careful distinction between commitments and understandings. The gist of it was that while there would undoubtedly be sympathy for the desire of the Japanese to retain their Emperor, there could be no advance commitment by the United States government on this point. The best way for Hirohito to ensure his continued reign would be for him to take the lead in proclaiming and enforcing the surrender, and in seeing to it that Japanese troops were brought home peacefully from China and other occupied foreign territory. In short, there was no guarantee, but there was a promise of sympathetic understanding.

Dulles told Jacobsson he should return to Switzerland at once to pass this on to Kitamura and Yoshimura. He put him in an Army auto that afternoon, with a sergeant from G-2 as an escort, and the Swede hurried home to Basel. The war-torn roads were in bad shape. Bridges were still smashed, pavements were broken and in many places there were still telltale white tapes to mark where "safe" lanes had been cleared through German mine fields. In spots, they had to leave the road and be helped across broken ground by G.I.s. One of these, peering at the strange civilian riding in the back seat, asked Jacobsson's escort: "Who is he? Some congressman they turned loose to run around Europe?"

Dulles, after a telephone call to Potsdam, decided he should report in person to Stimson, who had joined the President at the Big Three meeting. OSS headquarters in Wiesbaden called the big air base at nearby Frankfurt, and without difficulty, for Dulles' organization bore a very high priority for aircraft requisitions, lined up a flight. On the morning of July 20, Dulles and a few aides drove to Frankfurt, climbed into a bucket-seat C-47 transport and flew to Berlin. En route, Dulles reminded the group that it was the anniversary of the 1944 attempt on Hitler's life by a group of German officers—another project in which the OSS had played an important role.

When he landed at Berlin, Dulles drove at once to Potsdam and told Stimson of the Japanese overtures. The Secretary of War noted the conversation in his diary for that date: "Late in the afternoon Allen Dulles turned up, and I had a short talk with him. He has been in the OSS in Switzerland and has been the center of much underground information. He told us about something which had recently come in to him from Japan."

Stimson's diary did not indicate to whom, if anyone, he passed on Dulles' "something." Dulles returned to Wiesbaden, having fulfilled his immediate mission, which was to make sure the information about the surrender proposal was available to Truman before he made a final decision on the ultimatum which everyone knew would emerge from the Big Three sessions.

The Japanese in Switzerland were acting urgently. When Jacobsson saw the two bankers, he noted with surprise that for the first time in his long acquaintance with them, they dispensed with the customary ritual small talk at the opening of a conversation and jumped right at him for Dulles' answer. Within a few hours, both Minister Kase and military attaché Okamoto sent off the first in a series of strongly worded telegrams to the Foreign Office and Army General Staff in Tokyo. Kitamura added his voice in wires to top government financial figures.

But the Japanese in Switzerland got no encouragement from their government. Somehow, its intelligence service had failed to provide enough information on Dulles for the Foreign Office even to know who he was. ("A certain Mr. Dulles" was the way one official labeled him later. "We could not identify the Mr. Dulles in question.") In addition, the Japanese cabinet was already committed to a different line of action. It hoped to persuade Russia, still neutral in the Pacific war, to act as intermediary in arranging a peace agreement. Japanese Foreign

Minister Togo had already ordered his ambassador in Moscow, Naotake Sato, to raise the subject with Soviet Foreign Minister Molotov and to seek permission for a special Imperial envoy to come to the Russian capital.

Sato was a trained and seasoned career diplomat. From Moscow he could see quite clearly the hopelessness of his country's position, and his cables to the Foreign Office this summer reflected his hard-boiled assessment. On July 1, he advised his government to end the war in any way possible. Bluntly he pointed out that Japan, now alone and friendless, could look to no one for help or sympathy. Acceptance of any terms—including even unconditional surrender—seemed to Sato the only way to preserve the Emperor and the structure of the nation.

Sato's advice was sound, as both Togo and Prime Minister Suzuki knew very well. But they also knew what Sato, long absent from home, could not know: it was not so simple as that. While Japan was being publicly torn apart by American bombs and naval gunfire, there was also occurring a desperate private struggle, no less intense for the fact that it was scarcely visible outside the innermost circles of the government.

From the day he took office in April, 1945, Suzuki had been trying to arrange an end to the war. In this effort he had the backing of two other members of the Supreme War Council, the "inner cabinet" that really ran the nation. They were Togo and Navy Minister Yonai. But War Minister Anami and the chiefs of the Army and Navy General Staffs, General Umezu and Admiral Toyoda, wanted to fight on. There was thus a three-to-three deadlock in the council. The fact that Emperor Hirohito wanted to end the war, and had in fact been quietly sounding out the nation's senior statesmen on it as early as February, was not at this juncture decisive. The Emperor, though deified by his subjects, had in fact no solid political power. He could exert influence on individual leaders, but he could not dictate policy to the council.

In this stalemate the Army had seized the political initiative in early June and had rammed a fight-to-the-end plan through at an "Imperial conference" of the council, held in the presence of a mute Hirohito.

Suzuki could not stop this, but one of his allies, Koichi Kido, Lord Privy Seal of Japan and thus a man with constant access to Hirohito, could ignore it. On June 9, the day after the council action on the Army plan, Kido spent a half hour alone with the Emperor in the palace library. He showed Hirohito a memorandum he had written urging efforts to end the war. The Emperor seemed pleased. The Lord Privy Seal wrote that night in his meticulously detailed diary: "His Majesty commanded me to set my hand to the tentative peace plan immediately."

In the next few days, Kido talked to the members of the Supreme Council individually. This private persuasion paid off. On June 18, notwithstanding its earlier actions, the council agreed to propose, through neutral nations, that an effort be made to negotiate a peace. This could hardly be called a decision to surrender, but it was a beginning.

On that same day, in Washington, President Truman's inner council of war advisers also held a meeting, but with quite a different aim. At the end, the President put his stamp of approval on OLYMPIC, the invasion of the Japanese homeland. It was scheduled for November, and would be followed, in March, 1946, by CORONET, a landing on the Tokyo plain in the main island of Honshu. CORONET was designed as the death blow to the empire.

War, however, was not the only item on Harry Truman's agenda for June 18. In the United States as in Japan, the search for peace was under way even as both sides braced for the final decisive combat. That day Joseph C. Grew, Under Secretary of State, saw the President privately for the second time in three weeks to talk about peace. As he had in the first of these meetings, Grew urged the President to give Japan a chance to keep its Emperor if it surrendered, arguing that such an offer would greatly facilitate the surrender.

This same thought had been much on Stimson's mind too. These two men—one the Secretary of State during the years in the thirties when Japan first began to make war in Asia, the other the last U.S. Ambassador to Japan before Pearl Harbor— knew the mind and heart of the enemy as did few other Americans. Stimson complained later in his private diary that some influential officials at the White House and State Department knew little about the Emperor:

. . . There has been a great deal of uninformed agitation against the Emperor in this country mostly by people who know no more about Japan than has been given them by Gilbert and Sullivan's "Mikado," and I found . . . that curiously enough it had gotten deeply imbedded in the minds of influential people in the State Department. . . .

Certainly Stimson and Grew knew the Japanese better than Truman and James F. Byrnes, the incoming Secretary of State.

Grew, near the end of a long career, was especially urgent with the President. In a written memorandum he spoke as a diplomat, in measured words. Now, face-to-face, he spoke as an individual, and he spoke with a passion that his cultured voice could not entirely mask. His record of the conversation, set down later the same day, was this:

I said to the President that I merely wished to square my own conscience at having omitted no recommendation which might conceivably result in the saving of the lives of thousands of our fighting men so long as we did not recede an inch from our objectives in rendering Japan powerless to threaten the peace in the future.

Grew suggested that the President issue a statement calling for Japanese surrender, but holding out the possibility that the Emperor might be allowed to remain in power. He suggested this should be done as soon as Okinawa fell, or at least before the attitudes on both sides were so hardened by the inevitable heavy casualties of an invasion of Japan that the move could no longer be made. Truman told Grew he liked the idea, but wanted to hold it up until he could talk to his allies at Potsdam. He asked Grew to put the matter on the Big Three agenda.

Meanwhile, in Japan, things were moving at last after the Supreme Council's reversal on June 18. The next day Togo visited ex-Premier Koki Hirota, who had already been in contact with Soviet Ambassador Jacob Malik on Togo's behalf. The Foreign Minister asked Hirota to renew his efforts with Malik, an old acquaintance from the days when Hirota had been assigned to Moscow. The object of the talks would be to seek Malik's support for the attempt to persuade Russia to act as broker in peace talks.

Then, on June 22, the Emperor for the first time stepped into the Supreme Council's deliberations. He called the council into his presence and said flatly that it was time to consider the possibility of ending the war. When General Umezu, nicknamed "The Ivory Mask" for his cold determination and aloofness, spoke up in disagreement, the Emperor stepped even further out of character to rebuke him. The Army chief's arguments in favor of fighting on and his predictions of eventual victory rang hollow on June 22, the day the last Japanese resistance was wiped out on Okinawa.

But now, as the peace effort finally began to gain momentum inside the Japanese government, it was beginning to be stalled by people and events outside. Twice within a week, on June 24 and June 29, Hirota saw Malik. He got no encouragement from the taciturn Soviet, and when he sought a third talk, he was told the ambassador was ill.

Time was also running out for those in Washington who wanted to see peace without an invasion of Japan and believed it could be achieved. Stimson had been preparing proposals in response to Truman's desire to make absolutely sure there was no alternative before subjecting his Army to the inevitable heavy losses of OLYMPIC and CORONET. Truman simply could not order an invasion which might result in several hundred thousand casualties without satisfying himself there was no other way out.

Stimson drew up a paper after conferring with Grew and Secretary of the Navy James Forrestal. On Monday, July 2, he took it to the White House and handed it to Truman. The gist of his argument was that Japan could be made to surrender without invasion, thanks to the air and sea bombardment and blockade already under way—an operation that could be intensified horribly with a new weapon that Truman and Stimson, and a very few others, now knew would be available soon. On the other hand, in Stimson's opinion, a landing on the home islands would probably "cast the die of last ditch resistance." He predicted that any attempt to "exterminate [Japan's] armies and her population by gunfire will tend to produce a fusion of race solidity and antipathy which has no analogy in the case of Germany."

Stimson urged that a final warning be issued "before the actual invasion has occurred and while the impending destruction, though clear beyond peradventure, has not yet reduced her to fanatical despair."

As for the Emperor, Stimson proposed a statement expressing the determination of the Allies to wipe out "all authority and influence of those who have deceived and misled the country into embarking on world conquest." This would be enforced by a military occupation, with the occupying forces to be withdrawn only when "a peacefully inclined government, of a character representative of the Japanese people," was set up. Then he added this comment: "I personally think that if in saying this we should add that we do not exclude a constitutional monarchy under her present dynasty, it would substantially add to the chances of acceptance." With this in mind, his proposed draft of the ultimatum carried an additional sentence after the statement on the eventual establishment of a government "representative of the Japanese people." It read: "This may include a constitutional monarchy under the present dynasty if it is shown to the complete satisfaction of the world that such a government will never again aspire to aggression."

The Stimson paper went with Truman to Potsdam, and was the basis for the proclamation which was put into final form by Byrnes, with Truman and Churchill checking it and making minor revisions. But in that final form the ultimatum did not include Stimson's closing suggestion.

Grew had also tried to talk with Byrnes about the status of the Emperor before the Big Three meeting, but the new secretary, sworn in on July 3, was too busy preparing for the meeting to discuss the subject. It was not until late on July 6, as Byrnes was leaving his office to board the *Augusta,* that Grew was able to hand him a proposed draft statement. Byrnes put it in his pocket as he left for Potsdam.

Byrnes also took with him some advice from an old and trusted friend, Cordell Hull, now ill and retired but still available for consultation. Byrnes visited him several times before taking office, and just before leaving for Potsdam he telephoned him again. He said that high officials of the War, Navy and State departments—apparently meaning Stimson, Forrestal and Grew—had approved inclusion in the final ultimatum of a clause declaring that the "Emperor institution" could be preserved. He asked Hull's opinion of this.

The man who had been Secretary of State on the day that Japanese "peace negotiators" sat in his office while Japanese fliers killed more than two thousand Americans at Pearl Harbor replied that he thought it was "too much like appeasement," and that as Byrnes explained the proposed wording it also seemed to leave room for the perpetuation not only of the Emperor but also of the privileged feudal ruling caste. Ten days later, Hull amplified his views in a cable to Byrnes—forwarded, ironically, through the courtesy of Acting Secretary Grew, whose thinking ran the other way—in which he raised an additional question of American domestic politics. If the Japanese should reject the ultimatum despite a concession to the Emperor, he said, "the Japs would be encouraged while terrible political repercussions would follow in the U.S." He closed with the suggestion that no ultimatum be issued until Russia entered the war and Allied bombing reached a "climax."

Byrnes replied the next day, July 17, in a cable in which he agreed that the ultimatum "should be delayed," and when issued should contain no commitment to the Emperor. Later, explaining his view, he was to argue that he believed "it would hasten surrender," and perhaps bring it to pass before Russia entered the war, "to assure the Japanese that the form of their future government would be left to them." Thus Hull wanted to get the Russians into the war, while Byrnes said he wanted to keep them out. Hull was against "appeasement," while Byrnes wanted to let the Japanese select their own future government. For these sharply differing reasons, both men were opposed to making any commitment to the Emperor of Japan.

The reasoning of the Allied military leaders on the subject was equally complex. The American and British high commands were interested in the status of the Emperor for a single reason: his possible usefulness in making a surrender effective. On July 16 at Potsdam, Field-Marshal Sir Alan Brooke, Chief of the Imperial General Staff, raised the matter at a Combined Chiefs of Staff meeting. He spoke of the "unconditional surrender" policy and said that "from the military point of view there might be some advantage in trying to explain this term in a manner which would ensure that the war was not unduly prolonged in outlying areas." He made the point that the Emperor was the one person who, if kept in power, could order a surrender of scattered Japanese forces.

At a meeting of the U.S. Joint Chiefs of Staff the next day, General Marshall argued that "from a purely military point of view . . . nothing should be done prior to the termination of hostilities that would indicate the removal of the Emperor of Japan, since his continuation in office might influence the cessation of hostilities in areas outside Japan proper."

The views of the two Army chiefs were the only ones on this subject recorded in the secret minutes of the two meetings of July 16 and 17. On July 18, the military discussions culminated in a top-secret Joint Chiefs memorandum to Truman, signed by Fleet Admiral William D. Leahy, Truman's chief of staff. It is interesting to note that while Brooke and Marshall are recorded as prefacing their remarks with a disclaimer of anything but "military" considerations, this final paper dealt with political matters as well.

In it Leahy said that the Chiefs feared the Stimson draft (permitting "a constitutional monarchy under the present dynasty") could be misinterpreted in two ways: "extreme devotees" of the present Emperor might read in it a threat that Hirohito would be deposed or executed, while "radical elements" in Japan might see in it an Allied determination to continue the institution of the Emperor and Emperor worship. The Chiefs suggested changing the Stimson wording to provide simply that "the Japanese people will be free to choose their own form of government." The memorandum concluded with this statement:

From a strictly military point of view, the Joint Chiefs of Staff consider it inadvisable to make any statement or take any action at the present time that would make it difficult or impossible to utilize the authority of the Emperor to direct a surrender of the Japanese forces in the outlying areas as well as in Japan proper.

The military leaders, then, wanted to keep the Emperor in power so that he could surrender his scattered armies. But they apparently thought this could best be accomplished by not mentioning him in the ultimatum.

In the end, the heads of government accepted the advice of Byrnes, Hull and Leahy—though their parallel conclusions stemmed from divergent lines of reasoning—rather than the suggestions of Stimson and Grew.

In Japan, with the Malik-Hirota talks at a dead end, the Emperor was again intervening. On July 7, he ordered Suzuki to send a special envoy to Moscow to seek mediation. On July 10, the day the U.S. Navy opened its close-range air and sea bombardment of Japan, Suzuki and Togo told the full Supreme Council for the first time of the feelers that had been put out to Russia, and of the Emperor's new command. The council selected former Premier Prince Fumimaro Konoye for the critical mission. At 3 P.M. on July 11, Togo dispatched a cable to Sato:

Very Secret
Urgent
The foreign and domestic situation for the Empire is very serious, and even the termination of the war is now being discussed privately. Therefore . . . we are also sounding out the extent to which we might employ the U.S.S.R. in connection with the termination of the war. . . .

This was what Sato had been waiting to hear from home. But the rest of Togo's cable was a disappointment to the hard-boiled professional diplomat. Togo cautioned him:

. . . Please bear in mind not to give them the impression that we wish to use the Soviet Union to terminate the war.

And this was followed later that night by another cable, in which the Foreign Minister said:

. . . It is his majesty's heart's desire to see the swift termination of the war. In the Greater East Asia war, however, as long as America and England insist on unconditional surrender, our country has no alternative but to see it through in an all-out effort for the sake of survival and the honor of the homeland.

Sato's reaction was swift, precise—and negative. At 11:25 P.M. on July 12 he replied:

33

. . . I believe it no exaggeration to say that the possibility of getting the Soviet Union to join our side and go along with our reasoning is next to nothing. . . . The manner of your explanation is nothing but academic theory. . . .

The thinking of the Soviet authorities is realistic. It is difficult to move them with abstractions, to say nothing about the futility of trying to get them to consent to persuasion with phrases beautiful but somewhat remote from the facts and empty in content. . . . If indeed our country is pressed by the necessity of terminating the war, we ourselves must first of all resolve to terminate the war. . . .

In international relations there is no mercy and facing reality is unavoidable. . . . I beg for your understanding.

Despite his misgivings, Sato did as he had been ordered and the next day asked for an interview with Soviet Foreign Minister Molotov. But now again the clock was running out on Japan. Sato was told that Molotov was too busy preparing to leave for Potsdam to see him. Sato had to give his message and request for the Konoye visit to Alexander Lozovsky, the Deputy Foreign Minister.

The American government had Togo's message almost as soon as Sato, and before it reached the Russians. The cryptographers of the U.S. Navy had long before broken the Japanese codes, and had used the knowledge gained from their interceptions to good effect during the fighting. Now the intercepts dealt with peace, and again the Navy code room was providing advance information. Forrestal was handed the Togo-Sato message on July 13. In addition, he got an intercepted and decoded copy of Sato's reply. The messages were forwarded to President Truman, then approaching Land's End and the English Channel aboard the *Augusta*.

It was five days later, on July 18, before Sato could get an answer from Lozovsky. When it came, it was almost exactly as he had predicted. The deputy, using the formal phrasing of diplomacy, said:

> I have the honor to call your attention to the fact that the Imperial views stated in the message of the Emperor of Japan are general in form and contain no specific proposal. The mission of Prince Konoye . . . is also not clear to the government of the U.S.S.R.

Sato reported the rebuff verbatim to Togo, then followed with another piece of plain-spoken advice:

> . . . There is no other way than to present a concrete proposal when dealing with this government.

The clock was running faster now. On July 18, the cruiser U.S.S. *Indianapolis,* suddenly ordered from her overhaul berth in the San Francisco Navy yard two days earlier, was steaming westward across the Pacific at top speed. She carried a small, top-secret cargo. Her destination: Tinian Island in the Marianas.

The Suzuki government did not know how little time was left, but it was moving, its eye on the Big Three at Potsdam. New instructions were sent to Sato on July 21. Togo reiterated one earlier statement: "We cannot accept unconditional surrender in any situation." But in an accompanying separate message, he provided the more specific statement demanded by the Soviets:

> The mission of special envoy Konoye is to ask the government of the U.S.S.R. for its assistance in terminating the war and to explain our concrete intentions concerning the matter in accordance with the wishes of the Emperor.

Communications were slow. The new instructions did not reach Sato until July 24.

In Potsdam that day Stimson conferred with Truman for fifteen minutes. He had heard, from Byrnes, that it had been decided not to mention the Emperor specifically in the ultimatum which had been approved by Truman and Churchill and would be issued as soon as Chiang Kai-shek had cleared it. The final declaration would not go beyond a statement that the final form of government in Japan was to be left up to the Japanese people. Stimson nevertheless spoke again of his concern over the Emperor question. In his diary, he recorded the conversation this way:

I then spoke of the importance which I attributed to the reassurance of the Japanese on the continuance of their dynasty, and [said that] I had felt that the insertion of that in the formal warning was important and was the thing that would make or mar their acceptance, but that I had heard from Byrnes that they preferred not to put it in, and that now such a change was [made] impossible by the sending of the message to Chiang. I hoped that the President would watch carefully so that the Japanese might be reassured verbally through diplomatic channels if it was found that they were hanging fire on that one point. He said that he had that in mind, and would take care of it.

One day later, on July 25, an order approved by Harry S. Truman made final the most momentous decision he had yet had to make as President. That order was put into writing in Washington, then flown across the Pacific—to Tinian Island.

On July 26, the United States and Britain, with China as a co-signer and Soviet Russia an approving kibitzer, issued the Potsdam declaration.

The Japanese heard about it quickly. The text was beamed to Japan by a San Francisco short-wave transmitter of the U.S. Office of War Information three hours after it was received in

Washington. There was instant attention in Japan, as Stimson and Grew had warned there would be, to the fact that the ultimatum made no mention of the future status of the Emperor. Despite Hirohito's own statement to Suzuki that he found nothing in the ultimatum offensive to him in principle, the Supreme War Council and the cabinet could not accept it as written. The military wanted to denounce it outright, and when this was refused they insisted that two conciliatory clauses—promising that Japan's armed forces could go home and renouncing any intention of "enslaving" or "destroying" Japan as a nation—be censored before it was published in Japan. The cabinet, after long discussion, decided not to answer but to disregard or *mokusatsu* (literally, "kill with silence") the ultimatum. This decision was not intended, at least by the peace party, to be publicized, but somehow it leaked to the Japanese papers, and in addition Suzuki used the word on July 28 at a news conference. It was this word, broadcast by the Domei news agency, translated by U.S. monitors as "ignore," and interpreted by the American leaders as "reject," that was reported to President Truman at Potsdam as the Japanese response to the ultimatum.

Truman received this advice shortly after he had been told by Stalin that the Japanese proposals for mediation were still considered by the Soviets as "too vague" for consideration. Stalin's attitude, combined with the report that Japan had decided to "ignore" or "reject" the Potsdam ultimatum, left Truman convinced that he now had no choice but to let the order he had started toward Tinian on July 25 stand as it had been written.

Now all the efforts had failed. Dulles and Jacobsson and the Japanese in Basel had failed, their negotiations begun so late that it would have been difficult to change the course of events

37

before the ultimatum was issued. Grew and Stimson had failed, their suggestions opposed by Byrnes and Hull, blurred by the contradictory advice of the military chiefs, and overshadowed by the rising Russian obstructionism which was already emerging at Potsdam as an overriding problem. The Emperor of Japan and his Foreign Minister had failed, their hopes mistakenly pinned on the theory that Russia would be willing to mediate peace rather than grabbing for the last-minute spoils of war.

It was too late now. For a few more days, the desperate men in Tokyo would continue to seek a way out of the currents that seemed to be sweeping them inexorably toward either abject and total surrender or a final suicidal resistance. But already events were in motion, on the tiny island of Tinian in the Marianas, which would sweep away all subtleties of diplomacy and politics in a single overwhelming blow.

The clock had run out, although Japan's leaders did not know it. Neither did the more than 250,000 Japanese still living in a city that so far had been strangely untouched by the fiery blasts that had scourged the rest of the nation. This city was known throughout Japan as a place where exceptionally beautiful willow trees grew. It was largely unknown to the rest of the world. Its name was Hiroshima.

CHAPTER THREE

Twilight at Hiroshima

HIROSHIMA had been spared the most frightful results of the war. While almost every other urban area in the island kingdom had been seared by the incendiary mixtures dropped by the B-29s, this ancient river-mouth city had felt the concussion of only twelve enemy missiles in three and one half years of war. Two small bombs were dropped by a flight of U.S. Navy raiders in March, 1945, and six weeks later a single B-29, unable to reach its prime target, let go a string of ten 500-pounders. In all, about a dozen people were killed.

Otherwise, this big port and manufacturing city seemed to be an eerie backwater of the war. Enemy planes flew overhead night and day, causing continual air-raid alarms, but they went on elsewhere. All kinds of reasons for this strange immunity were advanced. Many said the Americans had crossed Hiroshima off their target lists because so many of the Japanese nationals in the United States were from Hiroshima prefecture. There was even talk in this summer of 1945 to the effect that some relative of President Truman—"perhaps his mother"—was in the area and that therefore he personally had ordered the B-29s to stay away.

This story may have seemed far-fetched even to those who started it. But this kind of extreme rumor reflected the confused situation in Hiroshima. Although they had not felt the blast and flames of Twentieth Air Force bombs, the city's people knew very well that the war was going badly. They were aware of it every time they sat down to eat, every day they went to work, every time they walked the city's streets.

Down by the docks, from which almost every Nipponese soldier who went to the southwestern Pacific fighting area had sailed, a deathlike quiet hung over the big embarkation facilities. The *Gaisenkan,* "Hall of Triumphal Return," where troops had listened to final instructions and exhortations, was now quiet and empty. Where the city in earlier years had bulged with as many as 100,000 troops en route to the front, it now held only one division, and that was preparing for defense, not attack. Including support troops, there were about 24,000 soldiers in Hiroshima. The once-busy harbor was dead. American planes had dropped so many mines into the waters of the Inland Sea that no shipping came to Hiroshima any more. There were no more civic celebrations of the sort that provided the big send-off for the "Ever-Victorious Fifth Army" in 1942. When it had sailed south to capture Singapore, thousands of Hiroshima citizens lined the docks and jetties of the harbor to shout "Banzai!"

The strange situation that insulated Hiroshima from the horrible blasts that had torn Tokyo, Yokohama and other cities worried some people. There were those in Hiroshima, describing themselves as "intellectuals," who feared, as they lay awake at night listening to the planes overhead, that the Yankees were saving them for some particularly dreadful fate.

The military authorities, who had lately established the defense command for all of southern Japan in the old, moated feudal castle in the northern part of town, were worried too. They ordered steps taken to secure their installations. Under the orders, ironically, the citizens of Hiroshima themselves did what the Americans had not done and destroyed great chunks of their city. Almost 70,000 dwellings were demolished in the spring and summer to make three broad east-west firebreaks through the city. It was assumed that the seven channels in which the Ota River flowed through the city, which was built on the river's fan-shaped delta, would provide enough north-south open space to stop fires. The demolition work was started by local building construction firms, but they did not move fast enough to satisfy the Army, which ordered the people drafted into labor battalions to speed up the work. By the first week in August, 30,000 adults and 11,000 students had been thrown into the work.

As a result of the destruction of homes, over 90,000 of the city's peak wartime population of 380,000 had been ordered to leave in five mass evacuations. A sixth forced exodus was under way in early August. The Army draft took more, about 5,200 men in the first half of 1945. Still others simply decided to get out. The flow of unauthorized evacuees reached the point in mid-summer where police had to man the major exit roads and turn back those whose departure had not been approved by the authorities.

The steady drop in population, coupled with the tightening food situation, had a marked effect on commerce in Hiroshima. Before the war there had been almost 2,000 food retailers in the city. By mid-1945, there were only 150 stores still open to sell food to the 250,000 civilians left in the city. With less of everything to spend money on, the banks found themselves doing a flourishing business in their savings departments; balances in July were 28 per cent above the same date a year earlier.

The people who were left in Hiroshima were busy. Thousands had been mobilized into "neighborhood associations" to tear down houses—sometimes including their own—in the firebreak program. Women and school children were assigned in big groups for such work or for labor in the city's factories. There were many of these, almost all producing for the war: military supply depots turning out cloth, uniforms, shoes; a repair yard for small ships, run by the Army, which was the largest in Japan; the Great Eastern Food Company, which canned beef for the Navy; the Kirin brewery, which made beer for both military and civilian use; and the sprawling plants of the Mitsubishi industries, which made many things, from airplane engines to the giant kites which were to be used as anti-aircraft protection for the few remaining warships of the Imperial Navy. The railroad yards were busy day and night. Since May, all available freight cars had been shunted onto the job of building up munitions stocks in the Western Defense Command, and by July incoming freight at Hiroshima was running three times as heavy as outgoing traffic.

The factories, warehouses and rail yards of Hiroshima were running hard, trying to turn out supplies and equipment for an Army that would soon have to meet a terrible American onslaught on the home islands. But their activity masked a deeper economic and military hopelessness that was painfully apparent to the top planners if not to the man in the street. The average citizen in Hiroshima might know only that his rice ration was smaller, or that the corner grocery store had gone out of business because it had little or nothing to sell. But the Japanese cabinet knew more. An official study in June had predicted that minimum requirements for rice to support the people on a subsistence-only basis would outrun supplies by a full fourteen million tons in 1945. It added that the first grim signs of starvation were already beginning to appear in more isolated sections of Japan.

The Hiroshima resident might know only that there were fewer trucks in his city's streets, that the seven rivers no longer echoed to the chugging of boat engines, that few planes took off from the new airport at the southern tip of the city. The cabinet, on the other hand, knew that the armed forces had been desperately short of fuel for almost a year. As early as the fall of 1944 the Navy was so pinched that some of the warships lost in the Philippine Sea battles might not have been able to regain their home ports even if they had escaped from the American bombs and torpedoes.

The Japanese Army was making shell cases out of dull gray substitute metals, for there was no more brass. Some regular military units were being issued bamboo spears. These were also to be the principal weapons of the "National Volunteer Fighting Corps," a sort of last-ditch home guard into which every Japanese male would soon be mobilized. Every foot of shoreline was being prepared for defense; but in most cases this meant only barbed wire (there was little cement for fortifications), machine guns (there were almost no artillery pieces available) and caves in the hills (it was obvious the Americans could not be kept off the beaches). The Navy, not only short of fuel but also decimated by U.S. guns and bombs, had finally adopted the *kamikaze* tactics of the Air Force. In July, seven hundred small craft, loaded with explosives and intended for one-way voyages only, were being prepared in southern Japanese harbors against the inevitable day when America's invasion fleets would appear over the horizon.

Even the Japanese propaganda machine was admitting the

hopelessness of the situation. "One Hundred Million People Die in Honor!" was the new slogan. "Better to Die Than Seek Ignominious Safety!" Those who still hoped for victory now talked of some "God Chance," a miraculous happening that would turn the tide at the last moment. An Army propagandist, conceding he was "shocked by the rapid change in the war situation," called on the people to "strengthen the citadel of the mind."

August 5, 1945, was little different in Hiroshima from previous Sundays in this year of shortages, defeats, evacuations, demolitions and forced labor. As in every wartime society, some felt the pinch more acutely than others. Some sacrifices were major, personal and immediate. Others were minor, generalized, more potential than actual.

One of those in Hiroshima whose troubles were not weighing especially heavily on him was Dr. Takuji Imagawa, who operated a small clinic and private hospital in the Nekoya precinct near the center of the city. He had evacuated his wife and three daughters, the oldest of them thirteen, to the relative safety of suburban Furue, high on the hills that overlooked the flat delta city from the west. The doctor stayed downtown and, with the help of three nurses, kept his little hospital open. Today he had a dozen people on his in-patient list, including both patients and the relatives who customarily stayed with the sick in Japanese hospitals to cook and care for them. These few customers kept Dr. Imagawa occupied during the day. Several air-raid alerts interrupted, and thus prolonged, his rounds.

About six in the evening he left the clinic in charge of his nurses and went to the neighboring Kawara precinct to eat dinner with a couple of medical colleagues. The host, a surgeon named Matsuo, spread out a dinner that was, for the time, quite lavish: fish, meat and wine adorned the table in addition to more mundane staples like rice. The doctors sat over their wine cups and talked of professional matters. They had been pondering giving up their private practices for the duration, since supplies were growing scarcer, and going into one of the public clinics where their income might be lower but where there would at least be medical supplies and drugs available. That night they made a final decision to do this, and Dr. Imagawa agreed to go to the prefectural authorities Monday on behalf of the trio.

Back at the clinic shortly after 10 P.M., he had a pleasant surprise. One of his patients, a not-so-young *geisha,* invited him to join her and her visiting daughter to share some rice-ball delicacies the girl had brought in. The three sat up until past midnight, playing at the game of flower-cards and finishing off two flasks of wine in the process. Imagawa's cheerful mood was further enhanced when the *geisha* offered to take his radio and listen for air-raid warnings so he could sleep undisturbed. The doctor went off to bed and fell sound asleep. So, apparently, did his patient, for she did not awaken him for either of the air-raid alerts announced that night on the radio.

Sunday was a good deal less comfortable for Hayano Susukida, whose husband was a war correspondent stationed in Java with the Japanese forces there. She was alone in Hiroshima with her thirteen-year-old son Shojiro. An older son had been sent, with one hundred classmates from the Higher Commercial School, to live and work at the Mitsubishi rayon plant at Otake, sixteen miles from Hiroshima, and her four-year-old daughter had been sent out of the city for the duration. In addition, only one room of the Susukida house was still standing, the rest of it having been torn down as part of the firebreak that passed behind it.

Mrs. Susukida was up early on Sunday, for she had to cook breakfast for Shojiro before attending a meeting of her neighborhood association. At the meeting, she was given her work assignment for the next day: to report to a spot just south of the Hijiyama bridge, where her group would start salvaging roof tiles from homes that had been torn down there. The air-raid alarm sounded periodically through the day, and she spent most of Sunday either in the shelter or in the wreckage of her own demolished house, trying to collect scrap wood and timber from it for firewood. She got little rest that night, either. Unlike Dr. Imagawa, she got up for both the air-raid alarms, the first shortly after midnight and another at about 2:30 A.M. She sat gossiping with her neighbors in the local shelter until about 3:00, only four and one half hours before she was due to report for her labor assignment.

The air-raid alerts which kept most residents of Hiroshima city running to and from their shelters on that Sunday night did not make so much of a stir in the suburbs. But life was complicated in other ways. Many there were city people who had sought a safer residence in the face of the expected eventual fire raids on Hiroshima, and were trying to resettle their households. A case in point was that of Yuko Yamaguchi. With her husband overseas in military service, she had taken her three small children to live with his parents. The father-in-law, head of the gas company in Hiroshima, was well-to-do. There would have been plenty of room for four more in his comfortable and spacious city house. But the government took the house for Army officers' quarters, and now the whole Yamaguchi family was living in a rented farmhouse in Inokuchi village outside the city. Yuko's own parents were still in the city. Her father, an eye specialist, preferred to stay close to the hospital where he worked. The net result of these dislocations was a good deal of coming and going to keep family and business running on something approaching an even keel.

On this Sunday, Yuko, her children and her in-laws breakfasted together at the farmhouse. The women spent all day unpacking boxes of household goods they had brought with them from the elder Yamaguchis' city mansion. About 3 P.M., a gas company car arrived to pick up the father-in-law, who had to attend a directors' meeting that evening and planned to stay on overnight in the city with other relatives.

Mother and mother-in-law worked together to feed the children, two daughters, eight and seven, and a five-year-old boy. The older woman, in what seemed to Yuko an unusual gesture, took it upon herself to put the youngsters to bed. In an uncharacteristic display of sentiment, she told her daughter-in-law that although it might seem difficult to have three children to care for in times like these, things would get better and then the young couple would be "better off for having the children." Apparently in an effort to cheer up Yuko, who was concerned for her husband's safety, she added that once the fighting ended they would be able to get back to their city house and life would be much easier. At the farmhouse that night, the women and children slept well, undisturbed by the air-raid alerts that spoiled the repose of those still in the city.

People rose early in Hiroshima. Despite the air-raid alarms that kept many awake until three o'clock in the morning, most people were up and moving by six or a little later. Dr. Imagawa,

refreshed by his unbroken rest, was up at six, and the first thing
he did was to telephone his wife. He told her to bundle up some
medical supplies which he had taken to the house in Furue and
to bring them downtown to the clinic. He had hardly hung up
when the telephone rang with an emergency call from a family in
Kannon precinct. Could the doctor come at once to look at a
sick child? He said he would be right along, and since he hadn't
bothered to eat breakfast for the last thirty years, he picked up
his bag, hopped on his bicycle and set off at once without waking
anyone at the clinic. On the way, he decided to look at another
patient who lived on the route to the house to which he had been
called. He turned off near the Kanzaki elementary school in
Kawara precinct and stopped at the sick man's home. It was a
new house, its windows glazed with wire-reinforced glass, considered more resistant to bomb blasts. He took off his shoes—they
were new ones—at the door and walked through the little garden, with its tiny pond, to the semi-detached room where the
patient, head of the household, was being attended by his eight-
year-old son. Dr. Imagawa greeted him, then set down his bag
and began a routine checkup of his patient.

Hayano Susukida had to hurry this morning, for she had to
feed her son breakfast and put together a lunch for him before
he left for his labor group. She herself was due at the Hijiyama
bridge for the tile-salvaging job. She got up a little before seven,
less than four hours after she came home from the small-hours
gossip session in the air-raid shelter, and got breakfast for
thirteen-year-old Shojiro. After fixing him his lunch too, she
gulped her own breakfast and left hurriedly to join her own labor
group, not stopping to clean up the one room in which they now
lived. To start the day's work she was put at the end of a long

line, taking the salvaged roof tiles as they were passed from hand to hand to her and piling them neatly. After half an hour, positions were changed and she found herself at the head of the line, stooping to pick up tiles from rubble piles and starting them along the human chain. Meanwhile, Shojiro was waiting on the military parade ground near their home, where his school class, drafted en masse for the labor crews, had been ordered to report for work. Mrs. Susukida's older son Junichiro, out at the Mitsubishi plant in Otake, was having a more leisurely morning. Breakfast was not served until 7:30. After barely nibbling at it, since his stomach was upset this morning, he went to his dormitory to change into school uniform for the classes that were held each day before the students went into the rayon factory.

There was less than usual in the way of early-morning work for Yuko Yamaguchi, since her father-in-law had spent the night in the city instead of returning to the family's temporary home in the suburban farmhouse. By 7:30, her two daughters were on their way to school. Her mother-in-law left a few minutes later to catch the commuter train into the city so she could pick up some additional belongings that were still sitting in the storehouse of their recently requisitioned city home. Five-year-old Ryuichi was sent out into the farmyard to play and Yuko got busy with her morning chores.

All over the city similar scenes could be found. Women in almost every house were cooking breakfast over the little charcoal burners that served most Japanese homes as combination stoves and heaters. Work parties were forming up or just starting their tasks. Among them were a number from outside the city, groups pulled together in each village in the surrounding hills and sent into Hiroshima in response to the military command's decision a week earlier to speed up the demolition and firebreak work. In all, including both city and country residents, there were over forty thousand persons—women, old men and children for the most part—in these "patriotic work parties" on August 6. This Monday's force included a new element. The day before, the prefectural government had ordered all able-bodied girls in the secondary schools to join the "volunteer" work groups.

In the moated grounds of the old castle built in 1594 by Terumoto Mori, the feudal lord who first started Hiroshima on its way up from primitive fishing village to flourishing city, the day shift reported for work at the Army communications center. The nineteen women and thirteen men in the group filed into the underground, reinforced-concrete bunker as the night shift left its machines and started home in the bright sunlight of the new morning.

Busy with morning routines of one kind or another, most people in Hiroshima paid little attention to the air-raid alert that sounded at nine minutes past seven o'clock. Those who looked up at the faint drone of engines found, if their eyes were sharp, a single B-29, flying very high. Probably it was a weather plane of the kind that often flew over in the morning. It crossed the city twice and then, at 7:25, flew out to sea. The warning system sounded the all-clear at 7:31.

CHAPTER FOUR

"99"

SIX MILES ABOVE Hiroshima, at 7:25 A.M., August 6, the B-29 was a speck against the sun. The lone Superfortress, named the *Straight Flush,* had flown west across the city, turned and flown back east. From this height clouds could be seen pillowing the sky in all directions. Only the city itself seemed exposed to the sun, as though a hole had been punched in a fluffy bedspread. Major Claude R. Eatherly ordered a message sent from the *Straight Flush.* Staff Sergeant Pasquale Baldasaro, the radio operator, tapped it out in Morse code: "Y 2. Q 2. B 2. C 1."

Almost two hundred miles away, over the Pacific southeast of the island of Shikoku, another American bomber received the message. The pilot, Colonel Paul W. Tibbets, Jr., leaned over the shoulder of his radio operator, Corporal Richard Nelson, as he jotted down the letters and numbers. Using a weather code sheet, Tibbets interpreted: "Low clouds, 1 to 3/10ths. Middle cloud amount, 1 to 3/10ths. High clouds, 1 to 3/10ths. Advice: Bomb primary."

A few minutes later, Major Ralph R. Taylor, pilot of the

B-29 *Full House,* circling over Nagasaki, and Major John A. Wilson, commander of the *Jabbit III* over the city of Kokura, ordered similar weather surveys sent. But all Tibbets was interested in was the first message.

The words from the sky over Japan that morning, "Advice: Bomb primary," wrote a death sentence for the city of Hiroshima, for it was the prime target of the Americans. Kokura and Nagasaki were alternates, in that order, in the event of bad weather at Hiroshima. Within a few hours an ancient but suddenly new and frightening word, "atom," would be on the lips of men and women all over the world.

The culmination of a centuries-old quest brought the *Straight Flush* over Hiroshima to measure the extent of cloud cover. Probably it began thousands of years ago when men clad in animal skins came out of their caves and pondered, of a morning, on the nature and texture of the sun. Eventually, as scholars probed the secrets of matter, the body of their knowledge took the name "physics."

The modern exploration of the tiny vastness of the atom began in 1896 when a Frenchman, Antoine Henri Becquerel, discovered radioactivity in uranium ore. In 1905 Albert Einstein, a German Jew whose deep eyes and shaggy hair became the symbol of the new science of the twentieth century, published his theory of relativity. For the next thirty years the physicists of Europe and North America sought to penetrate the atom. They were confident, in theory at least, that if these invisible particles of matter could be ripped open, huge stores of energy would burst forth.

In January, 1939, while Adolf Hitler's swastika and vaudeville prop mustache stirred Germany to mass hysteria, the world community of physicists was electrified by news from Berlin. At the Kaiser Wilhelm Institute, Otto Hahn and Fritz Strassmann had bombarded the uranium atom and succeeded in splitting it. The process came to be called nuclear fission, a name derived from the biological process of cell division. Although results of the achievement were published and a number of articles appeared in the general press, the statesmen and the military chiefs paid scant attention to the development. Excitement in the international clan of physicists, however, was keen. To these scientists it was as though a new continent suddenly had emerged from the Atlantic Ocean, exactly where geologists had predicted it would. A fretful restlessness agitated their ranks.

By this time the dictatorships of Hitler and Mussolini, together with the ranting Nazi doctrine of "Aryan" supremacy, had driven scores of scientists to England and to the shores of America. Many of them were Jews; others merely sought the freedom on which scientific inquiry feeds. Among these men were physicists who speculated on possible military applications of the energy which they now believed would soon be released from the atom. Some of them feared that German researchers, with their growing knowledge of atomic energy, might one day provide Hitler with a weapon of terrible proportions. A few went into action.

In March, 1939, two worried men took the train from New York to Washington. They were George B. Pegram of Columbia University and Enrico Fermi, an Italian who began bombardment of uranium atoms in 1934. Fermi won the Nobel Prize in 1938, but declined to return from the Swedish ceremonies to Fascist Italy. Instead he came to America to continue his work. Niels Bohr, a Danish physicist visiting New York, confided to a friend that in his laboratory in Denmark the uranium atom had been split with a release of energy calculated to be a million times as powerful as that from an equal amount of high explosive.

Fermi had learned of Bohr's feat and the knowledge lent urgency to his Washington mission.

Fermi and Pegram got a polite hearing at the U.S. Navy Department, but no commitment. Years later Ross Gunn, technical adviser to the Naval Research Laboratory, recalled that as a result of the Fermi-Pegram call, he obtained the grand sum of $2,000 to conduct research on chain reaction.

The atom scientists were frightened. That summer two of them went to see Einstein, by now a U.S. citizen revered by his fellow Americans as a genius with a key to the mysteries of the universe. Einstein received the men at his Long Island summer home, padding to the door in bedroom slippers. One of the men was Leo Szilard, a brilliant Hungarian who had fled German laboratories with the rise of Hitler. The other was Eugene P. Wigner, a fellow Hungarian and a mathematical physicist.

Their mission was political. President Roosevelt must be warned personally of the atomic progress in Germany and be persuaded to provide government sponsorship for an assault on the atom in the United States. Einstein's help was vital, not only for its impact on the President but because of his friendship with the Belgian royal family. The Belgian Congo was the chief source of uranium ore. Actually, Einstein was not abreast of the latest atomic developments, and he argued against use of the prestige of his name in an area in which he couldn't give personal assurance of the facts. At last, however, he assented and a letter was drafted over his name. It urged quick government action to develop an atomic weapon and to procure uranium from the Congo.

Then Szilard sought out Alexander Sachs, New York financier, economist, amateur mathematician and the owner of a wide-ranging mind that matched President Roosevelt's in its de-

light with new and bold ventures. Sachs already was an un-
official adviser to F.D.R., a kind of lower-echelon Bernard
Baruch. Szilard and Edward Teller, another refugee Hungarian
physicist, revisited Einstein and perfected a final draft of the
letter Sachs was to carry to Roosevelt. A memo by Szilard accompanied the letter.

Sachs saw Roosevelt at the White House on October 11,
1939. By this time Nazi Germany had swept through Poland
with motorcycle shock troops and dread Stukas which dive-
bombed civilians on the roads. Europe was plunged into the
World War II that was to massacre non-combatants as no other
conflict in history since the barbarian hordes of Genghis Khan
plundered and murdered westward from Mongolia.

Sachs read the Einstein letter and the Szilard memorandum as
Roosevelt listened, his head tilted back and his cigarette holder
cocked upward. The President asked few questions. It was obvious he was impressed, but he seemed reluctant to add a major
undertaking to the score of new defense projects just getting
started. Sachs wangled an invitation to breakfast the next morning. He spent a sleepless night at his nearby hotel. How could he
bait and trap the President's imagination? He paced his room,
took several walks through Lafayette Square, where that other
presidential adviser, Baruch, was wont to hold daytime court on
a bench. At last, not long before dawn, a scheme evolved.

F.D.R. was alone at breakfast in the second floor study of the
White House when Sachs called. "What bright idea do you have
this morning?" Roosevelt asked cheerily. Just a story, replied
Sachs.

He told of Napoleon Bonaparte hungering for a conquest of
haughty England to add to his string of military victories. But
Napoleon was frustrated. The erratic tides and currents of the

English Channel blocked an invasion by French sailing vessels. A young American inventor, Robert Fulton, gained an audience with Napoleon. He proposed that France construct a fleet of steamboats which could negotiate the Channel tides with ease. Napoleon rudely brushed the idea aside as the brain child of a visionary. How, asked Sachs, might the history of Europe have been changed if Napoleon had heeded the plea? And in the world of 1939, who would first sponsor the atom scientists as they sought to pioneer a weapon of untold force and fury?

The President rang for a servant and soon a bottle of Napoleon brandy was brought. He filled two glasses and touched his to Sachs'. The big Roosevelt grin creased his face.

"Alex," he said, "what you're after is to see that the Nazis don't blow us up?"

"Precisely," said Sachs.

The President summoned Brigadier General Edwin M. (Pa) Watson, an easy-mannered Alabaman who served as a secretary. Roosevelt handed the papers to Watson and briefly explained their import.

"Pa," he said, "this requires action."

The United States government had begun work on the atomic bomb.

But for the first two years the pace of research was slow as a snail on glass. Nuclear enthusiasts groaned at the lack of money and the torpid reflexes of Washington officials. Hitler conquered Europe, loosed a torrent of bombs on England and invaded Russia. Japan's armies rolled into Indo-China and Benito Mussolini's Italy joined the Axis powers in total war. Meanwhile unco-ordinated atomic research proceeded in a few American universities. Not until the summer of 1941 was a "uranium section" formed in the National Defense Research Committee in Washington.

The scientists, fearful always of German progress, threw a volunteer cloak of secrecy over their work. The federal government appeared less concerned. When Fermi built the first atomic pile of graphite and uranium oxide in the basement of Schermerhorn Hall at Columbia University in 1941, Pegram couldn't even persuade the government to post a guard near it. It was the end of 1941 before real government muscle was put into the effort to split the atom and fashion a weapon. Vannevar Bush, head of the Office of Scientific Research and Development, reported to President Roosevelt on progress and got a pledge of more men and money for the effort. On December 6, 1941, Bush announced the new all-out drive to his colleagues. It was not too soon. The next day Japanese carrier planes bombed Pearl Harbor in a surprise attack and the United States declared war on the Axis.

What followed on the atomic research front was an only-in-America miracle. A nation that had performed many industrial feats now undertook, in rigorous secrecy, the most prodigious scientific-industrial-military enterprise ever conceived by man. Fifteen years later many of those who played leading roles in it still could not quite believe that it really happened.

By the summer of 1942 the pace was swift. Secretary of War Stimson, the first atomic statesman, placed the Army Engineers in charge. Top secret mission: To make an atomic bomb. Code name: Manhattan Engineer District. Priority: AAA.

On September 17, 1942, Brigadier General Leslie Richard Groves, a forty-six-year-old West Point engineer who had helped build the Pentagon for thirty thousand war workers, took command of the Manhattan District. Nothing was ever quite the same afterward in Manhattan. In time Groves became almost more controversial than the bomb the physicists designed for him. "Most impressive ego since Napoleon," said an admirer. Groves lowered a curtain of secrecy, drafted industrial magnates like so many privates, harried the help, irritated the scientists, coaxed incredible sums of money from the Treasury, hired secret agents who swarmed over the project, upstaged Congress, trusted no one—and produced a weapon that changed the world forever.

Leslie Groves frequently said that he carried every detail of the coast-to-coast undertaking in his head, and few in Manhattan would dispute him. He was to the atom bomb what J. P. Morgan was to banking and what Carnegie was to steel. This was extraordinary in a military man, for the project of which he took command in 1942 was an invisible compound of equations, theory and scientific faith. It was his task to make an unknown something from almost nothing, without known tools, blueprints or materials—and to do it before the enemy did.

Manhattan's Washington headquarters in the new War Department building in Foggy Bottom was run out of a hat, or rather, out of a hat and a hat box. Groves' chief assistant was his secretary, a radiant thirty-four-year-old widow, Mrs. Jean M. O'Leary. She had landed the job by rebuking Groves for intimidating the other girls in the stenographic pool with his brusque and rapid dictation. Jean O'Leary was a blue-eyed beauty who wore her brown hair in a crownlike braid. No one knew more about Manhattan's vast operations except Groves himself, and when Groves traveled Mrs. O'Leary ran the headquarters. Some Manhattan officials called her "Jol," but many referred to her as "Colonel O'Leary" because of her importance at the atomic command post.

Groves was a large man with a trim mustache and wavy hair. When slim, he was handsome, but he had diet problems. Among the atomic secrets in his office safe, he kept a secret from Mrs. Groves—a box of forbidden chocolates. After a few months of hectic work without his usual tennis, but with the candy, he'd gain weight and add an unwarlike paunch. Then his wife would insist on the diet and he'd try to thin down again toward his West Point shape. But Groves worked a fifteen-hour day and the candy brought quick energy. He never won the waist line battle. One of the chores of an intelligence aide, Captain Fred B. Rhodes, was to make sure a two-pound box of candy was always in the safe.

The Manhattan District became the melting pot of American science. Refugees or immigrants from almost every country in Europe were in its laboratories: Fermi from Italy; Szilard, Teller, Wigner and John von Neumann from Hungary; Hans Bethe and James Franck from Germany; Bohr from Denmark; George B. Kistiakowsky from Russia. They mingled with the home-grown zealots of the new physics, such men as J. Robert Oppenheimer, brilliant son of a New York businessman; Isidore I. Rabi out of Manual Training High School in Brooklyn; James B. Conant, president of Harvard University; Ernest O. Lawrence of the University of California Radiation Laboratory; Arthur and Karl Compton, the dedicated brothers from Ohio, and Vannevar Bush of the Carnegie Institution. Ph.D.s outnumbered the clerical help in some facilities and a dozen Nobel Prize winners marched as privates in the ranks. A surprising number of the atom scientists, both American and foreign, had studied in the late twenties at the University of Göttingen in Germany. It was, said Oppenheimer later, "in a funny way an international effort."

The boyish trappings of war have always intrigued grown men —the guns, the uniforms, the parades and above all the secrets. Participating in the Manhattan District was like belonging to a national Greek letter fraternity with hidden ritual. Everyone who counted had a code name. Groves had several, including "Relief" and "99." The number came from Jean O'Leary's manner of writing "G.G." for General Groves. Some of the scientists, quite uncodesmanlike, called Groves simply "Gee Gee." Dr. Arthur Holly Compton was A. H. Comas or sometimes A. Holly. Eugene Wigner became E. Wagner. Commander Frederick L. Ashworth, a Navy atomic weaponeer, became "Scathe." Captain William S. Parsons, another Navy officer destined to arm the atomic bomb in flight, was "Judge." Niels Bohr was Nicholas Baker. Enrico Fermi was dubbed Henry Farmer for Manhattan purposes.

The first Manhattan code came from a package of cigarettes. Groves was out of town and Mrs. O'Leary had to telephone some important but secret information to him. "Go get what you always see me using," she said. She was a steady smoker. Groves got the idea, went out and bought her favorite brand. When he called back, she spelled out the message, referring to letters by their position in the words on the pack. A few days later a formal code was adopted for Groves and other officers at headquarters.

Major components of the project were referred to in the code language. The atomic work at the University of Chicago was known as the Chicago Metallurgical Laboratory. Uranium separation at Columbia University was done at "SAM," or "special alloyed materials" section. Manhattan itself was called "DSM" in the early days, for "Development of Substitute Materials." The New Mexico bomb laboratory, on a lonely mesa at Los Alamos once occupied by a boys' ranch school, was Site Y. K-25 was the huge gaseous diffusion plant at Oak Ridge, Tennessee. Y-12 was the electromagnetic plant at the same reservation. The British atomic bomb effort, which underwent somewhat truculent integration with the American program, was born in September, 1941, and known as the "Directorate of Tube Alloys." The most colorful name was assigned to the University of Chicago's early project to make plutonium. Here the first man in charge, Gregory Breit, was called by a few top echelon people "the Coordinator of Rapid Rupture."

Three years before it came into being, the bomb itself went by a variety of names: "the gadget," "the device," "the gimmick," "the thing," "the beast," "S-1" or simply "it." Later, when the probable dimensions of the weapon began to evolve, the scientists looked to President Roosevelt and Prime Minister Churchill for the source of their private language. The uranium bomb, since it was designed on the gun-barrel principle, was named the "Thin Man" after Roosevelt. The plutonium bomb would have to be the shape of a sphere inside and the bomb casing itself would therefore be wider. Thus it was called the "Fat Man" after the merry proportions of Churchill. The scientists reasoned that anyone overhearing conversations about the Thin Man and the Fat Man would conclude that it involved another Roosevelt-Churchill conference. Later, when the Thin Man's gun barrel was shortened, it became known as the "Little Boy."

Weird discussions ensued over the long-distance telephone lines of the nation. Oppenheimer was named director of the Los Alamos bomb laboratory, or Site Y, in early 1943. Groves' office was in Washington's Foggy Bottom. The two men conferred by phone frequently, sometimes as often as four or five times a day. In these conversations they used a quadratic letter code which each man carried in his wallet. They would refer to Conant, for instance, as "5-8, 3-9, 6-2, 0-9, 4-7, 8-1."

On the overcast and dreary afternoon of December 2, 1942, Fermi presided over an historic break-through of the dawning atomic age. In a squash court under the football stands of Stagg

61

Field at the University of Chicago, scientists of the youthful Manhattan District produced man's first controlled chain reaction. For the first time atomic fission was started, kept under control and stopped. It was a crude affair by today's standards, a pile of graphite laid on crossed timbers on the floor of the squash court. Blocks of uranium metal and oxide were embedded in the graphite. As the pile was built higher in layers, the neutrons increased in number. Before darkness blotted the winter skies that day the physicists knew that some day this swiftly multiplying chain reaction would be placed in a weapon of untold power.

Arthur Compton went to a phone and called Harvard's Conant in Cambridge, Massachusetts. He spoke in the code lingo of Manhattan.

"Jim," he said, "the Italian navigator has just landed in the new world. The earth was not as large as he had estimated and he arrived sooner than expected."

"Were the natives friendly?" asked Conant.

"Yes. Everyone landed safe and happy."

From the beginning the scientists grasped the essence of the problem clearly, even if they didn't know the outlines of it. "The most important answers are to unrecognized questions," said Szilard. Chain reaction occurred plentifully in a derivative of uranium metal called U-235. The trouble was that while uranium ore was available, only seven-tenths of one per cent of the ore was the precious U-235. Therefore the problem was to separate small amounts of U-235 from tons of uranium. The fact that they were chemical twins made the separation process even more difficult.

An alternative material was plutonium, a new, man-made element that also undergoes rapid fission or chain reaction.

Glenn T. Seaborg and his associates at the University of California Radiation Lab produced the first infinitesimal particle of plutonium in 1940. Plutonium could be manufactured, but first a reactor had to be built and the plutonium formed from the fission of U-235.

To produce the bomb ingredients was above all an industrial task, and soon many of the largest American companies were building enormous plants to turn out the raw materials for the bomb fabricators. The statistics were staggering. It cost $2 billion to produce less than one hundred pounds of fissionable material for the three bombs ready by the summer of 1945. After he left the White House, President Truman told the platform committee of the 1956 Democratic convention in Chicago that one of the bombs carried but thirteen pounds of fissionable material. Much of that early cost, of course, helped cut expenses later in the atomic factories and today fissionable materials are produced for about $7,000 a pound.

At the peak the Manhattan District and allied payrolls reached 539,000 persons, or enough for thirty divisions of infantry. For the Hanford Engineer Works in the state of Washington, General Groves acquired almost a thousand square miles. To build the plant—at a profit of exactly $1.00, of which only 66 cents was paid—E. I. du Pont de Nemours & Company had to sign up ten thousand subcontractors. Even after rocketing expenditures, no one could predict success with absolute confidence. One day in September, 1944, the first plutonium process was to start operation at Hanford. Granville Read, chief engineer for du Pont, had made a prior date to attend the annual rodeo at Pendleton, Oregon. A friend tried to dissuade him from leaving. "Aw," he said, "we might as well go. If the thing blows up, we can't do anything about it anyway." Read received a message at Pendleton, in code, of course, announcing that all had gone smoothly.

Hanford had troubles representative of those which plagued the rest of Manhattan. A steel mesh fence had to be placed around a women's dormitory to discourage overambitious swains. One night a male worker had a date to meet his girl friend at the fence. When she failed to appear, the frustrated lover clipped a hole in the fence with wire-cutters. Guards caught him before he entered the female barracks. At a more serious level, almost every production advance was studded with danger. Once it was feared that by-products of the fissionable material might poison the water supply. Arthur Compton discussed the problem by long-distance phone with Crawford H. Greenewalt, a du Pont chemical engineer who served as liaison man between the scientists and the production experts. Compton used Greek mythology as a vehicle for the discussion. Greenewalt not only understood, but replied in kind. Eventually the problem was licked.

To operate its gaseous diffusion plant for the separation of U-235 at Oak Ridge, the Carbide and Carbon Chemicals Corporation had to employ ten thousand people. Because not even the Nobel Prize winners knew which would be best, three different methods of separating U-235 were initiated. All were costly and all developed two new problems for every solution.

Colonel Kenneth D. Nichols, chief of production of Manhattan, got some of the offbeat jobs. In the spring of 1943 the electromagnetic separation plant under construction at Oak Ridge required a large amount of silver. Being a government man, Nichols thought of the U.S. Treasury. He called on Daniel W. Bell, Under Secretary of the Treasury.

"How much do you want?" asked Bell.

"Fifteen thousand tons," said Nichols.

"My God, man," said Bell. "You don't talk about silver in tons. You speak of it in ounces."

Nevertheless Bell wrote out a receipt and Nichols signed for fifteen thousand tons of silver. Then, using a slide rule, they tried to convert troy ounces to tons. Neither of them could do it and one of Bell's assistants had to be called in. The silver was stored in vaults at West Point, where Nichols had graduated from the U.S. Military Academy. He brought it south in a convoy of trucks to New Jersey, where the silver bars were pressed into ribbons. Then the Allis-Chalmers Manufacturing Company wound the ribbons into coils for the electromagnetic plant. Aftc the war Oak Ridge yielded its treasure back to government vaults.

Nichols figured earlier in a find more precious than silver or gold—uranium. The heavy, hard white metal was in short supply in the United States when the physicists began to accelerate their experiments. Chief source was the Belgian Congo. One day the War Department ordered Nichols to have a talk with Thomas K. Finletter, special assistant to the Secretary of State. Finletter said a man named Edgar Sengier in New York had notified him he had twelve hundred tons of uranium in case the government wanted it. Finletter had no idea what could be done with that much uranium, but the metal was scarce and the war industries seemed to want everything that came out of the ground. Nichols thanked him and took the train to New York.

Sengier, managing director of the Union Minière du Haut-Katanga, greeted him with a knowing smile at the company's New York office. When the Germans overran Belgium, Sengier rerouted a Congo shipment of uranium to New York, locked it in a warehouse and notified the U.S. Government. He waited many months, then sent another reminder to the government.

Neither Nichols nor Sengier mentioned the words "atomic" or "radioactivity," but both understood the purpose of the visit. Sengier asked only three questions: "Are you from the Army? Can I see your credentials? Is this for military purposes?" Assured on all counts, Sengier offered the shipment at $1.35 a pound, an extremely reasonable price, considering that 65 per cent of the bulk was uranium ore. (Later the government paid as much as $8 a pound for ore of a lower grade.) The two men signed an agreement on a yellow slip of paper which was converted into official typewritten copies only after Nichols returned to Washington. The whole transaction took half an hour. In the months and years that followed, about two dozen uranium-laden ships crossed the Atlantic; one was lost to a Nazi torpedo.

The theory of the bomb was developed long before the means of making it. It was quite simple for the physicists to calculate the theoretical total energy release from a pound of bomb material. One pound equals about nine thousand tons of TNT. However, there were two stubborn practical problems. First, a single pound of U-235, about the size of a golf ball, was too small to sustain a chain reaction. There had to be a certain amount, the "critical mass," before an explosion could develop. Moreover, the physicists had to keep the material separated enough so it was noncritical until the exact moment for firing. This led to the idea of a target piece of U-235 and a projectile chunk which would be rammed into the target at great speed. There was a second problem. Assuming they could fire the projectile properly, they knew the split-second process still could not be 100 per cent efficient. At best, only a fraction of the atoms would undergo fission. The rest would fly off into space unsplit. If only one out of ten split, then a single pound would yield nine hundred tons TNT equivalent instead of nine thousand tons. All this left many elusive answers. How large was the critical mass? What kind of housing material or "tamper" could be used to keep the atoms from skittering off into space? How could the pieces of U-235 be positioned and then forced together inside a bomb casing that would fit in an airplane? How could the bomb be planned with safety to the users of the weapon when the duration of the explosion was calculated to be less than one-millionth of a second?

Groves, Oppenheimer and Nichols decided to build a bomb laboratory to find the answers to these questions. They reached agreement on it as they rode in a compartment of the Twentieth Century Limited between New York and Chicago one night in the fall of 1942. A site committee selected an isolated mesa in New Mexico and laboratories of the nation were stripped to equip the Los Alamos research plant. Scientists at the remote station "twisted the dragon's tail," as they called it, by pushing two pieces of uranium toward each other with screwdrivers until the first fierce chain reaction began. Danger stood at the fingertips, not only in the laboratories, but in the plants. "The manufacture of fissionable materials," said Bush, "is by long odds the most dangerous manufacturing process in which men have ever engaged. The process is accompanied by the production of radioactive by-products as poisonous as the basic material itself."

Behind the secrecy barrier of Manhattan, some of the very scientists who had adopted a code of voluntary censorship in 1940 grew restive under the rigid compartmentalization and security imposed by Groves. Collaborators of years' standing in nuclear research couldn't find out what their associates were doing. Sometimes it was like "swimming in molasses," said Harold C. Urey, director of the SAM project at Columbia. Inside the barriers learned men began bootlegging information to one another behind Groves' back. They rebelled by nature against the security belt fastened on them and resented the roadblocks to personal movements.

Groves supervised some compartments personally outside the chain of command. Luis W. Alvarez, son of the Mayo Clinic physician who later wrote a syndicated health column, worked for a while on a special aspect of the bomb problem at the Chicago Metallurgical Laboratory. Groves would telephone Alvarez between trains in Chicago and the two men would sit on a terminal waiting room bench while Alvarez gave a whispered report.

Secrecy was most rigid at Los Alamos. There mail was censored, outgoing phone calls monitored and outside trips permitted only by special authorization. Plain-clothes security agents worked as desk clerks in the hotels of nearby Santa Fe. All incoming mail had to be addressed care of "Army Service Force, United States Engineer Office, P.O. Box 1539, Santa Fe, New Mexico." At this address counterintelligence officers opened the mail on a spot-check basis. Once located on the isolated mesa, the family of a scientist or official could not leave. Babies were born without relatives outside knowing of their whereabouts. When one wife came down with pneumonia as her husband was being shipped overseas, she had to be treated on the base with no visits from her parents. When the scientists traveled, some of them were shadowed from city to city by security operatives who sent secret reports to Manhattan headquarters. Hidden microphones caught certain conversations for tape recorders. Scientists had to lie about their place of work when away from Los Alamos.

The main objective was to prevent news of atomic progress

from filtering overseas to the Germans and the Japanese. The Japanese got intelligence reports of the American atomic effort in 1944, but details were meager and the Imperial high command paid little attention. Tokyo war office records show that military strategists questioned Japanese scientists about chances of America developing a new weapon and were told that it would be 1947 to 1949 before the United States could perfect a usable atomic bomb. With that answer, the Japanese military ceased to worry about the American physicists.

Although the Germans had less success in penetrating Manhattan secrets, the fear was always there. Incidents which were laughable later caused alarm at the time. As a sample, one night after late work in Manhattan's Washington headquarters, Mrs. O'Leary went to her car in the parking lot. She saw a man in the front seat, apparently prying at something on the dashboard. She screamed. William A. Consodine, a Newark lawyer and a top assistant to Groves, happened to be entering the lot. He ran over and the intruder fled. When police picked up the man later, he turned out to be a private enterprise thief, not a spy. The Germans, in fact, never learned much of anything about Manhattan.

Americans likewise knew little about German atomic progress until an intelligence mission followed Allied armies into Europe in 1944. Colonel Boris T. Pash, son of a Russian Orthodox bishop in San Francisco, and physicist Goudsmit headed this secret operation which functioned under the code name "Alsos," a translation of the word "Groves" into Greek. They found that the Germans were at least two years behind the Allies and had no hope of producing an atomic bomb during the war. This news was in the hands of U.S. military chiefs a good six months before the final capitulation of Germany in May, 1945.

Groves' security measures had a secondary objective: to prevent secrets from reaching the Soviet Union. This effort was far less successful. Although Communist Russia and the United States were allies against Germany, American leaders viewed Stalin's dictatorship with profound distrust. The Soviet Union masked its military operations and weapons in a manner that frustrated and angered other allies. Furthermore, the U.S. Communist Party was determined to overthrow the American system and supplant it with Communism. Despite herculean efforts to thwart Russian espionage in the Manhattan project, Stalin's agents did get important bomb information. David Greenglass provided the Soviet intelligence network with a rough drawing of the explosive mechanism of the plutonium weapon. Colonel John Lansdale, Jr., a Harvard Law School graduate and top security officer for the atomic bomb, termed the failure to intercept Greenglass "the outstanding blunder of the century." Later Klaus Fuchs, an introverted, mousy British scientist working at Los Alamos, divulged the principle of atomic bomb research to the Russian spy system and served a postwar term in a British prison as a result.

Groves permitted employment in the Manhattan District of some scientists suspected of association with Communist Party members, but kept them under constant surveillance. He viewed such employment as a calculated risk, always weighing the man's knowledge against the dangers of his political ties. In no case was this better illustrated than in the case of Oppenheimer himself.

Oppenheimer was the logical choice to head the Los Alamos laboratory. Not only was he a brilliant exponent of the new physics, but he possessed an executive talent, rare in a scientist, which inspired men to follow him with zeal and devotion. Tall, rangy and thin, he owned an intellect which combined the capacity for administrative detail with the vision and curiosity of an Einstein. Politically he was as naïve as a prep-school radical. No two men could have been more unlike than Oppenheimer and Groves, yet they worked well together as a team.

When Groves appointed Oppenheimer scientific director of Los Alamos early in 1943, he knew that Oppenheimer had been friendly, even intimate, with a number of Communists. Oppenheimer was married to a former Communist. His brother and sister-in-law had been Communists. Another woman member of the Communist Party had been in love with him. He had contributed to Communist-backed causes and joined Communist-front organizations. Despite this, Groves believed Oppenheimer essential to the success of the Los Alamos project and thought him fundamentally loyal to his country. He overruled his own security office with this letter:

> War Department, Office of the Chief
> of Engineers
> Washington, July 20, 1943
>
> Subject: Julius Robert Oppenheimer
> To: The District Engineer, United States Engineer Office, Manhattan District, Station F, New York, N. Y.
>   1. In accordance with my verbal directions of July 15, it is desired that clearance be issued for the employment of Julius Robert Oppenheimer without delay, irrespective of the information which you have concerning Mr. Oppenheimer. He is absolutely essential to the project.
>
> L. R. GROVES
> Brigadier General, CE

But the security agents weren't satisfied. Investigation of Oppenheimer was intensified. Agents tailed him. On September 6,

1943, Colonel Pash reported that "this office is still of the opinion that Oppenheimer is not to be fully trusted and that his loyalty to a Nation is divided. It is believed that the only undivided loyalty that he can give is to science. . . ." On September 12 Lansdale quizzed Oppenheimer in Groves' office. A concealed microphone recorded the conversation and Mrs. O'Leary typed it for the record.

Groves and Oppenheimer discussed the matter later in the month on a train ride from Cheyenne to Chicago. Oppenheimer told the general he had never been a member of the Communist Party, but probably had belonged to every Communist-front organization on the West Coast. Whether he said this jokingly later became a matter of dispute. At any rate, Groves kept Oppenheimer on the job and two years later this strange pair traded congratulations on producing the bomb.

Outside the tight confines of the Manhattan District, few Americans had a hint of the revolution in warfare taking place in their midst. The press operated under a system of voluntary censorship under guidance of the Office of Censorship in Washington. One day in June, 1943, Major General George Strong, Army intelligence chief, called on N. R. Howard, a Cleveland *News* editor on leave to work at the censorship office. He briefed Howard on the atomic weapon research, then asked how news of atomic installations could be kept out of the papers. Howard suggested an advisory memo to the nation's editors.

"How many would we have to tell?" asked Strong.

"Oh, about twenty-five thousand," replied Howard.

The general was stunned. At that moment, the secret was shared by only about 2 per cent of that number of people. As a compromise, newspapers were requested to omit news of experiments involving any one of nine elements. One was uranium. The other eight didn't matter.

Even at the highest policy level the "need to know" rule applied. Roosevelt's last Vice President, Harry Truman, was kept in the dark. Only three officers in the big war plans section of the War Department knew of Manhattan. Secretary of State Edward R. Stettinius, Jr., had been in office for months before he heard of Manhattan. General Douglas MacArthur, Pacific Army commander, was informed of atomic plans only five days before the first bomb fell. General Dwight D. Eisenhower, the supreme commander in Europe, got his atomic news by word of mouth only and then in sketchy form with admonitions of silence. Some of those privy to the secret regarded the potential weapon with disinterest and even skepticism. No less a person than Fleet Admiral William D. Leahy, chief of staff to Presidents Roosevelt and Truman, talked of Manhattan as a project in which he placed "no confidence." A month before Roosevelt's death, at a time when use of the weapon in war was only five months away, a close adviser warned the President that rumors of extravagance in the Manhattan project had reached him and that it appeared Roosevelt had been "sold a lemon" by Bush and Conant. Secretary Stimson had to review the recent advances with the President to ease his mind.

A Michigan Republican congressman, Albert J. Engel, once told Willard Edwards, a Chicago *Tribune* correspondent, that $2 billion was being washed down the drain in another instance of New Deal boondoggling. The newsman was engrossed in more immediate war news and did not press an investigation. At Oak Ridge a construction worker kept his eye on a smoke stack used as a vent for invisible radioactive waste. One day he quit.

"I'm going back to Knoxville," he told his superior. "Nothing ever comes out of that stack or anywhere else in this place. What a way to fight a war!"

Only a few congressional leaders knew. For the first several years, financing was completely hidden. When money was needed, Stimson diverted it from some other military appropriation. In 1944 Manhattan grew so large and its appetite for cash so keen that Stimson was forced to request specific appropriations from Congress. In February he, General Marshall and Bush went to Capitol Hill and divulged the secret to House Speaker Sam Rayburn, Democratic Floor Leader John W. McCormack and Republican Leader Joseph W. Martin, Jr. Later in the year Stimson took his case to top Senate leaders, including Democratic Leader Alben W. Barkley and Republican Styles Bridges. The congressional chiefs guided the money bills through the House and Senate without discussion. Not until May, 1945, two months before the first test of an atomic weapon, did Groves guide a party of ranking congressmen through Oak Ridge. Stimson once choked off an investigation of Manhattan by the Senate War Investigating Committee headed by Senator Truman. Stimson called on Truman after learning members of the committee staff had wind of the Manhattan project. The Secretary of War was then seventy-six years old and regarded as the most dedicated man in the cabinet. With his trim mustache, gray bangs hanging over his forehead and grave demeanor, he was the epitome of old-fashioned integrity. Truman listened respectfully.

"I can't tell you what it is," said Stimson, "but it's the greatest project in the history of the world." Truman called off his investigators without more ado.

Under Secretary of War Robert P. Patterson, however, became worried a bit later. One of his chores was to handle War Department funds for Manhattan. When the sum mounted toward the $2 billion mark, he dispatched his own assistant, Michael J. Madigan, a New York engineer, on a private sleuthing tour of the whole project. The degree of activity staggered Patterson and he braced himself for a full congressional inquiry should the bomb prove a dud.

Investigation in case of failure was viewed as a certainty within Manhattan. On Christmas Eve, 1944, Groves called a dozen of his top Washington aides and security men into his office. Privately this group called itself the "Society of the Stupid." Groves never swore, but when something went wrong he would run his hand through his hair and groan: "Oh, me. How could you be so stupid?" He told the gathering at this meeting that he was greatly encouraged. Things were going well and he believed a bomb of great power would be produced and ready by August 1 of the next year. But he warned this could be accomplished only through work. "If this weapon fizzles," he said, "each of you can look forward to a lifetime of testifying before congressional investigating committees." Manhattan's labors quickened from that day forward and its symbol, the turtle (he progresses only when he sticks his neck out), grew wings.

For the physicists, chemists and mathematicians, Manhattan was a tense world. Urgency and excitement frayed nerves and no clock had enough hours marked on it. Gone were the leisurely days of the university classroom. Perhaps worst of all were the fears: fear that Germany would produce a bomb first, fear that our bomb might not work and fear that, if it did, it actually might burn the whole world to a crisp.

"We were all scared to death that the Germans might get the atomic bomb before we did," said von Neumann. "Most of us hoped," said Pegram, "although we soon knew that it was a vain hope, that the bomb could not be constructed, so that no one would be able to use such a horrible weapon." Fermi, coolly scientific, figured either outcome—success or complete failure—would be a triumph in extending the frontiers of knowledge.

Once some early calculations at the Radiation Laboratory in California seemed to point to a terrifying possibility—that an exploding atomic bomb might ignite the nitrogen in the air and the hydrogen in the oceans and consume the earth. Oppenheimer made a special trip from California to the woods of northern Michigan, where Arthur Compton was vacationing, to discuss this cosmic peril with his colleague. They talked at length, then communicated a joint anxiety to others of the atomic fraternity. New calculations were ordered in a number of cities and laboratories. Fermi made some studies on atmospheric ignition that allayed the fears of his co-workers, but he conceded privately later that his figures did not embrace all technical aspects of the problem. Meanwhile Groves was already nursing along another secret project in another desert.

CHAPTER FIVE

Silver Plate

ON A FALL DAY in 1944, ten months before the solitary American weather plane appeared over Hiroshima, Brigadier General Frank A. Armstrong, Jr., of the Army Air Force, stalked into the office of Colonel Roscoe C. (Bim) Wilson in Colorado Springs. Armstrong was commander of the 315th Bomb Wing and Wilson commanded a sister wing, the 316th.

Armstrong was mad. Reports had reached him that some new Boeing B-29s under his authority, in the 393rd Bombardment Squadron at isolated Wendover Field in Utah, were being stripped of power turrets and armament. Only the twin .50-caliber machine guns in the tails of the planes remained. As a veteran of B-17 missions over Europe, including the first daylight raid on occupied France, Armstrong was beside himself.

"How do they expect to fight a war with no guns?" he demanded. "I'm going over to Wendover tomorrow. Somebody's going to catch hell."

Wilson didn't quite know what to say. For the past year he had been the personal representative in the secret Manhattan District of General Henry H. (Hap) Arnold, chief of the Army Air Force. He knew why the bombers of the 393rd were being stripped—among other things to lighten the planes and give them maximum getaway speed after releasing an atomic bomb. He commiserated with Armstrong, but otherwise held his tongue. As soon as Armstrong left, Wilson called Groves in Washington.

"General Armstrong is blowing his top," he reported. "He's heard they're stripping B-29s at Wendover and he's going over tomorrow to find out why."

"Tell him he can't go," ordered Groves.

"How am I supposed to do that?" asked Wilson. "He's a general. I'm a colonel."

"Tell him he can't go," repeated Groves. "Use the formula on him."

The "formula" had been Wilson's military credit card since Arnold named him air project officer of Manhattan in June, 1943. Arnold authorized him to divert all air equipment and men necessary to insure that any atomic bomb produced by Manhattan would be dropped on schedule on the designated target. "If you get any lip," said Arnold, "refer them to me."

After Groves hung up, Wilson went to Armstrong's office. "I can't tell you why, General," said the colonel, "but you're not permitted to go to Wendover." Armstrong was baffled. "If you don't believe me," added Wilson, "call General Arnold." The trip to Wendover was not made and it was ten months before Armstrong found out why.

Wilson began his atomic job under the code name "Silver Plate," and the title eventually became the military designation for the complicated effort of assembling fifteen hundred officers and men to drop the first A-bomb. The men were gathered into the 509th Composite Group, the only complete "do-it-yourself" unit in the Air Force. The 509th had everything it needed for combat and survival—transport, ordnance, food, maintenance and airplanes.

One of Bim Wilson's jobs for Arnold was to submit a list of the finest pilots in the Air Force, officers who not only could fly a delicate and precise mission, but who could lead men, handle administrative chores and keep their mouths shut. He combed the roster, culled personnel reports from every theater of war and handed Arnold a list of a dozen names.

Arnold picked Colonel Paul W. Tibbets, Jr., as his man. A handsome flier with wavy black hair, heavy eyebrows and somewhat sad eyes, Tibbets was twenty-nine years old at the time. Quiet, a gentleman and a pipe smoker, he was without flamboyance. He gave a reassuring impression of stability and reliability. Born in Quincy, Illinois, he spent his early boyhood in Des Moines, Iowa, then moved to Miami. He attended the University of Florida and the University of Cincinnati before going to Randolph Field as a flying cadet in 1937. During the war in Europe he was a crack bomber pilot. He had flown General Mark Clark from England to Gibraltar for his secret submarine mission preparatory to the invasion of North Africa. He had also flown General Eisenhower from England to Gibraltar to command that invasion.

In the summer of 1944 Tibbets and his co-pilot, Captain Robert A. Lewis, were test-flying B-29s at the Alamogordo Air Base in New Mexico. They were testing the new planes at thirty-eight thousand and forty thousand feet, an altitude record for four-engine bombers at the time. One day Tibbets was attending a technical briefing on phases of flight operation when he got a telephone call from Colorado Springs. It was Major General Uzal G. Ent, commander of the Second Air Force. Ent told him he had a new assignment and that he was to fly to Colorado Springs at once. The general said the job would take him overseas and that he would not return to Alamogordo.

When he arrived at Ent's office, Tibbets was taken into a side room by Colonel Lansdale. The two men had never met before, but the Manhattan security officer began asking the flier personal questions about his habits, beliefs and past. Tibbets was surprised at how much this stranger knew about him, including facts that even some of his close friends didn't know. Tibbets answered as frankly and as accurately as he could. Finally, Lansdale grinned, took him by the arm and escorted him to Ent's office.

"I'm satisfied, General," said Lansdale.

Tibbets was introduced to two men who came into the office, Navy Captain William Parsons and a civilian, Norman F. Ramsey. Deac Parsons was a tall, quiet man with a hairline that had receded halfway back on his head. A graduate of the Naval Academy, he had worked on the early proximity fuzes and tested them in Pacific battle. For the past year he had been an associate director of the Los Alamos bomb laboratory in charge of atomic bomb ballistics. Groves considered him indispensable, and long before had picked him to arm the first A-bomb in war. Ramsey was a twenty-nine-year-old Harvard physics professor, son of a West Point brigadier general. He had worked on radar and for the past year had been chief scientist of the bomb delivery group at Site Y.

For an hour the four men instructed Tibbets in the mysteries of the split atom. Ent opened the conversation with a sketch of the military hope and objective. Then Ramsey took over and gave a short history of the physicists' probings and the current state of the atomic art. It was a fascinating session for Tibbets, who felt as though he had been pulled off one pla·et and suddenly set down on another. Ent said he had selected the 393rd Squadron as the flying nucleus of the 509th Group. Tibbets was to take over the organization job and pick out a training field to his liking.

Throughout the Army Air Force about this time colored tabs began to be attached to the service records of hundreds of men. A young second lieutenant from Baltimore, Jacob Beser, pulled strings to see Major General James A. Ulio, Army adjutant general. Beser had gone through service radar schools after taking mechanical engineering at Johns Hopkins University. He wanted to go overseas, an ambition normally quickly satisfied in wartime.

"Sure," said the general. "I'll get you orders."

He called for Beser's service file, then apologized.

"I'm sorry," said Ulio. "You're flagged. I can't touch you."

Several months later Beser was at Wendover Field with the 509th Group.

Tibbets had set out in a B-29 to find the best training base. His first stop was at Wendover. He looked no further. Wendover was a barren expanse of Utah right at the Nevada state line. The broad, treeless flats and the bright skies made it ideal for big bomber operations. G.I.s of the 509th said Wendover was 125 miles from nowhere: that was the distance to Salt Lake City. The Manhattan District gave the field and its operations several code names, including "W-47" and "Kingman." Bob Hope called it "Leftover Field" when he arrived with a U.S.O. show. Bing Crosby knew it as "Tobacco Road with slot machines." Yet, save for the empty desert landscape stretching away to the horizon, it could have been any one of several hundred drab, wartime bases.

The 509th was different from the outset. Top officers were enjoined to secrecy by Tibbets without being informed what it was they weren't supposed to reveal. Enlisted men on three-day passes were warned to keep quiet. Security agents prowled the streets of Salt Lake City and reported men who talked too much. Once, two men in a group of six radar specialists suddenly were whisked out of the 509th and off to Alaska without explanation. Civilians on important business arrived continually at the base. When these atomic ordnance specialists and scientists aroused curiosity, questioners were told they were sanitary engineers. Commander Fred Ashworth, an Annapolis graduate and aviation ordnance expert, arrived at Wendover on a hot Sunday afternoon. That evening Norman Ramsey drove him to a remote part of the base. There, sitting in the front seat of the car, Ashworth learned about the atomic bomb effort. Technical shops were off limits except to a few men with special badges. Men were cautioned never to talk about their work outside the shop, not even in the barracks.

Each man was told only what he needed to know to perform his job. Major Charles W. Sweeney, a happy twenty-four-year-old pilot from Lowell, Massachusetts, checked into Wendover one night. The next morning a young intelligence officer asked Sweeney to ride out to the target area with him. They got out of the car and climbed a mesa. There, out of earshot of others, Sweeney was told he was one of the pilots selected for a top-secret mission. The word "atomic" was not mentioned, but nothing that occurred after that ever seemed peculiar to Sweeney.

Security followed 509th officers everywhere. When pilots and crews went to Inyokern Naval Test Station in California for training with new ballistic shapes, wives left at Wendover received letters with no cancellation marks, delivered by air courier from they knew not where. After the first admonitions of secrecy, most officers resisted speculation, but for those who questioned Bim Wilson had a ready answer. He thought, he said, they were practicing to drop land mines on Formosa.

When young specialists, newly graduated from radar school at Boca Raton, Florida, checked in at Wendover a few weeks later, Robert Brode, physics professor at the University of California, drove them around the base. "We're in the weapons business," he told them. "We make drops here." When the radar lieutenants were taken on trips to Los Alamos later, scientists discussed U-235 and fission with them, but never confirmed the shot-in-the-dark speculation of one of the youngsters—that an atomic bomb was in the making.

Flight operations differed from anything ever seen by airmen. Bombing practice was constant, from thirty thousand feet, with bombardiers aiming through the Norden bombsight at a five hundred-foot circle on the desert. But the bombs never fell in the ordinary clusters. Each plane dropped a single, ten thousand-pound bomb. Relentless emphasis was placed on visual bombing. This puzzled some of the bombardiers who were veterans of the air war over Europe, since a clear day for visual bombing had been rare there and was even rarer over Japan. The bombardiers wondered why the visual drop was more appreciated than the more difficult one by radar.

The reasons were clear to those initiated in Manhattan secrets. The practice with single bombs simulated the eventual atomic flight when only one precious bomb, worth hundreds of millions of dollars in production costs, would be in the bomb bay. Groves and his assistants already had decided the first atomic bomb must be dropped by visual means on a clear day. Bombing by radar could not be trusted. If results of an atomic bomb were to be accurately assessed, the bomb could not stray from its target.

Some of the pilots executed an unorthodox maneuver after dropping their dummy bombs over the Utah flats. They made sharp, 158-degree turns and nosed the planes down to gain speed. Early calculations by the scientists indicated that any plane dropping the atomic bomb should be at least eight miles away when the bomb exploded, not only to be clear of the blast but to avoid being damaged by the shock waves expected to follow. (The eight miles were measured on a straight line from the point of detonation, slanting up and away to the plane about six miles above the ground.) Tibbets had innumerable conferences on this point. Falling from thirty thousand feet, the bomb would explode about 3½ miles forward of the release point. Tibbets had been informed the A-bomb would be fuzed to explode about two thousand feet above ground for maximum blast effect and minimum radioactivity. This would give the escaping plane forty-three seconds between the moment the bomb dropped and the moment it exploded. Rolling out of the 158-degree turn, the plane would be just about eight miles from the point of explosion in that time. Tibbets and Sweeney, especially, practiced this steep, diving turn.

Some of the practice bombs dropped at Wendover, after previous secret testing at Inyokern, were called "pumpkins" by the men. They were fatter than the normal high explosive bombs then whistling down on Germany. Only Tibbets and a few scientists and weaponeers at Wendover knew the reason. What the 509th bombardiers were dropping was the shell of the "fat man," or plutonium bomb. Inside the bomb casing, blocks of plutonium were to be formed in a loose sphere, to be compressed by sixty-four detonators at the instant of "implosion." The fact that no such bomb ever had been assembled, except on the drawing boards of theoreticians at Los Alamos, made no difference. The entire Manhattan project was that way: one section was always learning to use something that another section was still not sure it would ever be able to make.

Actually the Fat Man was not shaped like a pumpkin, but like a tear drop. The bomb's forward end was bulbous, tapering away gradually to the fins. Each bomb weighed about thirteen thousand pounds and wore a casing of such highly polished metal that crew members could use it as a mirror to comb their hair. Each pumpkin drop was a lesson in ballistics. Cameras mounted in the bomb bay photographed the free fall of the Fat Man to determine just how it acted. In the Salton Sea in Southern California, ground stations took moving pictures of the drops and special equipment recorded radio data to check performance of the bomb's electronic gear. The bombs used at Wendover contained no fissionable material, of course, but they did contain the same conventional explosive charges to be used later and the fuzes were designed to duplicate those to be used on the real mission. One afternoon when Sweeney's bombardier, handsome Captain Kermit K. Beahan, pushed the toggle button, the fuze exploded the bomb prematurely beneath the plane. The B-29 lurched and rolled from the shock. Mrs. Sweeney, an Army nurse, happened to see the flash from thirty thousand feet below. After her husband landed, she questioned him. "Oh, that," lied Sweeney. "It's supposed to do that." Sweeney didn't know it at the time, but he was being groomed to fly the second atomic mission.

Tibbets knew from the beginning that if an A-bomb was ever produced, he himself would be the pilot to drop the first one. Accordingly he picked his crew with the utmost care. Lewis, his co-pilot, had helped him test B-29s in New Mexico. Lewis was a chunky, diligent twenty-seven-year-old from Ridgefield Park, New Jersey, who had played center in high-school football and taken three years of correspondence-school courses before entering the Air Force. For his atomic bombardier, Tibbets selected Major Thomas W. Ferebee of Mocksville, North Carolina, and for his navigator, Captain Theodore J. (Dutch) Van Kirk, a twenty-three-year-old from Northumberland, Pennsylvania. Both men had flown with Tibbets in Europe under fire. The flight engineer was Technical Sergeant Wyatt E. Duzenbury, whose steadiness under pressure had impressed Tibbets during B-29 test operations. Lewis served as pilot of the crew during Tibbets' frequent absences from Wendover. The bomber itself was picked with care. Tibbets tested it, calibrated it and put it through shakedown operations. No one but Tibbets and Lewis was permitted to fly it and only Duzenbury and a selected ground crew could put a wrench on it. "I pampered and babied that airplane to the fullest extent," Tibbets said later. The process was duplicated when the 509th got new airplanes early in 1945.

The 509th was different in many respects. The military police outfit had no less than ninety-three officers and men. The Composite Group had its own airline, five C-54s operated by the 320th Troop Carrier Squadron. It was nicknamed the "Green Hornet Line," after the popular blood-and-thunder radio program.

The 509th was christened officially in December, 1944, after several months of assembly, and the next month ten B-29s, led by Tibbets, flew down to Batista Field, Cuba, for practice bombing runs over the Atlantic and navigation flights to Bermuda, the Virgin Islands and Norfolk. Tibbets traveled constantly, flying from Wendover to Washington, Los Alamos, Wright Field and Inyokern. A hundred and one items had to be co-ordinated. No flight in history was ever planned with such meticulous care or so far in advance as this one to drop a bomb that hadn't been made yet. Tibbets commuted in a C-54 and kept winter and summer uniforms hanging in the plane to be ready for any climate.

On one of the trips, Tibbets took Lieutenant Beser with him. An interservice committee of generals and admirals convened in Washington to discuss the best means of getting a plane over the target with the utmost precision. Navy officers said that if the target was to be in Japan, a submarine could surface off the coast and lay down a directional radar beam for the plane to follow. The air officers rejected this, feeling confident of their own navigation. Beser, as a radar specialist, was briefed on operation of instruments to detect enemy jamming of radio wave lengths, for the bomb was to be triggered by proximity fuzes. Electronic impulses reflected from the ground would set off the mechanism at a designated altitude. Radio interference on the right wave length might thwart the explosion.

While the 509th trained at Wendover, Commander Fred Ashworth, by now a budding atomic weaponeer, was summoned to the Pentagon office of Admiral Ernest J. King, chief of Naval operations. It was time to inform certain commanders in the Pacific of the bomb. Guidelines for the availability of the new weapon had been laid down on December 30, 1944, in a memorandum from Groves to Marshall. On the same day, Secretary of War Stimson read the memo and underlined certain phrases. Then, memo in hand, Groves and Stimson went to the White House to brief President Roosevelt in one of the many war conferences he was holding in preparation for the Yalta meetings with Churchill and Stalin. Roosevelt approved the memo as Marshall had done a few hours earlier. As underlined by Stimson, it read:

War Department
Washington, Dec. 30, 1944

TOP SECRET

Subject: Atomic Fission Bombs

To: The Chief of Staff

It is now reasonably certain that our operations plans should be based on the *gun type bomb,* which, it is estimated, will produce the equivalent of a ten thousand ton TNT explosion. The first bomb, without previous full scale test, which we do not believe will be necessary, *should be ready about 1 August 1945.* The second one should be ready by the end of the year and succeeding ones at . . . intervals thereafter.

Our previous hopes that an implosion (compression) type of bomb might be developed in *the late spring* have now been dissipated by scientific difficulties which we have not as yet been able to solve. The present effects of these difficulties are that more material will be required and that the material will be less efficiently used. We *should have sufficient material for the first implosion type bomb sometime in the latter part of July.* This bomb would have an effect which would be equivalent to about *500* tons of TNT. During the remainder of 1945 it is estimated that we can produce . . . additional bombs. The effectiveness of these should increase towards 1,000 tons each as development proceeds and, if some of our problems are solved, to as much as 2,500 tons.

The plan of operations while based on the more certain more powerful gun type bomb also provides for the use of the implosion type bombs when they become fully available. The time schedule must not be adversely affected by anything other than the difficulties of solving our scientific problems. *The 509th Composite Group, 20th Air Force has been organized and it is now undergoing training* as well as assisting in essential tests.

The time has come when we should acquaint the Assistant Chief of Staff OPD and possibly one of his assistants and the Chief of Staff of the 20th Air Force, Brigadier General Lauris Norstad, with sufficient information so that the formulation of adequate plans and the necessary troop movements may be carried out without difficulty and without loss of security. It is proposed also that General Norstad, who is about to visit the Southwest Pacific, be authorized to give general information to the Deputy Commander 20th Air Force, Lt. Gen. M. F. Harmon, and limited information to the Commanding General of the 21st Bomber Command, Gen. H. S. Hansell, Jr. I also feel that it would be advisable for Admiral Nimitz to be informed of our general plans in order that we will be assured the essential Navy assistance in the area. This could best be accomplished by means of a letter from Admiral King to Admiral Nimitz to be delivered by one of the naval officers now on duty in my command.

The need for security will be emphasized to the officers whom it is proposed to alert.

I have consulted with General Arnold and he feels the above proposals are desirable.

Your approval is recommended.

L. R. GROVES
Major General, USA

The letter was interesting for its omission of MacArthur as one of those to be informed. A month later the data was embodied in a "Dear Chester" letter from Admiral King to Admiral Chester W. Nimitz, commander of the Pacific Fleet with headquarters on Guam. King handed the letter to Commander Ashworth on a day in early February. Ashworth folded it carefully and tucked it in a money belt. From Groves, Ashworth also carried instructions—to find the best spot in the Marianas for location of the 509th Group. Already the high military officers, as well as F.D.R. and Churchill, had ticketed Japan as the probable recipient of the first atomic bomb. Germany had been crossed off as a possibility. The first bomb wouldn't be ready until August and intelligence believed that the tottering Nazi regime would collapse long before that.

When Ashworth arrived at CINCPAC headquarters on Guam,

he had trouble burrowing through the layers of aides to reach the admiral. His orders required personal delivery to Nimitz and this provoked argument. Once closeted with the admiral, Ashworth had to help him with the reading, for the letter had become tattered and sweaty after a flight through tropical heat, and some of the words were blurred. Nimitz, who hadn't even heard that anyone was attempting to make an atomic bomb, was much impressed, but the August 1 date seemed far away. The Japanese were fighting tenaciously for every chunk of coral and the savage battles for Okinawa and Iwo Jima still lay before him. "This sounds fine," he said, "but this is only February. Can't we get one sooner?" Ashworth explained why that was impossible, repeating in detail the story about the difficulties with the plutonium bomb that Groves had outlined to Roosevelt.

Nimitz gagged on one section of King's letter. It ordered him to inform only one person on his staff. Nimitz named Vice Admiral C. H. McMorris, his chief of staff, as the atomic coordinator, but told Ashworth he'd have to get permission to tell another officer "to keep the wheels turning." As Ashworth was leaving, Nimitz put his hand on the shoulder of the young commander. "Son," he said, "I guess I was just born twenty years too soon."

Ashworth had carte blanche from King to pick any place in the Marianas that suited him for basing the 509th. He made a tour of the islands that were in American hands. Although Guam was the best developed, with superior port facilities, he picked the island of Tinian. It was several miles closer to central Japan than Guam and, being a small island, was more adaptable to secrecy of operations. More important, four-runway North Field was being built as the biggest bomber base in the world. Ashworth picked a site bordering North Field and spotted locations for three bomb assembly huts, prototypes of which already had been constructed and tested at Inyokern.

Tinian is a limestone ocean platform with high, pock-marked walls, about six miles wide in the middle and thirteen miles long, tapering to points at the north and south ends. Although its bluffs rise sharply from the sea, it is a level island. The highest point, Mount Lasso, is only 564 feet above sea level. It made an ideal anchored aircraft carrier. Shaped roughly like Manhattan Island in New York, Tinian had a network of good roads built by the Japanese. When the Americans landed, the roads were quickly named for Madison Avenue, Forty-second Street and other canyons of New York City. G.I.s fresh from the States called Tinian "The Rock," but veterans of Pacific fighting thought it a lush, pleasant haven with refreshing breezes.

The 509th village was built under the direction of Colonel Elmer E. Kirkpatrick next to North Field, where bombers stood almost wing tip to wing tip on their coral hardstands. Quonset huts, tents on wooden frames, skeleton hangars with canvas slung over the top for roofs, bomb assembly huts, a wooden mess hall and an outdoor movie theater, "Pumpkin Playhouse," comprised the town.

On April 5 the War Department operations section approved the code name CENTERBOARD for the actual mission of delivering the atomic bomb on Japan, but so secret was the project that the officer in charge of assigning code names was not even told what it was for.

The 509th began moving overseas late that month from Wendover Field. At the time, Germany was crumbling in flames on one flank of the Axis, but on the other American troops were fighting yard by yard for the island of Okinawa. Tibbets' pilots now had a full complement of fifteen B-29 bombers, all stripped of armament to give utmost speed at altitude and a fast getaway after bomb release. The huge Boeing Superfortress program had been born on paper in November, 1939, with production under way since 1943. The plane had a wing span of 141 feet, stood 28 feet high and was 99 feet long. It was driven by four 2,200 horsepower engines. Normal arms missing from Tibbets' planes included ten .50-caliber machine guns and a .20-millimeter cannon. Only protection remaining in the Silver Plate planes: two .50-caliber machine guns in the tail. Since February the 509th had been flying the latest B-29 model with fuel injection engines, the first electric reversible pitch propellers and pneumatic bomb bays on which were painted warnings: "Danger—Air Operated Door."

In the spring a new unit of two hundred men had been added to the 509th after intense, selective recruiting by Commander Ashworth. It was the 1st Ordnance Squadron (Special Aviation), most secret component of the group. Commanded by Major Charles F. H. Begg, the 1st Ordnance made security its byword. The men who were to handle the atomic bomb were subjected to a special loyalty check, then informed the duty might be hazardous in the extreme. A man would be expected to volunteer his life if necessary. No man was allowed to reveal his job either to his family or to other members of the 509th. First Ordnance men were not permitted to converse with one another outside the restricted work area. When the group traveled, 1st Ordnance was separated from the other units and accompanied by military intelligence officers. Once, on a railroad diner, no other passengers were allowed in the car until 1st Ordnance men finished eating. One of their number, First Lieutenant Morris R. Jeppson, was destined to help arm the first atomic bomb in flight.

As the 509th packed to leave Utah, another group at Los Alamos in New Mexico received overseas physical examinations and shots from Colonel James F. Nolan, physician and radiology officer at the bomb laboratory. These men were physicists, chemists, mathematicians and engineers who were to join the 509th as the 1st Technical Service Detachment, War Department Miscellaneous Group, at "Project A," as Tinian was dubbed at Los Alamos. In short, they were the scientists who were to put the bomb together and measure its performance overseas. In May, just before leaving, many of the Los Alamos scientists took part in a test shot of one hundred tons of TNT at Alamogordo Air Base. The purpose was to calibrate instruments and coordinate safety measures for the proposed test of the plutonium bomb, history's first atomic explosion, two months later.

The first section of the 509th landed at Tinian in Green Hornet C-54s on May 18 and each day thereafter added a few more men. Most of the group came by ship, debarking from the S.S. *Cape Victory* in Tinian harbor on May 29. The 1st Ordnance Squadron came in June, followed by the Los Alamos scientists.

Almost at once the 509th became the island curiosity. Tokyo Rose, punctual if not fully enlightened, greeted its arrival by radio from Japan, but that was the last official news the other B-29 crews had of this strange outfit. Its planes bore different markings: a huge black circle bisected by a black arrow on the tail section. Scientists (average age: twenty-seven) ornamented the group and played three dimensional tick-tack-toe in their heads. It was even rumored that when one scientist asked another if he'd like to play chess, the second replied: "With a board?" G.I.s of the 509th kept their distance from the youthful civilians, referring to them as "odd balls" or "long hairs."

The military police company promptly strung barbed-wire fences around certain areas and placed sand-bagged machine gun emplacements at strategic corners. To get into the restricted area, even a general had to show a pass, be convoyed to a second guard post and wait there until an escort came who knew him. Manhattan security agents, headed by Major William L. (Bud) Uanna, a Tufts College engineering graduate and Suffolk University law graduate, swarmed over the island. They were tagged erroneously as "F.B.I. men" by other outfits on Tinian. The Federal Bureau of Investigation never had a finger in Manhattan District operations, a fact Director J. Edgar Hoover emphasized with unrestrained vigor when it was discovered later that Russian spies had penetrated the bomb project. There were no Russian agents on Tinian, but there were Japanese prisoners and thousands of curious Americans. Uanna's men checked every stranger entering the 509th area.

It was chiefly the flying of the 509th that raised eyebrows among the other B-29 crews. Never did Tibbets and his men participate in the mass raids on the empire, nor did they ever share the sight of empty bunks at night after a raid. Instead they flew solo missions, occasionally bombing a Jap-held island and later making the round trip of almost three thousand miles to Japanese cities just to drop one bomb each—or so the rumor ran in Wing headquarters. Soon the elite and privileged status of the 509th became the standard gripe of the Twentieth Air Force in the Marianas. The muse captured an anonymous clerk at base operations:

> Into the air the secret rose
> Where they're going, nobody knows.
> Tomorrow they'll return again,
> But we'll never know where they've been.
> Don't ask us about results or such,
> Unless you want to get in Dutch.
> But take it from one who is sure of the score,
> The 509th is winning the war.

CHAPTER SIX

Decision for CENTERBOARD

TEN THOUSAND MILES from the coral outpost of Tinian Island, heat waves shimmered off the tops of thousands of car-pool automobiles outside the Pentagon in Washington, D.C. The time was late July, 1945, and the high officers at a meeting inside the world's largest office building were grateful for the air-conditioning, rare in Washington that summer.

General Carl Spaatz wasn't yielding an inch. Spaatz at leisure was a companionable soul, who listed bird-watching among his gentle pursuits, but as a military officer, he could be a gruff, stubborn Pennsylvania Dutchman. He had recently arrived from his headquarters in Europe and was anxious to shed Washington's paperwork war and be off to the Pacific, where he would command the Strategic Air Force. Besides, he didn't like the proposition he faced.

"Listen, Tom," he said, "if I'm going to kill 100,000 people, I'm not going to do it on verbal orders. I want a piece of paper."

General Thomas T. Handy, acting chief of staff of the U.S. Army, sympathized with Spaatz, but Handy, a Virginian with a drawl as wide as that of a Texan, had his job to do. The top brass, including his own immediate superior and fellow Virginia Military Institute graduate, General George C. Marshall, were in Potsdam, Germany, at the TERMINAL conference with the British and the Russians. This was no attempt to shift responsibility, Handy argued. It was just the normal Manhattan District procedure. The less in writing, the less chance of breaking security. Spaatz conceded this, but stood firm. Anything could happen with a weapon of such strange immensity.

"I guess I agree, Tooey," said Handy at last. "If a fellow thinks he might blow up the whole end of Japan, he ought to have a piece of paper."

The decision—to drop atomic bombs on Japan—that Spaatz and others then formalized by the written word had been months in the making. It was, of course, a decision of President Harry S. Truman, the commander in chief of the armed forces, but before a proposal became a decision many men wrestled soulfully with the idea of unleashing on human beings the elemental forces of the sun itself.

In the first years in Manhattan District there had been broad acceptance of the view that the bomb, if and when perfected, would be used against the enemy. Some physicists hoped the research would prove futile and one so confided to Admiral Leahy, the President's chief of staff. But most sided with President Roosevelt, who once said: "Pray God it works. It will save many American lives."

As early as August, 1943, when the atomic complex was still more blueprint than factory, Roosevelt and Churchill at the QUADRANT conference at Quebec agreed "that we will not use" an atomic weapon "against third parties without each other's consent." A year later at Hyde Park the two war leaders approved an *aide-mémoire* on Anglo-American atomic co-operation and initialed it on September 18, 1944.

"When a 'bomb' is finally available," the paper declared, "it might perhaps, after mature consideration, be used against the Japanese, who should be warned that this bombardment will be repeated until they surrender."

The apparent assumption of the two men that the bomb would be developed too late to use against Germany could be seen on the war maps of Europe. Germany was reeling back from the bastions of Fortress Europe before Eisenhower's armies, which had poured across the littered Channel beaches in June of that year. The end seemed only a matter of months. The intelligence mission, ALSOS, revealed to the Allies that Germany had no chance of making an atomic bomb before war's end. The fear of the refugee scientists that Hitler might use an atomic weapon to exterminate whole peoples had faded.

A few men began to change their minds about Allied use of an atomic bomb. In October, 1944, Groves briefed Admiral Leahy on the bomb that was still nine months away from completion. From then on Leahy had two distinct feelings about atomic weapons. First, he had scant faith they would work. Second, assuming they did, the prospect of employing them repelled him. Never in his official capacity as the top military officer of his country did Leahy ever argue against using the bomb, perhaps because he believed his task was to assay purely military, not ethical, problems. As an individual, however, he made no effort to mask his feelings.

In the winter of 1944-45, many of the atom scientists, particularly at the Metallurgical Laboratory at Chicago, began discussions on the atomic future which they now believed would be realized. The talks went forward in seminars and committees.

Most of the thought revolved around international sharing and control of the atom after the war and the prevention of an arms race. Discussion was stimulated by two formal committees on the subject, one headed by Zay Jeffries of the General Electric Company and the other by Richard C. Tolman, former graduate dean of the California Institute of Technology. From these discussions of the future, some scientists began to question use of the bomb in the present. Arthur Compton, director of the Metallurgical Project, heard of these qualms early in 1945.

Secretary of War Stimson took news of the scientists' debate to President Roosevelt at the White House on March 15, 1945. It was the last meeting of the grizzled old philosopher-warrior and the four-term President, for Roosevelt was about to leave for Warm Springs, Georgia, where he died a month later of cerebral hemorrhage. Stimson said that apparently one group of scientists wanted to withhold use of the bomb and keep it secret after the war, while another group sought international control and a free flow of atomic information.

In March, as the 9th Armored Division led the American thrust across the Rhine toward the heart of Germany, Japan began to be subjected to the mass bombardment of civilians which had been a commonplace in World War II ever since German bombers razed Rotterdam. On the night of March 9, sixteen square miles of Tokyo were set ablaze by the B-29s of General Curtis LeMay's bomber command. Two thousand tons of incendiary bombs, dropped from as low as five thousand feet, fired the city as though it were a forest in the American West. Planes careened upward on the fierce drafts of heat. Seventy-eight thousand Japanese were killed. With such obliteration of cities an accepted mode of warfare on both sides, it was difficult for most military chieftains to believe that a new weapon of destruction presented ethical questions not found in TNT and the fire bomb.

But the raiding bomber was not the laboratory. This same month Leo Szilard, the Hungarian physicist who first helped prevail on President Roosevelt to undertake atomic weapons research, wrote a memorandum which urged international control of atomic energy and pointed out that the United States was vulnerable to future A-bomb attack because of its huge metropolitan areas. While Szilard did not specifically oppose use of the bomb on Japan, the paper's tone tended to question the wisdom of initiating atomic warfare. Einstein sent a letter to Roosevelt, requesting him to let Szilard present these "considerations and recommendations." The letter arrived too late. It was in Roosevelt's office in Warm Springs when he died.

Niels Bohr, the refugee Danish physicist, also wrote a memo on the subject for Roosevelt late in March. At the Chicago laboratory, some scientists now spoke up, opposing use of the bomb against Japan, and Compton informed both Stimson and Groves of the varying views in the research halls. None of this, of course, reached the ears of the public or even of the thousands of workers in the Manhattan project. Only a few hundred men knew enough about the atomic bomb that hadn't been made yet to argue about it.

Harry Truman got his first inkling of the decision that would be his only an hour after becoming President of the United States on the night of April 12. He took the oath at 7:09 P.M. and held a brief cabinet meeting to assume the responsibility of office. As the Roosevelt cabinet members filed silently out, Stimson remained behind. He told the new President that the government he now headed was developing a weapon of enormous power. He provided no details. The next day, James F. Byrnes called on the President in the unaccustomed role of private citizen. Truman had summoned this many-officed man from Spartanburg, South Carolina, to offer him the post of Secretary of State. Byrnes told the President more of the awful force of the proposed bomb, but not until Vannevar Bush called a few days later did Truman get an extensive scientific explanation. Admiral Leahy, serving Truman as he had Roosevelt as chief of staff, immediately restaked his claim as the leading unbeliever. He told Truman after both listened to Bush that the bomb was a "fool thing" that would never go off.

In late April, statesmen of the allied world gathered in San Francisco to form the United Nations. Some scientists voiced concern that few of these political leaders were aware that the world they sought to remake was about to change forever. The conference was to open April 25. How could statesmen plan the world of tomorrow while ignorant of the enormous energy about to burst loose from the atom? This question propelled James Franck, a Nobel Prize physicist and refugee from Nazi Germany, to write a memorandum warning of the dangers the bomb held for mankind. Together with Compton, he called on Secretary of Commerce Henry A. Wallace in Washington, breakfasted with him and left the paper.

On the day the San Francisco conference opened, Stimson and Groves conferred at length with Truman on the bomb. Stimson, the intellectual of the cabinet and one of the wisest men in the whole war effort, had written a lengthy report. With the power of the atom unlocked in a weapon, as he assured the President it soon would be, Stimson pictured the world at the "mercy" of the atomic bomb unless steps were taken to control it. As for the war in the Pacific, Stimson said the bomb would enable the allies to dictate their own terms to Japan.

"Within four months," said Stimson in the paper, "we shall in all probability have completed the most terrible weapon ever known to human history, one bomb of which would destroy a city."

From that moment there was no doubt in Harry Truman's mind about the magnitude of his decision. Stimson's use of the phrase "within four months" was not guesswork. On December 30 Groves had predicted a uranium bomb would be ready August 1 and the huge Manhattan complex was adhering miraculously to the timetable.

Stimson urged President Truman to appoint a committee to advise him on atomic policy. The President assented and asked Stimson to get it under way. The panel constituted a few days later was called simply the Interim Committee. No group of men had more to do with Truman's decision to use the atomic bomb and no group did more to pave the way for postwar peaceful use of atomic energy and the prolonged effort of the United States to place atomic weapons under international control. Members of the committee were:

Secretary Stimson, chairman; George L. Harrison, president of the New York Life Insurance Company, assistant chairman; Byrnes, personal representative of President Truman on the committee and soon to be Secretary of State; Ralph A. Bard, Under Secretary of the Navy; William L. Clayton, Assistant Secretary of State; Vannevar Bush, director of the Office of Scientific Research and Development and president of the Carnegie Institution; Karl T. Compton, chief of the OSRD field office and president of the Massachusetts Institute of Technology; James B. Conant, chairman of the National Research Council and president of Harvard University.

Stimson named a scientific advisory panel composed of Arthur

Compton; Enrico Fermi, who managed the first controlled chain reaction at Stagg Field; Ernest O. Lawrence, head of the Berkeley Radiation Laboratory, and J. Robert Oppenheimer, director of the Los Alamos bomb laboratory.

Before the committee sessions began, Byrnes had a visit from three scientists at his home in Spartanburg. President Truman had forwarded to Byrnes the Einstein letter found in Roosevelt's office which introduced Szilard. While Szilard preferred to see Truman, the White House had referred him to Byrnes. Szilard went to Spartanburg accompanied by Walter Bartky, associate dean of physical sciences at the University of Chicago, and Harold Urey of Manhattan's SAM project at Columbia University.

Szilard and Byrnes did not hit it off, to put it mildly. Byrnes felt that Szilard was too aggressive and too critical of the cabinet. He got the impression that Szilard wanted the atom scientists to share government policy-making with the President and his cabinet. For his part, Szilard thought Byrnes failed to grasp the significance and potential of atomic energy. Byrnes got along better with Bartky and Urey and the session ended amicably enough with a general discussion of the atom. Szilard left a memorandum and a bad impression with Byrnes.

One of Groves' security agents had followed the three scientists to Spartanburg and Groves told Byrnes in Washington the next week that the agent had kept track of Szilard after the meeting. This was routine throughout the Manhattan District when key persons left reservation or laboratory, but it did nothing to endear Groves to the scientists.

The Interim Committee met in Washington May 31. Marshall and Groves sat in with the eight-man committee and its four-man technical panel. Chairman Stimson launched the meeting on a solemn note. He stated, simply but eloquently, the awesome nature of nuclear power and declared it was the committee's function to recommend action that might turn the course of civilization. He stressed that a prime consideration was how America's use of the revolutionary weapon would appear in the long march of history. Nuclear energy, he said, might mean the doom of civilization or its perfection. It might be a "Frankenstein which would eat us up" or it might be the means by which "the peace of the world would be helped in becoming secure." Most of the committee's deliberations concerned the postwar future of atomic energy and control, how and when the development should be announced to the public, the status of the bomb as of that day and whether fission facts should be revealed to the Russians.

The question of the bomb's use against Japan consumed less time, but discussion was vigorous. The doubts of some Chicago scientists were known to the committee. General Marshall tentatively questioned whether use of the bomb could be avoided. Could it be kept secret, thus concealing America's defense hand in the future? Scientists on the panel replied that too many men all over the world knew too much about the prewar experiments. Sooner or later the full secret would be discovered in other countries.

Oppenheimer forecast the shape and size of the bomb's destruction. He said that if exploded above ground it would be devastating to troops and war facilities. He predicted it might kill twenty thousand people, assuming that air-raid shelters were being used.

At the luncheon table Arthur Compton raised the possibility of a bomb demonstration before foreign observers. Talk went around the table. Would an international show persuade the

Japanese war lords to surrender? This was the "gut" question, and the more answers the committee sought, the more questions arose. What if the bomb proved to be a dud? What if the Japanese refused to send representatives? If the Japanese refused to quit after witnessing or hearing about the demonstration shot, wouldn't the chances multiply of having the atomic bomber shot down? Wouldn't any miscalculation in the complicated delivery and explosion of the bomb reinforce Japanese determination to fight to the end?

Another suggestion offered was to warn the Japanese explicitly of the murderous scope of the new bomb and then drop it only if surrender was not forthcoming within a stated number of days. What if Japan retaliated by moving Allied prisoners of war into key areas, then daring the United States to go ahead? Even if this didn't occur, wouldn't all the shock value be lost and fighters be sent aloft to intercept the atomic mission? No matter what the suggestion, the committee members felt that it gambled with the lives of thousands of American men already being staged on Pacific islands for the assault on Japanese shores. At this moment, American soldiers and Marines had been fighting bitterly for two months on Okinawa and it would be another month before the last Japanese resistance was quelled at a cost of forty-one thousand American casualties. The fanaticism of Japanese *kamikaze* pilots, who crashed bomb-laden planes into U. S. invasion ships off Okinawa, had made a deep impression on the American public. Would the nation look kindly on "invitations" and "warnings" to Nippon's militarists?

In the end all questions seemed to merge into a larger one— would the atomic bomb have a good chance of ending the war quickly and saving American lives? The answer to that appeared to be yes, but on the slim possibility that some type of demonstration could be arranged that would save both American and Japanese lives, the scientific panel was asked to prepare a report on the feasibility of an atomic bomb exhibition.

The committee then prepared its report. On the issue of the bomb's use, the White House received a unanimous recommendation that the bomb be dropped on Japan as soon as possible, without specific warning, and that it be delivered on a dual target comprising a military installation and surrounding houses and buildings susceptible to maximum blast damage. Implicit in this last point was the realization that many civilians would be killed.

Byrnes, as Truman's representative, reported the recommendation to President Truman on the afternoon of June 1, going directly to the White House from the Interim Committee session. After listening to Byrnes' account, Truman said that he had been thinking about the problem and had reached the same conclusion. Much as he regretted it, he told Byrnes, he must order the bomb used.

From the hour that President Truman voiced this tentative decision to use the bomb against the Japanese unless they surrendered first, government machinery moved swiftly toward the final assembly and delivery of the weapon.

Intelligence officers in the Pentagon began work on target charts. The choice was limited. MATTERHORN, the sustained bombing campaign against Japan, had reduced hundreds of square miles of metropolitan Japan to rubble. The atomic bomb, to make the maximum imprint, should explode over a relatively untouched city, the planners decided. Stimson confided to his diary that he was alarmed at the extent of conventional bombing, fearing the "S-1," code name for the A-bomb, would not have a fair background against which to show its strength. Groves and

Arnold conferred on the target list. Oppenheimer was consulted at Los Alamos. LeMay on Guam was asked for his selections and he radioed back: Kyoto, Hiroshima and Niigata in that order.

On the night of June 4 Byrnes went to Leahy's home to give him a report on the Interim Committee's work. They talked far into the night, Byrnes trying to convince the old Navy ordnance officer of the frightful power about to be unleashed by the A-bomb. Leahy was not persuaded. It wouldn't work, he said.

On that same day, at the Metallurgical Lab in Chicago, seven atomic scientists met under the chairmanship of Franck in search of a method to prevent use of the bomb against Japan. The other members were Donald Hughes, J. J. Nickson, Eugene Rabinowitch, Glenn Seaborg, Joyce Stearns and Leo Szilard. They conferred on and off for a week to prepare a document that might have impact at the White House.

While the Franck group met, the official scientific panel of the Interim Committee gathered at Los Alamos on the weekend of June 9-10 to carry out its instructions. Was a demonstration of the bomb feasible? All four members of the panel—Arthur Compton, Oppenheimer, Fermi and Lawrence—put their minds to the questions. Opinion was divided at the outset. They discussed the doubts of their colleagues. Lawrence pressed hardest for explosion of the bomb before international observers. Many locations were suggested: desert islands, New Mexico, even a sparsely inhabited area of Japan after an evacuation. But in the end, none of the propositions for an advance show seemed realistic and the committee wrote a report approving military employment of the bomb.

The Franck report was presented first. On June 11 Franck's document was given to George Harrison for Stimson. In a covering letter, Compton pointed out that the Franck report was at variance with both the Interim Committee's conclusions and those of the scientific panel. The summary of the Franck document reasoned that the United States could not keep the bomb secret and that, unless international control of the new forces could be obtained, other countries within ten years would have bombs which could lay waste as much as ten square miles of a city at a crack. In a nuclear war, the United States would be at a disadvantage because of its dense concentrations of people and industry, the scientists stated. Their report read in part:

We believe that these considerations make the use of nuclear bombs for an early unannounced attack against Japan inadvisable. If the United States were to be the first to release this new means of indiscriminate destruction upon mankind, she would sacrifice public support throughout the world, precipitate the race for armaments, and prejudice the possibility of reaching an international agreement on the future control of such weapons.

Much more favorable conditions for the eventual achievement of such an agreement could be created if nuclear bombs were first revealed to the world by a demonstration in an appropriately selected uninhabited area. . . .

Five days later, on June 16, Harrison received the official report of the Interim Committee scientific panel. Compton's group took account of the debate among its colleagues, but placed itself reluctantly in opposition to the Franck committee with these words:

Those who advocate a purely technical demonstration would wish to outlaw the use of atomic weapons and have feared that if we use the weapons now our future negotiations will be prejudiced. Others emphasize the opportunity of saving American lives by immediate

107

military use and believe that such use will improve the international prospects, in that they are more concerned with the prevention of war than with the elimination of this special weapon.

We find ourselves closer to these latter views: we can propose no technical demonstration likely to bring an end to the war; we can see no acceptable alternative to direct military use.

Two days later, on June 18, President Truman summoned the joint chiefs to the White House to formulate final strategy against Japan. Stimson, Secretary of the Navy Forrestal and Assistant Secretary of War John J. McCloy also attended the meeting. General Marshall described the plan to invade the Japanese home island of Kyushu on November 1 with a total force of 766,700 men. He predicted casualties would be relatively light. Leahy took issue with this, noting that losses on Okinawa had run to 35 per cent of the striking force. The other chiefs were far more optimistic than Leahy. "There is reason to believe," said Marshall, according to the official notes made by Brigadier General A. J. McFarland, "the first 30 days in Kyushu should not exceed the price we paid for Luzon." That Philippine operation had cost 31,000 Americans killed, wounded and missing. Marshall quoted a message from MacArthur: "I regard the operation as the most economical one in effort and lives that is possible." Marshall told Leahy the Kyushu landing would be easier than Okinawa; there were more beaches and there was more room to maneuver beyond the beaches. Admiral King said he thought U.S. casualties would be somewhere between Luzon's 31,000 and Okinawa's 41,700.

The chiefs unanimously decided, with President Truman's approval, on a twofold strategy to defeat Japan; first, intensification of the aerial bombardment and, second, invasion of Kyushu in November, to be followed by a landing in the spring of 1946 on the Tokyo plain. Stimson gave his assent too, but, apparently thinking of the atomic bomb, said he "hoped for some fruitful accomplishment through other means." After the meeting, some of the officials lingered. McCloy opened the subject of atomic bomb policy. He said the Japanese should be warned that we had a new weapon of destructive force which we proposed to unleash on them if they failed to surrender. His suggestion found no support.

The day after the signing of the United Nations charter in San Francisco, the first formal break occurred in the phalanx of Truman advisers supporting delivery of the bomb on Japan. Under Secretary of the Navy Bard sent a note on June 27 to Assistant Chairman Harrison of the Interim Committee. Ever since June 1 when he joined other Interim members in urging quick use of the bomb without warning, Bard had been having second thoughts. In the Navy headquarters, Rear Admiral Lewis L. Strauss, an assistant to Forrestal and a consultant on atomic matters, had quietly urged a demonstration of the bomb for the Japanese. He argued that residents of an area near Nikko, Japan, could be warned to evacuate and that a forest of cryptomeria trees there could be used to demonstrate the blast and heat. Strauss, who had visited Japan, shuddered at the thought of the bomb being dropped over narrow streets with their teeming population. Bard did not have such a precise suggestion, but as he looked at Japan from his Navy vantage point, he saw a nation already wrecked and surrounded. Accordingly, he felt it his moral duty to speak up. His message to Harrison follows:

Secret
Memorandum on the Use of S-1 Bomb
Ever since I have been in touch with this program I have had a feeling that before the bomb is actually used against Japan that Japan should have some preliminary warning for say two or three days in

advance of use. The position of the United States as a great humanitarian nation and the fair play attitude of our people generally is responsible in the main for this feeling.

During recent weeks I have also had the feeling very definitely that the Japanese government may be searching for some opportunity which they could use as a medium for surrender. Following the three-power conference emissaries from this country could contact representatives from Japan somewhere on the China coast and make representations with regard to Russia's position and at the same time give them some information regarding the proposed use of atomic power, together with whatever assurances the President might care to make with regard to the Emperor of Japan and the treatment of the Japanese nation following unconditional surrender. It seems quite possible to me that this presents the opportunity which the Japanese are looking for.

I don't see that we have anything in particular to lose in following such a program. The stakes are so tremendous that it is my opinion very real consideration should be given to some plan of this kind. I do not believe under present circumstances existing that there is anyone in this country whose evaluation of the chances of success of such a program is worth a great deal. The only way to find out is to try it out.

RALPH A. BARD

27 June 1945

But the pace of planning quickened. On July 4, Independence Day, joint Anglo-American agreement to use the atomic bomb was reached at a Combined Policy Committee meeting in the Pentagon. Five British and Canadian officials, led by the British ambassador, Lord Halifax, and Field Marshal Sir Henry Maitland "Jumbo" Wilson, and five Americans, led by Stimson and Bush, spent two hours working out formalities. In conformance with the Quebec agreement, requiring consent of both governments, "Field Marshal Wilson stated that the British government concurred in the use of the T.A. [tube alloy] weapon against Japan," according to the official meeting notes.

The following day, on the eve of his departure for the conference with Churchill and Stalin at Potsdam, Truman approved a statement to be released to the public following explosion of an atomic bomb over Japan. This statement, drafted by Stimson and Groves, was to give the world at large its first information on the atomic weapon and the mammoth undertaking to produce it.

In the shadow of the Potsdam conference, another high policy adviser to President Truman expressed reservations on use of the bomb. Hap Arnold, boss of the Army Air Force, had been to the Marianas, where LeMay convinced him that "we're driving them back to the stone age" with conventional bombing raids on Japan. Now Arnold had a talk with his deputy, Lieutenant General Ira C. Eaker. They believed the bombing of Japan, coupled with the blockade, had brought the empire to her knees. Japan was short of gas and oil, they agreed, most of her factories destroyed. Arnold did not believe an invasion would be necessary, although Eaker, as his stand-in, had attended the Joint Chiefs' meeting of June 18 and had agreed the invasion should be planned. Arnold told Eaker the official Air Force position had to be this: Whether or not the atomic bomb should be dropped was not for the Air Force to decide, but explosion of the bomb was not necessary to win the war. Eaker henceforth expressed this view at conferences he attended in Arnold's absence.

The Truman party split into groups for its journey to Potsdam. The President sailed on the *Augusta*. Stimson and his advisers crossed on the *Brazil,* a converted troopship. Each morning Stimson asked his aide, Colonel William H. Kyle, the same question: "Any news from Groves yet?" Stimson radioed George Harrison from the ship: "Please advise me if possible to this ship as soon as results are available from test, advising whether successful and whether results were equal to or greater or less than expected." Kyle was carrying a sheaf of secret atomic papers in a locked brief case inside a larger locked brief case. Aboard ship he stowed them in a safe in his stateroom. On the French Riviera, where the party paused for a day, Kyle requisitioned another safe from the Army and mounted a twenty-four-hour M.P. guard over it.

On July 12, when the Truman party on the *Augusta* was nearing the end of the Atlantic crossing, a poll was taken at the Chicago Met Lab on how the bomb should be used. Dr. Farrington Daniels, new director of the laboratory, polled 150 scientists at the request of Arthur Compton. Daniels circulated in the workshops, approaching the scientists one at a time. Five methods of using the bomb were listed on a typewritten sheet. Each man read the statement, then wrote the number most nearly corresponding to his views on a slip of paper and dropped the paper in an envelope. At the end of the day Daniels gave the poll results to Compton. The questions read as follows:

1. Use them in the manner that is from the military point of view most effective in bringing about prompt Japanese surrender at minimum human cost to our armed forces. (23 votes)
2. Give a military demonstration in Japan to be followed by renewed opportunity for surrender before full use of the weapon is employed. (69 votes)
3. Give an experimental demonstration in this country, with representatives of Japan present; followed by a new opportunity to surrender before full use of the weapon is employed. (39 votes)
4. Withhold military use of the weapons, but make public experimental demonstration of their effectiveness. (16 votes)
5. Maintain as secret as possible all developments of our new weapons and refrain from using them in this war. (3 votes)

In later years a dispute arose as to how the 46 per cent who voted for Choice Two interpreted "a military demonstration in Japan" and what those who received the poll results thought it meant. Did it mean dropping the bomb on an isolated area with military observers present or dropping it on a purely military target? At any rate, these scientific discussions and reservations about the bomb's use had little impact at the top-policy level. President Truman already had decided to use the bomb without specific warning, provided the New Mexico test proved successful and the Japanese did not respond to a formal demand that they surrender.

The New Mexico test of a plutonium bomb was slated for July 16 on an expanse of arid land fifty miles from Alamogordo. Oppenheimer tipped off Arthur Compton and Lawrence in Manhattanese, wiring them this invitation: "Any time after the 15th would be good for our fishing trip. Because we are not certain of the weather, we may be delayed several days. As we do not have enough sleeping bags to go around, we ask you please not to bring anyone with you."

The atomic age opened at 5:30 A.M., New Mexico time, July 16. A flash that lighted the skies 250 miles away brightened Point Zero with the dazzle of many suns. Men who looked directly at it, against orders, were temporarily blinded. A giant sphere of fire, laced with hues of deep purple and orange, spread out for a mile. The earth shook. A blast of hot air rolled out in a wave. The hundred-foot tower on which the bomb rested was vaporized. At observer posts ten miles out, the roar of the instant chain reaction came many seconds later. A column of white smoke shot straight up, then flowered into a mushroom that finally climbed to forty thousand feet. All over the Southwest inhabitants marked the clap of thunder and the strange way the sun

seemed to rise and then go right back down again. Miles away a
blind woman cried out that she had seen a light.

A press release had been prepared in advance by Manhattan
officers, giving a necessarily fake explanation for the unearthly
eruption. Each word of the release was numbered. Groves had
one copy and an aide in Albuquerque the other. After the blast
Groves telephoned the aide, making slight changes by use of the
number code. Philip F. Belcher, an Army intelligence officer,
carried the release to the press in Albuquerque. It provided this
lead paragraph for the Associated Press:

> An ammunition magazine exploded early today in a remote area
> of the Alamogordo Air Base reservation, producing a brilliant flash
> and blast which were reported to have been observed as far away as
> Gallup, 235 miles northwest.

Groves promptly phoned his girl Friday, Mrs. O'Leary, in
Washington, using a prearranged code. "Don't tell anybody except George Harrison," he said. Two of Groves' aides were
standing expectantly by her phone. "Well," she replied for their
benefit, "I guess anybody can see by my smile what happened."
Groves gave her the size of the blast, as best it could be approxi-
mated in a hurried survey of the scientists around him.

Jean O'Leary drove to the Pentagon at once and went into
conference with Harrison, who kept his injured left leg, stiff at
the knee joint, propped on a chair while they talked. They
worked out a message for Secretary Stimson at Potsdam. It read:

Top Secret
War Department
Classified Message Center

Secretary General Staff
Col. Pasco, 16 July 1945

Urgent
War 32887. To Humelsine for Colonel Kyle's Eyes Only from Harrison for Mr. Stimson:

OPERATED ON THIS MORNING. DIAGNOSIS NOT YET COMPLETE BUT RESULTS SEEM SATISFACTORY AND ALREADY EXCEED EXPECTATIONS. LOCAL PRESS RELEASE NECESSARY AS INTEREST EXTENDS GREAT DISTANCE. DR. GROVES PLEASED. HE RETURNS TOMORROW. I WILL KEEP YOU POSTED.

                    End   161524 Z

Back came a message from Potsdam:

                    Top Secret   16 July 1945
From: Terminal
To: War Department
   To Secretary General Staff for Mr. George L. Harrison's Eyes only. From Stimson. Top Secret, SVC 384
   I SEND MY WARMEST CONGRATULATIONS TO THE DOCTOR AND HIS CONSULTANT.

The next day Mrs. O'Leary met Groves at the Washington airport. They went to Harrison's office, where all three worked out a message that would give Stimson an idea of the explosion's scope. They gauged the flash in terms of the 250-mile distance between Washington and Stimson's "Highhold" estate on Long Island, and related the blast thunder to the fifty miles between Washington and Harrison's farm at Upperville, Virginia, in the shadow of the Blue Ridge Mountains. The message read:

                    Top Secret
                    War Department
                    Classified Message Center
                         Office, Special
                         Consultant George L. Harrison
                         17 July 1945

115

To: Terminal
Number: War 33556
Secretary of War from Harrison.

DOCTOR HAS JUST RETURNED MOST ENTHUSIASTIC AND CONFI-
DENT THAT THE LITTLE BOY IS AS HUSKY AS HIS BIG BROTHER. THE
LIGHT IN HIS EYES DISCERNIBLE FROM HERE TO HIGHHOLD AND I
COULD HAVE HEARD HIS SCREAMS FROM HERE TO MY FARM.

End

172017 Z

The comparison between the baby and the older brother related the plutonium test in New Mexico to the U-235 bomb
which had never been tested, but which all were confident would
work. Groves and a top assistant, Brigadier General Thomas F.
Farrell, a blue-eyed and peppery power expert, worked through
the night to write full descriptions of the Alamogordo explosion
for Stimson and President Truman. Working in the Foggy Bottom office, Groves wrote a semiofficial dispatch and Farrell a
more colorful, emotional one. Farrell wanted to use a Biblical
quotation to reflect the doubts before the test. A fragment stuck
in his mind, but he couldn't quite remember it. Groves called his
daughter, who was studying Bible at a girls' school, but she
couldn't find the verse. Captain Fred Rhodes called his sister, a
Sunday-school teacher at Washington's Temple Baptist Church.
He told her to look it up in the concordance, the Bartlett's of
the Bible. Five minutes later she called back with the citation:
Mark 9:24. Farrell's letter to Potsdam read in part:

The scientists felt that their figuring must be right and that the
bomb had to go off, but there was in everyone's mind a strong
measure of doubt. The feeling of many could be expressed by, "Lord,
I believe; help Thou my unbelief." We were reaching into the unknown and we did not know what might come of it. It can be safely

116

said that most of those present—Christian, Jew and Atheist—were praying and praying harder than they had ever prayed before. . . . Dr. Kistiakowsky, the impulsive Russian [interpolated note by Groves: "an American and Harvard professor for many years"] threw his arms around Dr. Oppenheimer and embraced him with shouts of glee.

Groves gave a detailed report of the extent of blast and the crunching damage to steel test structures which had been erected on the desert:

The test was successful beyond the most optimistic expectations of anyone. Based on the data which it has been possible to work up to date, I estimate the energy generated to be in excess of the equivalent of 15,000 to 20,000 tons of TNT; and this is a conservative estimate.

This official estimate, buttressed by calculations of the scientists, had a curious prelude. Before the test the physicists established a pool at the Los Alamos laboratory. Each entrant guessed the expected explosive yield in terms of tons of TNT. The overwhelming majority of men guessed under a few thousand tons. Some estimated in the mere hundreds of tons. Two late-arriving visitors, Lee DuBridge and I. I. Rabi, almost bracketed the pool. DuBridge picked zero and Rabi picked eighteen thousand tons. Rabi won. The final estimate made after the shot and after Groves worked up his paper was twenty thousand tons.

Some critics of the decision to use the bomb contended later that Groves underplayed the blast effect for the authorities at Potsdam. The actual messages, as preserved in the long-secret Manhattan files, give no support to this view. If anything, Groves went out of his way to stress the immensity of the explosion.

The general, in his long letter to Potsdam, wrote:

Drs. Conant and Bush and myself were struck by an even stronger feeling that the faith of those who had been responsible for the initiation and the carrying on of this Herculean project had been justified. I personally thought of Blondin crossing Niagara Falls on his tight rope, only to me this tight rope had lasted for almost three years, and of my repeated confident-appearing assurances that such a thing was possible and that we could do it.

Groves noted, as an aside, that he no longer considered "the Pentagon a safe shelter from such a bomb." But, he concluded, the "real goal" still lay ahead: "The battle test is what counts in the war with Japan."

Observations of physicist Ernest Lawrence were included in the package which an air courier carried to Potsdam on July 18. Lawrence wrote in part:

The grand, indeed almost cataclysmic proportion of the explosion produced a kind of solemnity in everyone's behavior immediately afterwards. There was restrained applause, but more a hushed murmuring bordering on reverence in manner as the event was commented upon. . . . Dr. Charles Thomas (Monsanto) spoke to me of this being the greatest single event in the history of mankind. . . .

The President, Byrnes and Leahy were motoring through the ruins of Berlin when the Alamogordo explosion occurred. Berlin's shattered buildings, standing like tombstones, the heaps of stone and splintered lumber, the long lines of homeless Germans, all testified to the effectiveness of Allied bombers and Russian shells. Stimson received Harrison's first message at 7:30 P.M. in Berlin and hurried at once to the "Little White House" at No. 2 Kaiserstrasse in suburban Babelsberg. Byrnes was also there with Truman. After Stimson's translation, they knew that now one bomb could do what it had taken thousands to do to once-beautiful Berlin. The next day, with the receipt of the second message, Stimson again called on President Truman and explained how, had the plutonium bomb been exploded in Washington, its flash could have been seen on Long Island and its roar heard almost as far as the Blue Ridge Mountains.

This second message, with its seeming reference to the birth of a baby, was discussed with less gravity by the young decoding officers at the Potsdam communications center. They surmised that Stimson, then almost seventy-eight years old, had become a father and they wondered if the Big Three would adjourn for a day to celebrate.

The day after the mushroom cast its shadow on New Mexico, Arthur Compton forwarded a number of scientists' petitions to George Harrison in Washington. One of them, written by Leo Szilard, urged President Truman not to use an atomic bomb against Japan unless it was preceded by a specific warning. Szilard had first offered a petition requesting that the bomb not be dropped on Japan at all. This attracted some signatures, but Szilard then modified it to urge that it be used only after a warning as to its nature. Sixty-seven atom scientists signed this version. Another petition urged use of the bomb if Japan refused to surrender. Still a third asked quick use of the A-bomb to end the war and spare American lives. The scientists were clearly divided as to what should be done.

That same day, in Potsdam, Stimson called on Churchill in his quarters and showed the British Prime Minister the "Highhold" message. In a conference with Byrnes, Stimson urged a prompt warning to Japan in light of the New Mexico shot, but Byrnes said the timetable already had been worked out with President Truman. Stimson did not press the matter further.

On July 21, at 11:35 A.M., the courier arrived at Potsdam

with Groves' lengthy Alamogordo report, complete with damage photographs. Stimson found it "an immensely powerful document," revealing "far greater destructive power than we had expected of S-1." He hurried with the papers to the Little White House.

Truman and Byrnes were in the second-floor sitting room of this three-story stucco house on the banks of Lake Griebnitz. The house had no screens and the three men occasionally had to swat mosquitoes. Stimson, his careful enunciation somewhat blurred by excitement, read portions of the report aloud to Truman and Byrnes. The President was elated and left for a formal Potsdam session in a jaunty mood.

Stimson later took the report to Churchill, but the Prime Minister had time for only a cursory examination before an evening conference session. The next morning Stimson returned and this time Churchill read everything.

"Now I know what happened to Truman yesterday," said Churchill. "When he got to the meeting after having read this report, he was a changed man. He told the Russians just where they got on and off and generally bossed the whole meeting."

Colonel Kyle was waiting for Stimson when he returned from seeing Churchill.

"What did he say about it?" asked the colonel.

"He called it the Second Coming in wrath," said Stimson.

At an all-American session in Truman's quarters, once the home of a German movie producer who was now in a Russian forced-labor battalion, Truman, Byrnes, Stimson, Arnold, Leahy, Marshall and King reviewed war strategy in light of the new weapon's success. Leahy's moral reservations were well known. Arnold stated that his Air Force thought the war could be ended with conventional bombing. Marshall, however, felt that an invasion would still be necessary, with more American losses, if the bomb was not used.

Churchill, invited to take part in one session, found himself of a mind with Truman—that the bomb should be used as soon as ready. He believed it would deliver the world from a war that had bled his country for six years. He also pointed out that now Japan might surrender without a last-minute entry of Russia into the Far Eastern conflict. In the end, Truman reaffirmed his decision to use the bomb. Agreement was also reached that no mention of the nuclear weapon would be made in the forthcoming ultimatum to Japan.

Once the decision was reaffirmed by the President, a dispatch was sent to Washington—where General Spaatz had expressed his unwillingness to use an atomic bomb without "a piece of paper"—ordering preparation of a "tentative directive for submission to the Secretary of War" and stating that Spaatz should be given copies of it.

Huddles at Potsdam on use of the bomb were sandwiched between formal conference sessions. Stimson conferred with Arnold after receiving this message from Harrison in Washington:

All your local military advisers engaged in preparation definitely favor your pet city and would like to feel free to use it as first choice if those on the ride select it out of four possible spots in the light of local conditions at the time.

Stimson's "pet city" which Washington commanders wanted to put at the top of the atomic target list was Kyoto, the ancient capital of Japan and cultural center of the empire. It was an old argument. Stimson's earlier intervention had spared the city and its renowned Buddhist monasteries. On July 2 the debate had reopened. The air staff had prepared a memorandum for General

Arnold, declaring that it did not agree with Stimson and urging that "Kyoto be reserved as a target for the 509th Composite Group." On July 3 the Joint Chiefs of Staff, after hearing Arnold, had radioed MacArthur and Nimitz, ordering that there be absolutely no bombing of four cities: Kyoto, Hiroshima, Kokura and Niigata. The message did not say so, but this was the first atomic reservation list. Stimson now argued the matter with Arnold at Potsdam. He believed that "the bitterness which would be caused by such a wanton act" as the atomic destruction of Kyoto might turn the Japanese against America in the postwar era should trouble develop with Russia in the Far East. Finally, the Secretary of War gained Truman's emphatic approval to strike Kyoto from the atomic list. "My decision has been confirmed by the highest authority," Stimson cabled Washington. He told Harrison that the preferred list in Potsdam was "Hiroshima, Kokura, Niigata."

President Truman was anxious to know when the bomb would be ready on Tinian Island, and messages zipped back and forth across the Atlantic on the subject. Harrison cabled on July 21:

Patient progressing rapidly and will be ready for final operation first good break in August.

Two days later Harrison gave more specific dates:

Operation may be possible any time from August 1, depending on state of preparation of patient and condition of atmosphere. From point of view of patient only, some chance August 1 to 3, good chance August 4 to 5 and barring unexpected relapse almost certain before August 10.

General Eisenhower, the supreme European commander, was not an official member of the Potsdam delegation. Nevertheless he consulted with delegation members. Stimson briefed him on the atomic project and the Alamogordo shot. Eisenhower frankly told the War Secretary that he hoped the bomb would not have to be used against Japan because he hated to see the United States be the first to employ a weapon with such incredible potential for death and destruction.

Thus, in the many weeks in which the decision evolved, no less than six U.S. war leaders had expressed reservations about use of the bomb: Admiral Leahy, Generals Arnold and Eisenhower, Rear Admiral Strauss, Assistant Secretary of War McCloy and Under Secretary of the Navy Bard. Of these, however, only Bard flatly and formally opposed the use of the bomb without an advance demonstration and warning.

On the other side, a score of influential White House advisers supported use of the bomb, including Stimson, Marshall, Groves, seven of the eight members of the Interim Committee and all of its scientific advisers, plus many other top scientists.

Yet within the framework of decision, some qualms persisted. On July 23 Groves, in Washington, telephoned Colonel Nichols, his Manhattan production chief, who was in Oak Ridge. Groves had seen some of the scientists' petitions on use of the bomb, but not the results of the Chicago Met Lab poll of July 12. Groves asked Nichols to contact Arthur Compton at Oak Ridge and get the poll tabulation. Nichols did so. Groves then asked for Compton's personal opinion. Compton said he believed the bomb should be used, but only to the extent necessary to force surrender of Japan. Nichols relayed this to Groves. The Manhattan chief wanted the poll results in hand, he said later, in case "somebody got to the White House with a claim that all the scientists were against using the bomb."

The next day, July 24, Truman informed Russia's Stalin at Potsdam of the bomb in a manner best described as "studied casual." Churchill, Truman and Byrnes had worried that Stalin might open fire with a volley of questions, which Truman was prepared to deflect. At the conclusion of the afternoon session, Truman walked up to Stalin. He said simply that the United States had developed a new and powerful weapon and intended to use it against Japan. Stalin appeared unimpressed. He smiled and said he hoped good use would be made of it. The exchange lasted only a moment. Byrnes and Churchill were eager to hear Stalin's reaction from Truman's lips. They discussed it on the sidewalk outside while waiting for cars. "He never asked a question," said Truman.

Back in Washington at the Pentagon, Handy, Spaatz, Eaker, Farrell and Major General Howard A. Craig wrestled with the details of exploding a nuclear weapon on enemy territory. Colonel John N. Stone arrived from Potsdam with verbal instructions from Arnold. Among other things, he brought word that Nagasaki should be added to Hiroshima, Kokura and Niigata on the target list. Farrell argued against Nagasaki, contending that its hilly terrain was unsuited for a full demonstration of the bomb's power. Besides, it had been pummeled by conventional bombs. Farrell lost the round and Nagasaki was added. In late afternoon a directive, largely based on a draft by Groves, was typed out, ordering that a series of atomic bombs be dropped on Japan. The directive read:

Top Secret

War Department
Office of the Chief of Staff
Washington 25, D.C.

To: General Carl Spaatz
Commanding General
United States Strategic Air Force
1. The 509 Composite Group, 20th Air Force will deliver its first

special bomb as soon as weather will permit visual bombing after about 3 August 1945 on one of the targets: Hiroshima, Kokura, Niigata and Nagasaki. To carry military and scientific personnel from the War Department to observe and record the effects of the explosion of the bomb, additional aircraft will accompany the airplane carrying the bomb. The observing planes will stay several miles distant from the point of impact of the bomb.

2. Additional bombs will be delivered on the above targets as soon as made ready by the project staff. Further instructions will be issued concerning targets other than those listed above.

3. Dissemination of any and all information concerning the use of the weapon against Japan is reserved to the Secretary of War and the President of the United States. No communiqué on the subject or release of information will be issued by commanders in the field without specific prior authority. Any news stories will be sent to the War Department for special clearance.

4. The foregoing directive is issued to you by direction and with the approval of the Secretary of War and the Chief of Staff, USA. It is desired that you personally deliver one copy of this directive to General MacArthur and one copy to Admiral Nimitz for their information.

THOS. T. HANDY
General, G.S.C.
Acting Chief of Staff

At 6:35 that evening the directive was radioed to Potsdam for clearance by Marshall and Stimson. There was a "notice to code clerk" at the start: "This message is of the greatest secrecy and urgency and should be seen only repeat only by those people necessary to get it early Wednesday morning to McCarthy for General Marshall for his eyes only from Handy." Handy also asked approval to send this directive to the Pacific commanders:

The injunction against attack of Hiroshima, Kokura and Niigata covered by Joint Chiefs of Staff action WARX 26350 of 3 July 1945 is removed and the targets are released to the commanding general,

U.S. Army Strategic Air Forces for attack only by the 509 Composite Group, 20th Air Force.

Six hours later, early on July 25, came a priority message from Potsdam:

S/W approves Groves directive.

The order to drop the first atomic bomb on an enemy city had, in effect, been signed.

The next day, July 26, President Truman and the new British Prime Minister, Clement Attlee, issued the Potsdam Declaration, with China's Chiang Kai-shek as a third signatory. It was an ultimatum to Japan to surrender unconditionally or face "prompt and utter destruction." No mention was made of the atomic bomb. Two days later Japan rejected the ultimatum even as Spaatz and Farrell were flying out to the Pacific to prepare the death blow for the empire.

Farrell arrived at Guam on July 31 to function as the voice of the Manhattan District in the Marianas. After a quick survey, he sent a message to Groves and other authorities at the Pentagon. Using prearranged code words—"Scale" for himself and "Cannon" for LeMay—Farrell reported the bomb would be ready for delivery the next day. Both "Scale" and "Cannon," he said, interpreted the directive, ordering the bomb dropped "after about 3 August," to mean that it could be dropped on the first if weather permitted. Washington took no issue with this interpretation, which could advance the bomb drop by two days, but soon after the telecon message was sent, a typhoon swept toward Japan and thwarted operations for a week.

On the same day in Washington, Stimson, who had flown back

from Potsdam, debated with Groves and Harrison as to what should be done about the views of the scientists. Before them was a two hundred-page statement by a group of scientists who wanted to explain the bomb's workings to the world. Groves felt a compromise might be for the War Department to issue a carefully worded statement at the proper time. When consulted, Robert A. Lovett, Assistant Secretary of War for Air, strongly opposed publication of the scientists' document, contending we were becoming "a nation of blabbermouths." In the end, it was not released, although the official Smyth report, remarkably revealing, was made public after the bomb fell.

While President Truman slept in the Little White House in Babelsberg after the Potsdam conference ended at 3 A.M. on August 2, top-secret field order No. 13 was being typed at Twentieth Air Force headquarters on Guam, half a world away:

Twentieth Air Force attacks targets in Japan on 6 August. Primary target: 90.30—HIROSHIMA URBAN INDUSTRIAL AREA.

By the time the President was eating breakfast, thirty-two copies of the order were being distributed to command posts on Guam and Tinian islands. Operation CENTERBOARD was under way.

Thirty minutes before the President left Babelsberg to return to Washington that morning of August 2, a courier arrived with a Stimson revision of the White House announcement to be released after the bomb exploded. Truman tucked it among the papers he was taking back with him. Accompanied by Byrnes and Leahy, he flew from Berlin to England, then boarded the *Augusta* in Plymouth Harbor. King George VI entertained the Americans aboard H.M.S. *Renown,* anchored nearby, at lunch.

Jovial small talk predominated, but the British monarch and Leahy fell to discussing the atomic bomb. The admiral predicted the first explosion in war would fail to meet expectations. The king, fully informed on the bomb, offered to place a small wager to the contrary.

Back aboard the *Augusta,* President Truman, anxious to get home before the first atomic bomb fell on Japan, requested Captain James Foskett, the skipper, to lay on all possible speed. Task Force 68—the *Augusta* plus the U.S.S. *Philadelphia,* which served as escort—set course for Newport News at 26.5 knots. When night lowered over the Atlantic on August 2, the *Augusta* was pounding westward on rolling seas. Two months had passed since Harry Truman decided to use the bomb unless Japan surrendered. Japan had refused. Now the President of the United States would say no more until the bomb fell.

CHAPTER SEVEN

Little Boy on Tinian

AS THE ALLIED STATESMEN journeyed home from Potsdam, a flight surgeon on Tinian Island puzzled over the word "radiation." He was Lieutenant Colonel Harold A. (Spike) Myers, a native of Des Moines and a graduate of the University of Iowa who was surgeon of the 313th Bomb Wing. In his Quonset hut office Myers received three callers on the night of August 4. The trio was attached to the mysterious 509th Composite Group. The men were Dr. James F. Nolan, an Army reserve physician who had trained in civilian life in X-ray therapy of gynecologic cancer, and two physicists from the university campus via Los Alamos, Robert Serber and twenty-nine-year-old Philip Morrison.

"We could have a plane crash at North Field in a couple of days," Nolan began.

Myers knew that. He had tried to help several times recently when B-29s, carrying two thousand-pound mines with which to seal off Japanese harbors, crashed on take-off. The ugly explosions had left nothing for a doctor to do and precious little for the burial squad.

"We could have one hell of an explosion," said Nolan. "If that happens, don't send any first aid into the area before it's been tested for radiation. Otherwise the people who go in may die too. We just don't know."

Crazy talk? It sounded a bit that way to Spike Myers. He had heard rumors of a new-type bomb and knew that the 509th had undergone special training in Utah, but that was all.

"You know what this is, don't you?" asked Nolan.

"No," said Myers. "Frankly, I don't."

"Well," said Nolan, "it's a new kind of bomb, and because of the possibility of an accident on take-off, we have to do some planning."

Serber and Morrison pulled out a case of measuring instruments and explained the workings to Myers. If the radiation got above a specified level, they said, he was to keep everybody out of the crash area. Otherwise he could follow S.O.P. and rush in medical and rescue equipment. They promised that one or more of them would come back at the time of take-off and sit it out with him. They left Myers pondering this new hazard called radiation.

All over Tinian Island somewhat similar oblique conferences took place that week. Little Boy, the shortened version of the Thin Man U-235 bomb, had been assembled August 1 in an air-conditioned bomb hut where the humidity was kept between 40 and 50 per cent.

Little Boy didn't appear outwardly strange for a weapon that was about to revolutionize warfare and raise a question mark over civilization itself. It had a familiar bomb casing of steel about 14 feet long and about 5 feet in diameter. It weighed, over-all, just under 10,000 pounds. Inside, the bomb had a proximity fuze, set for 1,850 feet. When the falling bomb reached this point, the proximity fuze would touch off an explosive charge in the tail of the bomb. This in turn would shoot a small chunk of U-235 forward at a speed of 5,000 feet per second. In the nose, surrounded by a "tamper" of heavy metal to reflect chain-reacting neutrons, was a small cup of U-235. The hurtling chunk, shaped to fit the cup precisely, would strike the forward piece of U-235. At that instant, within a segment of time too small to measure, the atomic explosion would occur. The fissionable core of the bomb was far less than one half of one per cent of the total weight.

What Nolan and the scientists feared, and what they couldn't tell the medical officer, was a take-off crash of a plane carrying a live atomic bomb. There was the possibility that burning gasoline would ignite the explosive charge, thus sending one piece of U-235 flying at the other to produce a "critical mass" and a violent chain reaction that could wipe out half of Tinian Island.

Although Little Boy was the result of six years of atomic research and its complex mechanism had taken thirty months to design and produce, so well had Oppenheimer's team performed that the core of Little Boy had been fitted in the waiting bomb case only a few hours after it arrived on Tinian.

"Bowery" shipments, code name for the movement of U-235, had begun three weeks before. In the second week of July, Major Robert R. Furman, a thin, sandy-haired Princeton engineering graduate, was summoned to Manhattan headquarters. "You're going to take a package to Tinian," Groves told him.

Furman flew to Los Alamos, where he got his instructions from Oppenheimer. Together with Dr. Nolan, then serving as hospital physician at the laboratory, he would take the target chunk of U-235 to Tinian Island. They were to take it by ship from San Francisco aboard the U.S.S. *Indianapolis,* a heavy cruiser. The mission was vital, for if anything happened to this piece of uranium, the bombing would be delayed for weeks. No replacement in that amount was in sight from the production plants at Oak Ridge. The orders to the two men were explicit: under no circumstances were they to save a life before the U-235. If the ship sank, the U-235 was to have the first motor launch or life raft.

To mask their mission, Nolan and Furman purchased collar insignia of the field artillery. Nolan further equipped himself with some of the new atomic gear, several pocket ionization chambers, a large and heavy ionmeter and a portable Geiger-Mueller counter.

On the morning of July 14 Furman signed a receipt for the U-235 (then representing an investment of about $300 million) and then, when Colonel Lansdale's security team decided something extra was needed, he signed a receipt for a copy of the receipt.

The charge they were to chaperon turned out to be a lead cylinder about the size of a potato chip can, measuring some eighteen inches in diameter and a bit less than two feet high. It had a curved metal handle on top like a bucket or garbage pail, but when Nolan tried to lift it the can wouldn't budge. It contained about two hundred pounds of lead insulation.

A caravan of seven cars escorted Nolan, Furman and the cylinder to Kirtland Air Base at Albuquerque. They flew to Hamilton Field at San Francisco and were met by another swarm of security agents. Under heavy guard, they drove to Hunters Point Navy Yard and delivered the lead bucket to the office of the commandant, where a Marine took post outside the door.

The two escorts checked in with Rear Admiral William R.

Purnell, who was keeping a watchful eye on the proceedings. Purnell had long been connected with the atomic project and would soon fly to Tinian. He had consulted with Captain Charles B. McVay of the *Indianapolis* and impressed him with the importance of his secret cargo. Of its nature he said not a word.

A few hours before dawn on July 16, the day of the Alamogordo test, a 15-foot crate was swung aboard the *Indianapolis*. While the crane creaked over the deck and the crew watched the operation, Nolan and Furman boarded the ship by a rear gangplank followed by two sailors who carried the lead cylinder swaying from a crow bar on their shoulders. In the vacant quarters of the flag lieutenant, the can was attached to eyebolts which were welded to the deck. Straps were criss-crossed over the cylinder and Furman snapped a padlock on them and dropped the key in his pocket. The room contained a double-decker bunk, and for the duration of the voyage, Furman and Nolan kept four-hour alternate watches beside their cargo.

The cruiser raced for Tinian, pausing only a few hours at Pearl Harbor to refuel. Captain McVay asked no questions. Nolan confided to the skipper that he was really a medical, not an artillery, officer, but this only confused McVay. Linking the heavy cylinder, the doctor and the only weapon that came to mind, McVay said: "I didn't think we were going to use B.W. [bacteriological warfare] in this war." Nolan did not enlighten him. Sailors were curious about the long crate stowed on the deck. Some seamen poked fingers through the wrapping paper inside the wooden frame and speculation had it that the crate contained a secret weapon. Indeed it did, for this was one of three alternate casings for Little Boy.

The *Indianapolis* on the morning of July 26 dropped anchor in Tinian harbor about a half mile offshore. The big crate was lowered to the deck of an LST and again, while all eyes followed this operation, Nolan and Furman transferred their cylinder to a motor launch at the stern of the ship. Ashore, they stowed the can in a pick-up truck and drove to the bomb assembly hut near North Field, where they got a receipt for the U-235.

The ill-starred *Indianapolis,* torpedoed and sunk four days later, brought the only U-235 ready at the time it sailed. Shortly before the little lump arrived at Tinian, more of the fissionable material was started on the long journey from Oak Ridge. The second shipment was divided into three parts so that the loss of any one would not retard the first bomb too many days before a replacement could be readied. Three suitcases, each with a little piece of U-235, were assigned to Captain Rhodes, Groves' aide from Washington, and an assistant. They placed their luggage in the middle car of a three-auto convoy. Rhodes, a short, stocky Maryland University law graduate, had grown accustomed to security platoons in his days at Manhattan, but this one topped them all. About fifteen intelligence officers piled into the cars. They carried enough arms to invade a Jap-held island— .38-caliber pistols, tommy guns, shotguns and carbines. The arsenal covered the floorboards. They drove to the Knoxville airport, then switched to a C-54, which flew them to Santa Fe. There another motor convoy escorted Rhodes and his suitcases up the twisting mountain road to the Los Alamos bomb laboratory.

On the night of July 25 at the laboratory, Major Claude C. Pierce, Jr., a Harvard-trained lawyer, signed a receipt for Oppenheimer and took custody of the three parcels of U-235. This time they were placed in three containers. The pail-like receptacles were about two feet high and one foot wide, made of thinly rolled steel with a high nickel content. The top of each container was screwed down and made flush with the sides. Two eye-screws, each about two inches across, were fitted to the top for handles.

A Manhattan security agent took charge of each container. Instructions: Don't let it out of your sight until delivered on Tinian Island. Pierce took one pail. First Lieutenant Nicholas Del Genio took another. The third was placed in the hands of Captain Charles O'Brien. Lieutenant Commander Francis Birch, a young Harvard professor in civilian life and a group leader for making and testing Little Boy at Los Alamos, was assigned to accompany Pierce. Oppenheimer had a parting plea for Birch that night: "Make it work."

Pierce and Birch flew with their can to San Francisco, to Honolulu, then to Kwajalein and finally to Tinian. At each stop, they changed pilots and had to caution each one not to mention or discuss with anyone the unusual circumstances of the trip. Leaving Honolulu, their plane lost an engine soon after take-off. The pilot returned and was assigned the only transport available, a plush-seat command plane. As they taxied out to the runway for the second try, a transport bearing General Spaatz was warmed up and ready to roll down the runway. Spaatz, carrying in his pocket the first war directive to drop an atomic bomb, was on his way to Guam to assume command of the new Strategic Air Force. To the surprise of those who heard, the tower ordered Spaatz' plane to wait until the one transporting an Army major, a Navy lieutenant commander and a steel can took off. So tight was Manhattan security that no one on the field knew why a four-star general was held up for a plane with nothing much aboard except a priority. Spaatz, of course, would have understood had he known. The first airborne shipment of U-235 arrived on Tinian July 29. Captain Parsons met the two men with a jeep and the cylinder was safely deposited in the bomb hut.

Del Genio and O'Brien also arrived with their U-235 without mishap, but two of the later "Bowery" shipments almost came to grief. One agent, guarding a metal container with fissionable material, rode in a plane that lost an engine out of Hamilton, sprang a gas leak at Kwajalein and flew through a tropical storm near the Marianas that forced rain between fuselage joints of the transport.

Most harrowing trip of all was that flown by Captain Edward M. Costello, pilot of a B-29 of the 509th which carried a bomb casing for the atomic mission as well as a gray wooden box loaded with component parts for a Little Boy bomb. While his plane, the *Laggin' Dragon,* was loaded at Kirtland Field at Albuquerque, a ground crew guard was posted at the plane and a double line of M.P.s paced back and forth about fifty feet away. Bomb-bay doors were kept closed and the small round windows in the doors leading to the bomb bay inside the aircraft were covered with paper and taped down. These precautions were duplicated at each stop en route to Tinian. The *Laggin' Dragon* carried a Manhattan security agent, wearing quartermaster corps insignia, as custodian of the shipment. His disguise did not fool crew members, who were accustomed to the security "creeps," as they called them, and who knew they changed names, ranks and branch of service as the job required.

When Costello's plane landed at Mather Field, Sacramento, base officials insisted that the seven-man life rafts carried on the plane be removed and inspected prior to the overseas flight. The rafts were carried in the B-29 in two boxes near the top of the fuselage between the wings. The boxes were covered by a door fitting flush with the fuselage skin. In an emergency, a handle in the cockpit would unlatch the door and simultaneously inflate the rafts with gas, causing them to pop out. When the Mather officials returned the rafts after inspection, they attempted to safety wire the rotary latches on the raft door. The Manhattan security agent refused to let them, but offered to tell the air crew to do the job. Unfortunately he forgot, and the plane took off from Mather at noon on July 29 with the raft door unfastened.

The plane was very heavy. In addition to a bomb casing weighing five tons, a box filled with bomb parts and the gas load for the flight to Hawaii, Costello was transporting his full ground crew as passengers. He had masked the real weight by turning in a spurious weight-and-balance sheet as a means of safeguarding the security of his cargo.

Fifty feet off the ground Costello heard a loud "Whap!" The plane started to nose down. Costello pulled back on the wheel and rolled trim tab, but couldn't bring the nose up. "Help me, Harry!" he yelled to his co-pilot, Second Lieutenant Harry B. Davis, a hefty six-foot-three, 220-pounder. The plane began to level after Davis pulled back too, but Costello was sure the *Laggin' Dragon* would crash anyway. He turned ten degrees left to line up a less cluttered crash area. The turn was just enough to dislodge a life raft from the plane's tail. It had burst out of the hatch, inflated and wrapped itself around the right horizontal stabilizer, blocking movement of the elevator.

Costello called the tower for emergency landing instructions. The tower said to stand by. Then came word to cruise around until enough fuel had been consumed to reduce landing weight under 120,000 pounds. Costello estimated this would take five hours. Just then the tail gunner reported that fabric, ripped by the blow of the raft, was tearing off the elevator in shreds. Costello told the tower he was coming in. The *Laggin' Dragon* landed hot, the tires screeched and the plane ate runway. It was saved by its new reversible pitch props, which braked the aircraft to a halt just in time.

When the plane taxied back to the line, hydraulic stairsteps were shoved up to the right wing and four maintenance men, led by a major, scrambled up. A bald Manhattan security agent, who had been standing by, climbed up on the wing after them.

"Get down off this wing," ordered the agent, a captain.

"I'm director of maintenance here," replied the major. "You get down off this wing."

"I'm representing General Arnold," retorted the captain. "Here are my credentials and I'm telling you to get down."

With that, the agent "pulled a potsy," as police lingo has it. He yanked out a small wallet, adorned with a miniature gold badge and enough signatures of the Pentagon high command to start a school in handwriting analysis. The Mather major retreated to the ground. Costello finally got a new right elevator and the plane took off thirty hours later.

All Bowery shipments arrived safely, despite the narrow escapes, and each time another plane landed at Tinian an announcement was flashed to "Morose" and "Misplay," code names respectively for Manhattan headquarters in Washington and the Los Alamos laboratory.

By the end of July, 509th planes had been bombing Japan with single practice pumpkins for more than a week. The Japanese understood it no more than did the B-29 crews of other outfits on Tinian. After a 509th plane dropped one bomb of ordinary explosive on Tokyo July 20, Radio Tokyo complained:

The tactics of the raiding enemy planes have become so complicated that they cannot be anticipated from experience or the common sense gained so far. The single B-29 which passed over the capital this morning dropped bombs on one section of the Tokyo metropolis, taking unawares slightly the people of the city and these are certainly so-called sneak tactics aimed at confusing the minds of the people.

Unknown to Radio Tokyo, or for that matter to Twentieth Air Force headquarters, the lone bomb on Tokyo indicated what happens when democracy rears its unruly head in a military operation. The B-29 *Straight Flush* had found its assigned target hidden by cloud. Sergeant Jack Bivans, assistant flight engineer, suggested that they bomb the Emperor's palace and forthwith end the war. A vote was taken over the intercom and the plane headed for the palace. The area was partly cloud-covered and the bomb was dropped by radar. That evening the crew of the *Straight Flush* received a severe reprimand, although crew members were never quite sure whether they were rebuked for aiming at the palace or missing it.

Farrell, official eyes and ears for Groves, flew into Guam July 31 accompanied by Group Captain G. Leonard Cheshire, Churchill's observer for CENTERBOARD, and Major John F. Moynahan, a former reporter on the Newark *Evening News,* who was serving as public relations officer for the operation. Moynahan's job was a cinch at the start, since newspaper correspondents on whom to practice public relations were not permitted near the 509th Group. The plane landed shortly before 6 A.M. and Farrell went immediately to LeMay's quarters. The stocky bomber general was about to take a shower, and the only thing he had on at the moment was his first cigar of the day jutting from his mouth. While LeMay splashed in the shower, the two men yelled atomic news at each other. Farrell left a copy of orders for

LeMay, one of a number he had worn in a chest pouch slung from his neck on the flight from the States.

"If anybody refuses you co-operation," said LeMay, "come back and see me."

Farrell reported later in the morning to Nimitz at CINCPAC headquarters. The white-haired admiral pointed out his office window toward the island of Rota. Several thousand Japanese soldiers, by-passed by the war, were living there, subsisting on a home-grown vegetable diet. Although they had no more ammunition with which to harass Guam, they did have radios on which they reported daily to Tokyo.

"You don't have a small atomic bomb to drop on those fellows, do you?" asked Nimitz. Farrell replied he had only two sizes, one incredible in its power, the other slightly larger.

A short hop took Farrell up to Tinian, where he went into consultation with what soon became known as "the Tinian Joint Chiefs of Staff": Farrell; Admiral Purnell, Navy co-ordinator; Navy Captain Parsons, head of the technical crew from Site Y and weaponeer for the flight, and Norman Ramsey, chief scientist. Ramsey knew everybody and checked everything with a cheerful, efficient confidence that did as much for morale as the 509th's habit of promoting seventy-five enlisted men and six officers every month.

Ramsey and Parsons informed Farrell that the casings for three Little Boy bombs, practically identical, were on hand. The two pieces of U-235 had been tried in Little Boy No. 3 and fitted nicely. LB-3 was ready to go any time. Farrell, using his prearranged code, quickly got off a message to Groves in Washington, reporting that the bomb could be dropped August 1, the next day, or any time thereafter. Before leaving Washington, Farrell had a verbal understanding that Kokura, not Hiroshima, would be the No. 1 target, but LeMay's intelligence officers reported a new prisoner-of-war camp on the outskirts of Kokura. After an exchange of messages with Washington, the priority was shifted back to Hiroshima.

The tent and hut city on Tinian had its problems as the hours ticked off toward A-day. Sudden and violent cloudbursts drenched the oiled coral roads several times a day and a hot rain invariably fell during the evening movie at the outdoor "Pumpkin Playhouse." The men sat through the shows with water sliding down their necks inside raincoats. Mail for the scientists in the 1st Technical Service Detachment was missent to a unit with a somewhat similar title in the Philippines. The 509th suffered its first and only casualty of the war when an M.P. tried to disarm an old Jap shell he found buried. It exploded, mangling a hand.

The only ordnance mishap in line of duty during the 509th's entire stay overseas occurred when a practice bomb broke loose from the shackles of a plane piloted by Major James I. Hopkins. The plane was just about to taxi away from its hardstand when the bomb thudded to the ground. Captain George W. Marquardt, standing nearby, froze and involuntarily closed his eyes. With information so sketchy on Tinian, no one could be sure which bomb was the "beast."

"If it doesn't explode now," thought Marquardt," it never will."

Nothing happened. The bomb lay quietly until replaced in the bomb bay. All hands breathed easier, for a rumor had swept the group that it was about to drop a bomb so powerful it would take "four bulldozers five days to fill in the hole."

Spaatz flew into the Marianas from Washington, paused briefly and then flew on to the Philippines to brief General Mac-

Arthur on CENTERBOARD. Spaatz met the commanding general of the Pacific ground forces on August 1 in MacArthur's Manila headquarters. It was not a pleasant mission for Spaatz. Mac-Arthur had led his forces for three and a half years in bitter fighting while the great bulk of American arms was being shipped to Europe to crush Hitler. Now a weapon of epic proportions had been sent to the Pacific and MacArthur was one of the last commanders to know of it. But if his pride was hurt, he did not show it. MacArthur listened intently while Spaatz talked of the bomb and the directive.

"This will completely change all our ideas of warfare," said MacArthur.

On Tinian on August 1 Captain Joseph D. Buscher, a Maryland lawyer and intelligence officer of the 393rd Squadron, and Lieutenant Colonel Hazen J. Payette, a Detroit lawyer serving as intelligence officer for the whole group, began briefing bomber and photo-reconnaissance crews on what the atomic target cities looked like from thirty thousand feet up. They went over and over the aerial photographs until the bombardiers, pilots and navigators could draw the outlines of the cities in their sleep.

Parsons, Farrell, Tibbets and Commander Ashworth met with LeMay to plan details of the attack. It was decided to eliminate Niigata, one of the cities in the July 25 directive, as being too distant and too small. The strike force, they agreed, would have seven planes. Three B-29s would leave early and take stations over Hiroshima, Kokura and Nagasaki to report weather to Tibbets and to headquarters on Guam and Tinian. LeMay assigned his best meteorologists to this task. Tibbets would have enough time approaching Japan to select the clearest city for a visual drop. Insistence that the bomb be dropped visually rather than by radar was the last plea Oppenheimer had made to security agents who left Los Alamos with the U-235. The Washington directive itself ordered visual bombing. Two B-29s would escort Tibbets to the target, one to carry scientists with instruments to measure the blast and the other carrying cameras. A seventh plane would fly to Iwo Jima, less than halfway to Japan, and stand by for a transfer of the bomb in case Tibbets' plane developed engine trouble.

American planes at the time were dropping streamers and flakes of aluminum, called rope and chaff, to hamper Japanese radar. On the one in a million chance that the aluminum foil would react on the bomb's proximity fuze, causing a premature detonation, it was agreed that all rope and chaff would be banned from the south end of Japan that day.

As the conference broke up, a message from Groves asked Farrell: "Query is there anything left undone either here or there which is delaying initation of first table five line 28 [Little Boy] operation question." Farrell could think of nothing

At 3 P.M., August 2, top-secret field orders for Special Bombing Mission No. 13, the first atomic attack in history, were mimeographed at Twentieth Air Force headquarters. The date was set: 6 August. Targets: Primary, Hiroshima urban industrial area. Secondary alternate, Kokura Arsenal and city. Tertiary alternate, Nagasaki urban area. Special instruction: "Only visual bombing will be accomplished." Bombing altitude: 28,000 to 30,000 feet. Air speed: 200 mph, or five miles faster than normal because of the lack of turrets on the 509th B-29s. The aiming point was near Japanese Second Army Corps headquarters, but the radius of damage was expected to include almost the entire city save the dock area. Planned for elimination were the Ube Nitrogen Fertilizer Company, Ube Soda Company, Nippon Motor Oil Company, Sumitoma Chemical Company, the Sumitoma Aluminum Company and an unknown number of inhabitants. Oppenheimer had estimated 20,000 casualties—if the city was using its air-raid shelters.

"No friendly aircraft," said the orders, "other than those listed herein, will be within a fifty-mile area of any of the targets for this strike during a period of four hours prior to and six hours subsequent to strike time." Although the scientists believed an air explosion—1,850 feet above ground—would reduce radioactivity to a minimum, they weren't sure and no chances were being taken on an American plane coming home sprayed with radiation. Thirty-two copies of the orders were distributed to commands on Guam, Tinian and Iwo Jima.

The next day, August 3, the word began to get around among the uninitiated. Captain Louis Schaffer, the M.P. commander, was sitting on the edge of the bomb pit at a North Field hardstand. This was the special pit where the bomb would be hoisted into the plane. A detail of M.P.s was waiting for another dry run. Schaffer hadn't the foggiest notion of the special weapon's nature, although he had become a close friend of Phil Morrison, the crippled physicist whose brilliant conversational gambits had seized Schaffer's imagination. One of the Manhattan (Schaffer had never heard that word either) security agents sat down beside him on the edge of the pit.

"You know what the beast is?" he asked.

"Nope."

"Well, it's going to end the war."

Then for two hours, Schaffer listened, fascinated, as the agent told the history of the atomic bomb project. At last things made sense to Schaffer, especially the conversation he'd heard that noon in the mess hall when Tibbets led a discussion as to whether the whole north end of Tinian should be evacuated when his mission plane took off.

LeMay flew up to Tinian for a last look. At the bomb hut to inspect Little Boy, he put out his cigar. Security agents at the door also divested him of matches and lighter.

Farrell, who had been ordered by Groves: "Don't let Parsons get killed. We need him," sent a message to Washington on the third, reporting that several Little Boy-type practice bombs had been dropped with ordinary explosives and that assembly was now also under way on the first Fat Man, or plutonium, bomb. He thought it would be ready August 7.

Kirkpatrick flew six hundred miles up to Iwo Jima to inspect the duplicate arrangements for bomb loading. Unknown to the men on Iwo, Kirkpatrick had to plan for the remote possibility that the atomic bomb plane might become badly crippled and that a crash on landing might explode the bomb. In that case, it was only military prudence to let Iwo, with a few thousand men, take the risk rather than Tinian with its military population of almost thirty thousand men and its priceless piece of ordnance, the plutonium bomb. In less perilous circumstances, the Iwo bomb pit would permit transfer of the bomb to a new plane in case Tibbets' plane lost an engine within range of the little island. Kirkpatrick also had to arrange for a communications center, for relay of messages between the bomber and Tinian.

Three scientists began transforming the *Great Artiste,* commanded by Chuck Sweeney, into a flying laboratory. They installed equipment to measure the blast pressure of the bomb. Essentially the gear consisted of radio receivers and automatic film recording devices in the plane. Three parachutes carrying cylinders about the size and shape of fire extinguishers would be dropped near the target and radio transmitters in the cylinders would send data back to the plane. Leader of the trio was Luis Alvarez of the University of California. He was assisted by

Harold M. Agnew of the National Bureau of Standards and Lawrence H. Johnston, a twenty-seven-year-old physicist who had worked at Los Alamos.

Tibbets and Parsons, key men of the mission, put their heads together to decide what to do in event something went wrong with the plane. Parsons had flown to Tinian directly from the Alamogordo test, which he had observed from a bomber. The two men agreed that as long as their plane held together and could be flown, Tibbets would try to make the target and release the bomb. If the plane lost engines or was hit by flak over Japan, forcing it to lose altitude, they would try to make open water. As the plane descended, Parsons would go into the freezing bomb bay and dearm the bomb. The plane would be fairly near to water at all times, but if the crew had to abandon the plane over land, an attempt would be made to put the aircraft on automatic pilot and send it down toward the target.

On the morning of August 4, seven of the fifteen B-29 crews met in the briefing hut. Parsons showed movies of the first atomic blast at Alamogordo. The awful majesty of the scene chilled some viewers and now every man there knew why pilots had practiced steep, breakaway turns at high altitude. Parsons stated frankly that no one could be sure exactly what would happen. Perhaps, he said, even exploding at the planned altitude of 1,850 feet, Little Boy might crack the crust of the earth. Pilots were warned not to fly through the cloud because of the danger of radioactivity. Some of the men whispered of the possibility of sterility, the bugaboo of servicemen since the invention of radar. Deac Parsons warily avoided use of the word "atomic"; it was a new weapon, period. Tibbets rehearsed details of routes, timing, fuel load. All possible air-sea rescue facilities were laid on, including Navy subs, Navy PBYs and planes from other groups prepared to drop life rafts.

After the meeting Parsons and Farrell prepared a private code for communications between plane and ground. It was simple enough. Twenty-eight items were listed in order on a sheet of paper and each line was numbered. The items covered every eventuality they could think of for the time of the drop. If the bomb failed to explode, there was a line for it. If the blast was as great as Trinity, another line. If the plane returned, bomb intact, still another line. Parsons was to flash Farrell immediately after the explosion over Japan and Farrell, using another code, would relay word to Groves in Washington.

Tibbets and his crew bomb-tested their plane, No. 82, that day. They climbed to thirty thousand feet. Tinian, far below, looked like the hole in a frosted doughnut as the white surf etched the island. Tibbets made a four-minute level bomb run, then banked sharply to the right after Ferebee toggled the practice pumpkin away. The plane's bombing system functioned perfectly.

August 5 on Tinian was a Sunday, hot with a glaring sun. All over the island men briefly bowed their heads to God, but the business of war did not pause long for worship. In the camp of the 509th, the arming of the warriors went forward amid the small annoyances and noises with which soldiers have always adorned the task of killing. First, higher echelons had to be informed. Edward B. Doll, another college professor and one of the few men who got into the Manhattan project by hearing about it and then applying, sent a message to Los Alamos. He reported that Jake Beser, in charge of radar countermeasures for the bombing plane, had detected no Japanese jamming of the frequency on which the bomb's radio proximity fuze would operate. All records had been searched since April, he said, and no jamming on that frequency could be discovered. Kirkpatrick, in another message, said that "Air Bronx" shipments had failed to arrive for the plutonium bomb. He wondered, jokingly, whether "covetous people" at Los Alamos wanted to hoard the precious stuff.

After church that morning Chuck Sweeney took a B-29 up to thirty thousand feet and loosed an unarmed Fat Man over the ocean while scientists on Tinian watched through binoculars. This was the first full dress rehearsal in the Pacific for the plutonium bomb, although a similar test of the bomb's electrical and fuzing mechanism had been made in New Mexico two days before.

The proximity fuze was rigged to emit a puff of smoke when it triggered the detonators. The knot of scientists followed the fall through their glasses, but the Fat Man plunged smokeless past the detonation altitude and disappeared into the ocean.

"Oh, great," said Alvarez to his colleagues. "Here we are about to unload on Japan and we're not sure the fuze will work."

But preparations went forward for Little Boy. Bernard Waldman, a physics professor on leave from Notre Dame University, went to work in George Marquardt's No. 91. This B-29 was to serve as a photo escort plane for the U-235 bomber and Waldman, under instructions from Oppenheimer, was to take movies of the blast. Waldman supervised the work of taking the Norden bombsight out of 91 and installing his fast camera in its place.

Tibbets had a quiet sense of history. He surmised this Sunday that the plane he was about to fly might be remembered for generations. Thus far it had been simply "82," the number on the tail, or more technically, Army Air Force serial No. 44-86292. It was time to christen his B-29 and he thought of a name both distinctive and with special meaning for him: *Enola Gay*. His mother, from the small Iowa town of Glidden, had been Enola

Gay Haggard before her marriage. Tibbets had never known or heard of anyone else named Enola Gay. Although he was married at the time (subsequently he was divorced and remarried), he had a reason for thinking first of his mother on this day. He had always wanted to fly and when he was a college student, studying to be a doctor, he decided to leave the campus and enter flight training. The announcement of his intentions provoked a family crisis. Members of the immediate family, relatives and close friends all argued against it. The consensus seemed to be that he was giving up a solid profession for a hare-brained gamble that might cost his life. Only his mother stood by him. "You go ahead and fly," she said. "You'll be all right." He had taken confidence from her, and even in the tight spots it never occurred to Tibbets that any plane he piloted would crash.

Both Tom Ferebee, his bombardier, and Dutch Van Kirk, his navigator, had met his mother. He broached the idea of naming the plane after her, and both agreed. He wrote the name on a slip of paper and instructed a painter to letter it on the left side just under the pilot's window.

Little Boy swung from its chain hoist in the bomb assembly hut. A selected group gathered about it: physicists, 1st Ordnance Squadron men, M.P.s, security agents, the brass. Notes were scrawled on the bomb in crayon. Most were good luck to the Tibbets crew or bad luck to the empire and Hirohito. One legend saluted the men of the *Indianapolis*. "No white cross for Stevie," wrote Major Moynahan, thinking of his small son at home. The men who had assembled Little Boy told Parsons they couldn't believe it was anything but one of the old practice bombs. It looked the same and in truth, as Oppenheimer once remarked, the fissionable material was tucked away in the interior "like a small diamond in an enormous wad of cotton."

The chain hoist gently lowered Little Boy to a trailer. A tarpaulin was placed over it and a tractor pulled it out of the hut toward the newly named *Enola Gay*. An imposing procession of command cars and jeeps formed. Admiral Purnell, General Farrell and Group Captain Cheshire rode in a staff car. Security agents, scientists and G.I.s climbed into the other vehicles. Captain Schaffer and seven of his M.P.s stood on the sides of the trailer, much as Secret Service men ride the running boards of the President's open touring car. M.P.s cleared the route fore and aft and two jeeps swept the shoulders of the road. At the hardstand, half a mile away, the five-ton bomb was hoisted off the trailer and lowered into the bomb pit. The *Enola Gay* was towed over the pit and the hoist lifted the weapon into the forward bomb bay, where it was clamped to the shackles.

As the fifteen-foot bomb-bay doors closed, the B-29 stood like a great bird over a nest, the radome protruding between the forward and after bomb bays like some kind of atavistic pouch. NO SMOKING WITHIN 100 FEET warned one of many signs on No. 82. Four armorers had painted their names on the side as had seven members of the ground crew. The tail now sported a big R instead of the 509th black arrow and circle. Tibbets at the last minute had decided the plane should be indistinguishable from other Marianas-based planes, in case inquisitive Jap fighters should get close enough for a look.

As the crowd scattered, Deac Parsons drew Tom Farrell aside. The two members of the "Tinian Joint Chiefs" were worried over the recent B-29 take-off crashes. In addition to the explosions of mines in several smashed planes, one bomber had burned like a torch as machine-gun bullets sprayed wildly about the runway, shooting down rescue teams racing to help the trapped crew.

"If that happens on take-off tomorrow morning," said Parsons, "we could get a nuclear explosion and blow up half the island."

"I know it," said Farrell, "but what can we do about it?"

Parsons pushed his overseas cap back on his balding head. He squinted in the sunlight.

"If I put off the final assembly until after take-off, the island wouldn't be in any danger in case we crash."

"Oh, fine," said Farrell. "We lose the crew, the plane, the bomb and you, but we don't blow up. Besides, you've never done such a job. Do you know how?"

"No," said Parsons, "but I've got all day and night to learn."

God, thought Farrell, if you have to go to war, what a great guy to do it with. "O.K., Deac," he said aloud. "Go ahead and good luck."

Two months earlier, at a Los Alamos conference, Lieutenant Commander Birch, Parsons' ordnance deputy, had proposed arming the bomb in flight. Groves, Oppenheimer and Parsons had vetoed the idea, fearing it would be too easy for something to go wrong. But Birch had developed a "double plug" system on his own anyway. This permitted insertion of the conventional explosive in the rear of the bomb while in flight. Without this explosive charge, the two pieces of U-235 could not be driven together. Separated, even under crash conditions, there was no danger of an atomic explosion. Now Parsons decided to experiment with the "double plug" device. He worked in the stuffy heat of the *Enola Gay*'s bomb bay all that afternoon and into the evening. There was just enough room for him to squeeze into squatting position behind the bomb. He practiced the maneuver over and over, working in the dark of the bomb bay by aid of a flashlight. That evening, when Farrell stopped by to check on the progress, Parsons' hands were black and bleeding from handling the sharp-edged and finely tooled parts.

"For God's sake, man," said Farrell, "let me loan you a pair of pigskin gloves. They're thin ones."

"I wouldn't dare," said Parsons. "I've got to feel the touch."

Parsons and Birch had developed a lubricant heavily loaded with graphite for the bomb's double plug. It blackened Parsons' hands and he couldn't get them clean. While he joked about going over Japan "with dirty hands," Birch noted that this bothered him more than any other phase of the task. At last he announced himself satisfied and ready to do the job the next day in flight. It was agreed that Birch, Ramsey and several other scientists would stand by in the communications center the next morning in case anything went wrong in the bomb bay after take-off and Parsons had to question them by radio. At 7:17 P.M. Farrell got off a message to Groves: "Judge [Parsons] to load bomb after take-off, using Birch's double plug. . . ."

While Parsons worked in the bomb bay, First Lieutenant Morris R. Jeppson, a twenty-three-year-old, piano-playing Mormon from Carson City, Nevada, and three other young lieutenants of the 1st Ordnance Squadron, Leon D. Smith, Bruce G. Corrigan and Philip M. Barnes, spent the day installing an electronic console in the crew quarters just forward of the bomb bay and just aft of the engineer and pilot compartments. The black box stood about two feet high and about thirty inches wide and contained meters, lights and switches, each to monitor a separate item in the bomb. Inch-thick cables, each holding twelve or more wires, ran from the box to a removable plug connection in the bomb. The purpose was to keep an electronic watch on all parts of the complex bomb. If the console showed a failure anywhere, the bomb either had to be repaired or it couldn't be dropped. As the two seniors of the black-box brigade, Jeppson and Smith had the call on the next day's mission. They flipped a coin to see who would go on the flight to assist Parsons. "We're expendable," cracked Jeppson. He won.

That Sunday men of the 509th worked, played and talked as they had for months. The soft-ball tournament of the shack league ran through its schedule of games and several men of the *Enola Gay* pitched horseshoes in the shade. A knot of officers, khaki shirts open at the neck, lolled on the steps of their bunk hut. Now that the big mission was on, the injunctions of secrecy seemed to have lost meaning. They fell to discussing the nature of the weapon and its frightening results as shown in Parsons' movies. Several thought it was a kind of souped-up TNT, but Ralph Taylor offered to bet a month's pay that it had something to do with splitting the atom. Nothing had been printed on the subject for four or five years, he said, a strange silence for something that once so interested the scientists.

On another part of the base, a dozen ground officers met in the office of Lieutenant Colonel Thomas J. Classen, deputy commander of the 509th, for a briefing on their duties the next day. They were told the scope of the bomb's power and what each man had to do to make sure the Tibbets crew took off exactly on schedule. Scientists and key military personnel were assigned particular dispersal areas away from North Field at the time of the *Gay*'s take-off. This was double insurance to prevent loss of irreplaceable bomb specialists in the remote chance of a nuclear explosion. News of Deac Parsons' all-day practice hadn't spread far.

As the tropical night fell with the suddenness of a blanket over a light bulb, the *Enola Gay* stood on her hardstand with three M.P.s pacing back and forth beneath her great wings. By the two tires of the nose wheel, a little metal sign had been placed, G.P. LOADED, the routine announcement that a raider was bomb-hung and ready. Suddenly an air-raid alarm, the first since the 509th arrived, shattered the night. Even though it was a mistake, the alarm did nothing to soothe strained nerves.

Some men of the seven mission crews dozed, but others couldn't force sleep, much as they knew they needed it for flights of more than twelve hours and almost three thousand miles. Dutch Van Kirk took two sleeping pills, but still stayed wide awake. He sat on the edge of his bunk, playing poker with Tom Ferebee, the bombardier with the bristling overseas mustache, Chuck Sweeney and Kermit Beahan, Sweeney's bombardier and the man for whom the *Great Artiste* was named.

George Marquardt hadn't slept since Friday night. He had been married only ten days before coming overseas and the thought of a bomb that might kill thousands of people nagged his conscience. Sleep wouldn't come.

First Lieutenant Michael Angelich of Indian Harbor, Indiana, thought more of home than others did that night. His sister, First Lieutenant Mary E. Angelich, was an Army nurse sta-tioned on Tinian and had cared for him during a severe eye in-fection. Now, about to ride the *Full House* as a weather scout for the secret-weapon mission, he paid an early evening visit to his sister. They chatted of family and home, but never a word of the flight. Back on his bunk, he stripped to his shorts in the hot, muggy night and chain-smoked and sweated until briefing time.

At 11 P.M. about one hundred men trooped into the Quonset assembly hut and sat on wooden benches for the final briefing. It was hot and the lights added to the discomfort. A few men wore long khaki pants, but most wore the homemade Tinian shorts—

pants scissored off above the knees. The frayed ends gave them a beachcomber appearance. A weather officer made an effort to break the tension with a wisecrack. It fell flat. The mood for laughter had passed.

"We are going on a mission," said Tibbets, "to drop a bomb different from any you have ever seen or heard about. This bomb contains a destructive force equivalent to twenty thousand tons of TNT."

The session was short, covering the weather forecast, flying altitudes, communications frequencies, positions of rescue ships and planes. Rendezvous point: Iwo. Targets by priority: Hiroshima, Kokura, Nagasaki. Fuel: 7,000 gallons for the *Enola Gay,* 7,400 for the others.

The chaplain of the 509th, William B. Downey, strode to the briefing podium. He was a husky, dark-haired pastor who stood six feet one and weighed 175 pounds. He was a Lutheran, from the Hope Evangelical Lutheran Church in Minneapolis, and at the age of twenty-seven he preached the gospel with a youthful fervor suited to fighting men. He wore his khaki shirt open at the neck and the sweat glistened on his forehead as he bowed his head.

"We pray Thee," he said, "that the end of the war may come soon, and that once more we may know peace on earth. May the men who fly this night be kept safe in Thy care and may they be returned safely to us. We shall go forward trusting in Thee, knowing that we are in Thy care now and forever. In the name of Jesus Christ, Amen."

In the mess hall a few minutes later, the tension broke with the clatter of tin plates in "Dog Patch Inn." The crew munched real eggs, the prize entree of all flight breakfasts, oatmeal, sausage, apple butter, bread and coffee.

At 1:37 A.M., with no fanfare, the three B-29 weather scout

planes took off on separate runways, rushing into a wall of black. In the tail gunner's position of the *Straight Flush,* Gillon Truett Niceley, twenty-one, of Elizabethtown, Kentucky, said his own private prayer as the ship roared down the packed coral. He asked God to please be as kind to him and the rest of the crew as He had been for the past two and a half years. Major Claude Eatherly's *Straight Flush* headed for Hiroshima, Major Ralph Taylor's *Full House* for Nagasaki and Major John Wilson's *Jabbit III* for Kokura.

A half hour later searchlights played on the *Enola Gay.* Some fifty men gathered under the wings as Army photographers took pictures of the fliers, ground crew, plane and crowd. The nine-man crew of the *Enola Gay* wore their flight coveralls. Tibbets, Ferebee and Lewis had donned baseball caps. Staff Sergeant George R. Caron, the tail gunner, wore a Brooklyn Dodgers cap. The rest wore G.I. work caps. There were three special passengers, Parsons for the bomb, Jeppson for the black box and Beser for the radar scanning device.

Other members of the crew who twisted up into the hatch behind the *Gay*'s nose wheel were Dutch Van Kirk, the navigator; Technical Sergeant Wyatt Duzenbury, flight engineer; Sergeant Robert H. Shumard, assistant engineer; Sergeant Joe A. Stiborik, radar operator; and Corporal Richard Nelson, radio operator.

The civilian scientists waddled clumsily in the full combat flying suits. Underneath was the survival vest with fish hooks, drinking-water kits, first-aid packages and food rations in case of being forced down at sea. Over this was the parachute harness with clips for a chest chute and a one-man life raft. On top came the armorlike flak suit for protection against flying shell fragments over Japan.

All hands were uneasy. The four civilians had not the slightest fear of the bomb, but worried over whether the planes could make the long flight to Japan and back. The airmen had no qualms about the airplanes, but had no confidence in the huge bomb resting in the *Enola Gay.*

Every man wore a pistol and holster, as required by regulations. Deac Parsons, who usually thought of everything, had forgotten to draw a weapon from supply. Nick Del Genio, the security agent, unstrapped his Colt .45 automatic and gave it to Parsons. Good-bys and good lucks said, Tibbets waved from the pilot's window and taxied the *Enola Gay* to her runway. On the runway to his right was Sweeney's *Great Artiste.* On the runway to his left was George Marquardt, piloting No. 91, the photographic plane.

Planes of the 509th had been using the voice radio call sign "Victor," but on a hunch that afternoon, Tibbets changed the sign, just in case the Japanese were monitoring the tower frequency. Now it was "Dimples."

"Dimples Eight Two to North Tinian Tower. Ready for take-off on runway Able." "Dimples Eight Two. Dimples Eight Two. Cleared for take-off."

Down the runway went the *Enola Gay,* slowly at first, then accelerating swiftly to 180 miles an hour. Tibbets held the plane to the ground, but Lewis thought, "It's gobbling a little too much runway," and began easing back on the wheel. Near the end of the oiled coral, with only a few yards to spare, the *Gay* left the ground. The time was 2:45 A.M., August 6, by the clock and calendar on Tinian. Sweeney, wearing his good luck religious medal around his neck, and Marquardt followed at two-minute intervals and then Captain Charles F. McKnight's *Top Secret* rumbled off for its stand-by chore at Iwo Jima. Special Bombing Mission No. 13 was on the way.

CHAPTER EIGHT

The Flight of the "Enola Gay"

THE *Enola Gay* struggled into the night under full throttle. She grossed sixty-five tons, sixteen thousand pounds over the normal bombing weight, and her skin rattled with the strain of the lift. Several loose cans slid along the deck with the sharp, upward thrust and banged against fittings in the after compartment. Tibbets kept the nose down to build speed while Co-Pilot Lewis milked the flaps. In his little greenhouse in the tail gunner's position, George (Bob) Caron said a swift prayer as the runway fell away behind and the ocean spread below like a piece of rumpled black velvet.

The crew breathed easier. The "moment of truth" had passed and the *Enola Gay* shuddered with the thunder of her four 2,200-horsepower engines as she gained altitude and the familiar reddish-blue flames streaked out from the exhausts. Tibbets swung left at a few hundred feet altitude and sought his compass heading for Iwo Jima, 622 miles to the north. Cradled in a steel embrace in the bomb bay, 10,000-pound Little Boy was off and away without mishap.

Following the *Gay* by a few minutes, the *Top Secret*, the

stand-by bomber assigned to Iwo Jima, gathered speed on the runway under the control of Charley McKnight. An operations officer from Wing headquarters, crouching in the cockpit, yelled: "Cut engines!" He pointed to the tachometer needle, which was fluttering wildly. McKnight shook his head. "No pain," he said. The tachometer always fluctuated in the *Top Secret*. He kept the throttles on full power and the plane rose effortlessly from the ground.

In the North Field control tower, Tom Farrell, watching the fading glow of the *Gay*'s engines, realized he had been trying to push the plane off the last few feet. He turned to Admiral Purnell.

"I never saw a plane use that much runway," he said. "I thought Tibbets was never going to pull it off."

Farrell scribbled a dispatch to Groves in Washington, telling him the mission was off the ground. He handed it to a security officer, who took it by jeep to the communications center at 313th Wing headquarters. Then the dozen men in the control tower pounded down the steps, jumped into a fleet of waiting jeeps and drove three miles to the range shack, where voice radio contact could be maintained with the *Enola Gay* for the first forty-five minutes of flight. Ramsey, Birch and other scientists were ready in case Parsons should request verbal assistance from the *Gay* on arming the bomb. Growls and stutterings of static thwarted contact. It was many minutes before Farrell could raise Tibbets. The conversation told him little except that Parsons was at work.

To fill the void until news should come, Farrell proposed that Norman Ramsey be relieved of his heavy financial responsibility. Ramsey was still the official custodian of the U-235, now on its way to Japan. The metal, product of three years' work by hundreds of thousands of people connected with the Manhattan project, had a value of something more than $500,000,000. Farrell expressed doubt that Ramsey could raise the price in event of loss. A receipt was typed out. It read in part:

I have personally received from Dr. Norman F. Ramsey, Jr., A.P.O. 247, c/o Postmaster, San Francisco, California, the material as identified below. I assume full responsibility for the safe handling, storage and transmittal elsewhere of this material in accordance with existing regulations. The material, including inclosures and attachments, is identified as follows: Projectile unit containing (x) kilograms of enriched tuballoy at an average concentration of (x).

Farrell signed the receipt and twelve men, including Ashworth, Birch, Purnell, Doll and *New York Times* reporter Bill Laurence, witnessed it with signatures scrawled over the paper like a short-snorter bill. At the bottom, Farrell wrote in ink:

The above materials were carried by Parsons, Tibbets & Co. to Hirohito as part of "Doomsday," leaving Tinian at 051645 Z (Greenwich time).

Use of the word "tuballoy" for the U-235 was a salute to the British observers on the island. "Tube Alloy" was the British code name for the atomic effort.

The group waited in vain for definite word from Tibbets. Static cut his voice into meaningless sounds. Then the plane faded out of range. The men in the range shack dispersed for breakfast. Some tried to sleep, but it was no go. Soon they headed for wing headquarters to await the strike message.

Out over the Pacific the *Gay* climbed to four thousand feet and Tibbets throttled back to cruising speed. Parsons, his khaki shirt unadorned save for the silver eagles of rank on his open collar, knocked out a cold pipe and lowered himself into the bomb bay. His assistant, Jeppson, wore tattered shorts and shirt and a dangling parachute harness. The *Gay*'s forward bomb bay had been equipped with heaters, but they didn't work. It was cool and fresh in the bomb bay, but not cold at this low altitude. The time was 2:52 A.M. Tinian time or 1:52 A.M. Japanese time.

While Jeppson held a flashlight and passed him tools, Parsons carefully inserted the explosive detonating charge through the tail of the bomb. He used the double-plug system developed by Birch. Again Parsons' hands became black with the graphite lubricant and he nicked his fingers on the sharply tooled steel edges. The intercom system extended into the bomb bay and Parsons spoke several times to Tibbets to reassure him. The entire job took only about twenty-five minutes.

"Okay," Parsons told Jeppson. "That'll do it."

Jeppson then pulled a green plug from the side of the bomb and replaced it with a red one which fitted snug, flush to the bomb's skin. The plugs were identical except for the color of their wooden handles and the number of aluminum prongs on each. The socket cut into the electrical circuit which connected with the explosive detonator. The plugs were about one and a half inches in diameter and slightly more than three inches long, shaped at the handle like a large automobile cigarette lighter. With the green plug in, two electrical channels were shorted so that the bomb could not detonate. The red plug which Jeppson now inserted completed the electrical circuit. The bomb was now completely armed and ready to go. Parsons and Jeppson climbed out of the bomb bay into the forward crew compartment and locked the door behind them.

As it rode in its steel shackles in the forward bay (the after bomb bay carried extra fuel tanks), Little Boy was a maze of electronic ingenuity in addition to its revolutionary fissionable material. When it was dropped from the plane, intricate timers in the bomb would shut off for the first fifteen seconds. These said, in effect: "Whatever else happens, you can't detonate until you have been falling at least fifteen seconds." There was a series of timers. If one failed, the bomb was still safe. No minority vote could set off the system. Another series of instruments prevented the bomb from exploding above 10,000 feet. There were several of these, too, to insure against a premature signal by a single one of the devices. After fifteen seconds of fall, barometric gauges would alert the radio proximity fuzes. These were set to explode the bomb at 1,850 feet above ground. There were four of the fuzes, at least two of which had to agree on the exact altitude. If one fuze signaled, "We're at 1,850 feet," but the bomb actually was still at 2,200 feet, the other three would veto the signal and the system would fail to respond. All these devices had to operate within an interval of only forty-three seconds, the estimated time from the moment of bomb release to the instant of explosion. The complex intertiming of the proximity fuzes at the end of the fall would take place within a fraction of a second.

In the crew compartment Parsons and Jeppson seated themselves in front of Jeppson's console, the two-by-two black box through which he monitored the bomb's electrical circuits. Every instrument on the panel had to read correctly or the bomb would have to be brought back to Tinian undropped. Every half hour of the flight, Jeppson reviewed each instrument.

Bob Caron, the twenty-five-year-old tail gunner from Long Island, fired a few rounds to clear and check his twin .50s, the only guns on the plane. Then he crawled forward into the rear crew compartment, where he chatted with Stiborik, the radar operator, and Shumard, the assistant flight engineer. Jake Beser, radar countermeasures officer, was stretched out on the deck asleep.

Tibbets turned over the controls to Lewis and "George," the automatic pilot, and went aft to survey his command. The colonel crawled through the thirty-foot padded tunnel, a tube eighteen inches in diameter which ran past the two bomb bays and connected the forward and rear compartments.

"Say, Bob," Tibbets asked Caron. "You figured out what we're doing yet?"

"Hell, Colonel," said Caron, "I don't want to get shot for breaking security."

"We're on our way. You can talk now."

"Is it some kind of chemist's nightmare?"

"No, not exactly," said Tibbets.

"How about a physicist's nightmare?" Caron had heard that some of the scientists at North Field were physics professors.

"Yeah," said Tibbets, grinning. "That's about it."

Tibbets tried to nap in the after compartment. He had been twenty-four hours without sleep. He kept his eyes shut for about fifteen minutes, hoping the vibration of the plane would lull him to sleep. It didn't. He started to crawl back through the tube. Caron plucked at his shirt.

"Say, Colonel," he asked. "Are we splitting atoms today?"

"You're pretty close, Bob," said Tibbets.

Lewis was weaving the plane around the cumulous clouds which towered about the *Enola Gay,* their fluffy sides occasionally painted with moonlight. Jeppson, a ground officer who had flown less than one hundred hours, climbed into the navigator's astrodome. There, alone in the Pacific sky, as though racing onward in an open cup, he marked the strange beauty of the moon as it flashed into view and then disappeared behind another cloud. He could see the ocean below and periodically the stars above and all his life he would remember the grandeur of the night as it stretched between Tinian and Iwo Jima.

Navigator Van Kirk estimated they would reach Iwo Jima and the rendezvous point with the other two planes at 4:55 A.M., Japanese time. Tibbets took over the cockpit and Lewis went back for a sandwich and pineapple juice. He paused behind the black box of Jeppson and Parsons. Tiny green lights glowed on the panel. "What the hell do those green lights mean?" he asked. They meant all parts of the bomb were satisfactory, explained Parsons. When red showed on the console, it was time to worry. But, cross your fingers, there had been no red light yet.

The first lonely gray of dawn lighted the horizon at 4 A.M. and the night swiftly folded back minute by minute after that. By the time little Iwo Jima, the Marines' island of blood, appeared off to the right, the whole sky was bright and shafts of the infant sun probed at the cockpit windows. Van Kirk had pegged the estimate exactly. The island hove into view at 4:52. The *Enola Gay* began climbing to the new altitude for the flight to Japan. At 4:55 Sweeney's *Great Artiste* and Marquardt's No. 91 circled at nine thousand feet and the three planes swam into formation. Tibbets took the lead. Sweeney and Marquardt flew several hundred yards off the wings and slightly to the rear. The big V altered course to the left and flew almost due northwest toward Shikoku, the large island off the southeast coast of Japan.

"Bud," said Tibbets over voice radio to Iwo Jima, "we are proceeding to target."

Bud was Major Uanna, the 509th security chief. He and Colonel Kirkpatrick had flown up to Iwo in a Green Hornet C-54 to take charge of the emergency stand-by base. Tibbets, Sweeney and Marquardt had been chatting by intercom radio on the way up from Tinian. Now a wing officer in McKnight's *Top Secret* cautioned them to begin radio silence as per orders. For the next three hours and fifteen minutes, the duration of the leg to the target, the formation would fly in silence.

McKnight landed his stand-by bomber on little, pork-chop-shaped Iwo Jima and taxied to a point directly behind the specially prepared bomb pit. Now if an emergency forced Tibbets to return to Iwo, the bomb could be unloaded and transferred to the *Top Secret* within a few minutes. A dozen M.P.s who had flown up from Tinian ringed the B-29. Curious G.I.s stood at a respectful distance and gawked. McKnight, following instructions, didn't leave the plane, but sat in his pilot's seat while the *Enola Gay* winged toward Japan.

In the *Gay,* Dutch Van Kirk and Stiborik measured the wind, taking sights through drift meters on the ocean whitecaps below, then checking their estimates with each other. Beser, still corking off on the deck, was awakened by an orange which rolled down the padded tunnel and popped him softly on the head. It was the signal from the forward compartment to rise and shine. Beser downed a cup of black coffee and began "winding up the gear," as he called it. Beser had his own black box in the rear on which he monitored the frequencies of the proximity fuzes in Little Boy. However remote the possibility, any evidence of Japanese jamming would mean the bomb couldn't be dropped. Also he had to be on the lookout for forbidden rope and chaff.

In Sweeney's plane, Luis Alvarez roused himself from a snug sleeping spot inside the padded tunnel. Once the planes were airborne, a curious calm had settled on the civilian scientists as the steady drone of the engines drummed away their apprehensions.

Alvarez, a tall, thin and intense man, discussed this with crew members and they assured him it was always this way. The worst part of a mission, they said, was sweating it out on the ground before take-off. Alvarez, Johnston and Agnew began checking their blast measuring gear. Three parachutes hung ready in barrel-like containers inside the bomb bay. In the after crew compartment, delicate cathode ray oscilloscopes would record radio signals from the chute transmitters on 16-millimeter movie film.

An oil leak in the No. 2 engine of the *Great Artiste* bothered Sweeney and his flight engineers. It was a small leak, but it had been in evidence for two hours. Sweeney decided it was not serious enough to put back to Iwo Jima.

As Tibbets set his compass course for the coast of Japan, two stripped B-29s of the 3rd Photo Reconnaissance Squadron on Guam flew the short hop to Tinian. In the briefing room at North Field the pilots were given their instructions by the two 509th intelligence officers, Payette and Buscher. They were told they were to photograph an explosion of unprecedented size, but they were not to fly through the debris clouds. The secret weapon might be exploded over any of three cities, depending on the weather. They were to check by voice radio with Iwo Jima control tower to see which city had suffered the blast. The pair of camera-laden B-29s took off from Tinian four hours behind the *Enola Gay*.

Tibbets' formation headed for Japan from Iwo on top of an undercast. Clouds tumbled toward the horizon like a field covered with bright fleece. The sun shone with dazzling intensity and not a fleck of upper cloud marred the endless blue above. Every man in the three planes was awake now and some felt the first gathering of the tight knot in the stomach that usually precedes combat.

Tibbets called all hands over the intercom. From here on in, he said, every man must be at his station. At the coast of Japan, Beser would begin recording the intercom conversation on green celluloid disks.

"This is for history," said Tibbets, "so watch your language. We're carrying the first atomic bomb."

It was the first time that most of the crew had heard the phrase.

At 6:40 A.M. the *Enola Gay* was pressurized and began her climb from nine thousand feet to the bombing altitude of thirty-one thousand feet, almost six miles above the Pacific. Parsons and Jeppson checked instruments on the bomb console. Parsons did not re-enter the bomb bay. It was freezing cold there now as the *Gay* reached for the upper sky. The bomb bay was unpressurized. The Navy captain had his oxygen mask ready, in case the console showed something wrong in Little Boy and he had to climb down to remedy it.

Up ahead of the *Gay*, Major Eatherly's *Straight Flush* approached the outskirts of Hiroshima at 7:09 A.M. The plane's name had been picked by the crew and referred not to the premier poker hand, but to the action of a toilet bowl. A cartoon on the side depicted a Japanese soldier being flushed down the drain. The *Straight Flush* flew the identical course to be followed later by Tibbets. It took a heading of 265 degrees, almost straight west from the Initial Point of the bombing run. A solid undercast covered Japan as far as the eye could see. Minutes later, however, First Lieutenant Ken Wey, the observer-bombardier, saw the entire city of Hiroshima open up through his bombsight. At the point where the *Enola Gay* would release its cargo, the city was so clear below that the crew could see patches of green grass.

The *Straight Flush* flew across Hiroshima at thirty-two thousand feet. Captain Francis D. Thornhill, the navigator, took a double drift reading to get the exact wind for transmission to Tibbets' plane. After flying west for about ten miles, the *Flush* made a full turn and came back across the city on a heading of ninety degrees. The cloud bank rimmed the city, but a great hole with a diameter of more than ten miles marked Hiroshima as though fate had driven a spike into the city's heart.

At the same time Major Taylor's B-29, the *Full House,* was high over the city of Nagasaki to the southwest. The *Full House* flew across the city at thirty thousand feet and turned back for a return pass. Nagasaki was fairly clear too, with only about 30 per cent drifting clouds at twenty thousand feet.

The *Jabbit III,* with Willie Wilson in the pilot's seat, flew over the secondary target, Kokura, at thirty-three thousand feet. The *Jabbit III* was a bit early, and after one pass, it headed out to sea. The sun beat down on the cockpit as on a greenhouse and Captain Ellsworth T. Carrington, the twenty-year-old co-pilot from Short Hills, New Jersey, dozed off in the heat. Wilson kicked him on the leg, but soon Carrington's head began to nod again. Willie had to kick his co-pilot several times before he came fully awake. The plane returned for a second look at Kokura. The city spread under the plane with only a few clouds hovering on the flanks. All three target cities lay open for the *Enola Gay* that morning.

It was 7:25 A.M. when the *Straight Flush* left Hiroshima and headed for Tinian. Gil Niceley, the tail gunner, breathed a bit easier as the plane rushed east and the undercast reappeared, shutting off his view of the city. Not a single Japanese fighter had risen to challenge the *Flush* and the few bursts of flak had puffed harmlessly two miles below the plane. Radio Operator Baldasaro

168

tapped out the weather report on 7310 kilocycles, using the scramble code.

At that moment the *Enola Gay* was flying northwest over the Pacific with the full morning sun glinting off the aluminum skin of her right side. Paul Tibbets had left his pilot's seat and was bending over Dick Nelson's radio table. He decoded from the scramble sheet as Nelson jotted down the letters and numbers sent from Eatherly's plane. Cloud cover less than $\frac{3}{10}$ at all altitudes. "Advice: Bomb Primary." Tibbets turned to Dutch Van Kirk, standing at his elbow.

"It's Hiroshima," he said.

Under Field Orders No. 13, Tibbets had been instructed to make a pass over Hiroshima, regardless of what the weather reports indicated, on the chance the city might be clear by the time he arrived. Now, however, he could forget about Kokura and Nagasaki and concentrate on a single city. Nelson later announced the weather messages from *Jabbit III* and *Full House,* but they were of academic interest only.

At 7:50 A.M. the *Enola Gay* passed over the edge of Shikoku Island. Crew members pulled on their cumbersome flak suits. The radar and IFF (Identification, Friend or Foe device) were turned off. The automatic pilot was relieved of duty and Tibbets took over manual control. Van Kirk, rechecking the wind drift, gave the heading. At 8:06 over Fukuyama Bay, Caron made a note of a convoy of surface vessels heading north. Beser reported from his scanner: No Japanese jamming evidenced on the bomb's proximity fuze frequency. Jeppson made a thumb-and-forefinger circle for Parsons. The console showed all of the bomb's electrical circuits in perfect order. Parsons relayed the word to Tibbets: The bomb's O.K.

Parsons came up to stand behind Tibbets in the cockpit. Soon they noted a large opening in the clouds ahead and the outlines of a city below. "Do you agree that's the target?" asked Tibbets. "Yes," said Parsons, nodding.

"We are about to start the bomb run," said Tibbets at 8:09 on the intercom. "Put on your goggles and place them up on your forehead. When you hear the tone signal, pull the goggles over your eyes and leave them there until after the flash."

Each of the twelve men aboard had been supplied goggles that resembled those worn by arc welders. They were full extinction polaroid glasses in which quinine crystals would admit only one color, purple, through the lenses. The side cups fitted snug to the skin, admitting only a feather of light. The goggles had been made under a Manhattan AAA priority months before, another example of the million and one items produced over the past three years for the single bomb that was now six minutes away from its fall.

Jeppson stepped to the corner of the crew compartment, picked up his parachute and buckled it to his harness. Then he hooked his oxygen mask to the emergency oxygen bottle. Several members of the crew eyed him with dismay. Jeppson suddenly had thought: "The blast from this bomb might blow out the windows of the pressurized cabin. If that happens, I'm not going to be caught without oxygen." He kept the mask handy at his side. No one else followed his example. The time was short and there was much to do.

Van Kirk's navigation had been accurate to a fraction of a minute. At 8:11 the *Enola Gay* reached "I.P.," the initial point of the bomb run. The aiming point in Hiroshima was now about seventeen miles dead ahead. Sweeney's *Great Artiste* dropped back about a thousand yards. Marquardt's photo plane already had fallen back and now made a full 360-degree turn to consume time before its photo job. In the *Gay* Tom Ferebee leaned forward on his little bombardier's chair and put his left eye fast to the Norden bombsight. Most bombardiers took over control of the plane at the start of the bomb run, but Ferebee and Tibbets had worked out their own system through long practice. Tibbets retained control until the last ninety seconds. Now Ferebee, his baseball cap thrown aside and his mustache brushing the bombsight, gave a heading adjustment to Tibbets. "Roger," said the plane commander. At 8:13 plus thirty seconds, Tibbets gave the plane to Ferebee. "It's yours," he said.

The *Enola Gay* flew west at 31,600 feet at an indicated air speed of 196 miles an hour. Her actual speed in relationship to the ground was 285 miles an hour. Ferebee's heading was 265 degrees, just slightly south of due west. The *Gay's* crew had seen no fighters in the sky. Japan, desperately short of war supplies, wasted no fuel or ammunition on high-flying observation planes.

Hiroshima lay open and bare beneath the plane. Only a few small clouds hung over the untouched Japanese city and these stamped occasional dark spots on streets and docks under the flood of sunlight funneling down from the east. Save for Tibbets, Lewis and Ferebee, who were too busy for vagrant thoughts, the men in the *Enola Gay* had a curious sense of unreality, as though time stood still on a beautiful August morning and they were floating idly on an aerial sightseeing excursion. The land and the plane seemed linked in harmony, lulled by the steady pulse of the engines.

Through his bombsight Ferebee saw the city unroll as though it were the same target photograph he had seen a dozen times. Everything appeared so familiar, the three great oblongs of land pushing into the bay, the seven fingers of the Ota River, the main roads crisscrossing the city like veins in a leaf. A slight lower haze lent a shimmering quality to the scene. The aiming point, the center of a main bridge over the Ota's widest branch, moved to the cross-hairs of Ferebee's bombsight. "I've got it," he said and started the automatic synchronization for the final minute of the bomb run. Forty-five seconds later, he turned on the bombing radio tone signal which meant: in fifteen seconds the bomb will drop from the plane.

The men of the *Enola Gay* heard the continuous tone in their radio headsets and each man pulled his goggles over his eyes. In the *Great Artiste* and No. 91, goggles were pulled down off foreheads and men began counting to themselves along with the hum in the earphones. From the *Gay's* height of six miles, the signal could be heard by radio hundreds of miles away. It was heard in the *Straight Flush,* the *Full House* and *Jabbit III,* all flying home to Tinian. It was heard by Charley McKnight as he sat in the pilot's seat of the stand-by *Top Secret* behind the emergency bomb pit on Iwo Jima. McKnight slid open the cockpit window and called to several crew members standing outside.

"They're dropping on Hiroshima."

In *Jabbit III,* co-pilot Carrington turned to pilot Wilson.

"How about that, Willie?" he exclaimed. "Tibbets is less than twenty seconds off schedule."

At 8:15 plus seventeen seconds the *Gay's* bomb-bay doors sprang open automatically from the preset signal on the bombing panel. Ferebee kept a finger near the toggle button. Had Little Boy failed to leap out, he would have pressed the button instantly for a manual drop. But looking back through his legs and the plexiglass on the underside of the *Gay's* nose, he could see the long shape fall. The radio tone stopped as the departing bomb broke a circuit. Little Boy tumbled out broadside, then promptly righted itself, nose to the earth.

The *Enola Gay* lurched up, suddenly ten thousand pounds lighter. The head of every man in her snapped with the jolt. At the same instant Kermit Beahan, bombardier of the *Great Artiste*, toggled the plane's bomb doors open and three bundles plummeted out to become free swinging parachutes several seconds later.

In a co-ordinated sweeping movement, the two forward planes broke off sharply from the westward run. Tibbets nosed his plane over to the right in a 60-degree bank and tight turn of 158 degrees. The fuselage screamed with the violence of the maneuver. Caron in the tail felt like the last man on a giant crack-the-whip. Sweeney performed the identical turn, but to the left.

Little Boy was calculated to explode forty-three seconds after leaving the plane. In the *Great Artiste*, Luis Alvarez kept his eyes glued to the blast recording gear. In the *Gay*, Joe Stiborik stared straight at his radar scope. Tibbets spoke fast on the intercom: "Make sure those goggles are on. Caron, keep watching and tell us what you see."

Tibbets measured the seconds mentally and slipped his own goggles down from his forehead after about thirty-five seconds. Each moment now seemed endless.

"See anything yet, Bob?" Tibbets asked.

"No, sir."

Jeppson had started his own count when the tone signal ceased. Now he was nearing the end. 39 . . . 40 . . . 41 . . . 42 . . . 43. Jeppson stopped the count. The thought flashed through his brain: "It's a dud."

At that instant, the world went purple in a flash before Caron's eyes. His eyelids shut involuntarily behind his goggles. I must be blinded, he thought, remembering in a split second that when he had looked directly at the sun a moment earlier, it had shone only faintly. He was too stunned to report on the intercom.

Bob Caron had been looking directly at an explosion which, in a slice of time too small for any stop watch to measure, had become a ball of fire eighteen hundred feet across with a temperature at its center of one hundred million degrees. Such was Little Boy at precisely 8:16 on the first Monday morning of August, 1945, over the Japanese city of Hiroshima.

CHAPTER NINE

The Face of Death

THE SOUNDING of the all-clear signal in Hiroshima at 7:31 A.M. on August 6 made little change in the tempo of the city. Most people had been too busy, or too lazy, to pay much attention to the alert. The departure of the single, high-flying B-29 caused no more stir than its arrival over the city twenty-two minutes earlier.

As the plane flew out over the sea, Michiyoshi Nukushina, a thirty-eight-year-old fire-truck driver at the Hiroshima Army Ordnance Supply Depot, climbed onto his bicycle and headed for home. He had received special permission to quit his post half an hour before his shift ended. Wearing an official-duty armband to clear himself through the depot gates, and carrying a new pair of wooden clogs and a bag of fresh tomatoes drawn from the depot commissary, he headed home through the narrow streets of Hiroshima.

Nukushina crossed two of the seven river channels that divided the city into fingerlike islands and finally arrived at his home in Kako-machi precinct a little more than half an hour after leaving the firehouse. Propping his bicycle by the entrance to his small combination home and wineshop, he walked inside and called to his wife to go get the tomatoes.

At this same instant, in a comfortable house behind the high hill that made Hijiyama Park a welcome variation in the otherwise flat terrain of Hiroshima, a mother named Chinayo Sakamoto was mopping her kitchen floor after breakfast. Her son Tsuneo, an Army captain fortunately stationed right in his home town, had left for duty with his unit. His wife Miho had gone upstairs. Tsuneo's father lay on the straw mat in the living room, reading his morning paper.

Off to the east and south of the city, a few men in air defense posts were watching the morning sky or listening to their sound-detection equipment. At the Matsunaga lookout station, in the hills east of Hiroshima, a watcher filed two reports with the air defense center. At 8:06, he sighted and reported two planes, headed northwest. At 8:09, he saw another, following some miles behind them, and corrected his report to include it.

At 8:14, the telephone talker at the Nakano searchlight battery also made a report. His sound equipment had picked up the noise of aircraft engines. Unidentified planes were coming from Saijo, about fifteen miles east of Hiroshima, and were heading toward the city.

The anti-aircraft gunners on Mukay-Shima Island in Hiroshima harbor could now see two planes, approaching the eastern edge of the city at very high altitude. As they watched, at precisely seventeen seconds after 8:15, the planes suddenly separated. The leading aircraft made a tight, diving turn to the right. The second plane performed an identical maneuver to the left, and from it fell three parachutes which opened and floated slowly down toward the city.

The few people in Hiroshima who caught sight of the two planes saw the parachutes blossom as the aircraft turned away from the city. Some cheered when they saw them, thinking the enemy planes must be in trouble and the crews were starting to bail out.

For three quarters of a minute there was nothing in the clear sky over the city except the parachutes and the diminishing whine of airplane engines as the B-29s retreated into the lovely blue morning.

Then suddenly, without a sound, there was no sky left over Hiroshima.

For those who were there and who survived to recall the moment when man first turned on himself the elemental forces of his own universe, the first instant was pure light, blinding, intense light, but light of an awesome beauty and variety.

In the pause between detonation and impact, a pause that for some was so short it could not register on the senses, but which for others was long enough for shock to give way to fear and for fear in turn to yield to instinctive efforts at self-preservation, the sole impression was visual. If there was sound, no one heard it.

To Nukushina, just inside his house, and to Mrs. Sakamoto, washing her kitchen floor, it was simply sudden and complete blackness.

For Nukushina's wife, reaching for the bag of tomatoes on her husband's bicycle, it was a blue flash streaking across her eyes.

For Dr. Imagawa, at his patient's city home, it again was darkness. For his wife, in the suburban hills to the west, it was a "rainbow-colored object," whirling horizontally across the sky over the city.

To Yuko Yamaguchi, cleaning up after breakfast in the

rented farmhouse where she and her in-laws now lived, it was a sudden choking black cloud as the accumulated soot and grime of decades seemed to leap from the old walls.

Hayano Susukida, bent over to pick up a salvaged roof tile so she could pass it down the line of "volunteer" workers, did not see anything. She was merely crushed to the ground as if by some monstrous supernatural hand. But her son Junichiro, lounging outside his dormitory at Otake, saw a flash that turned from white to pink and then to blue as it rose and blossomed. Others, also at a distance of some miles, seemed to see "five or six bright colors." Some saw merely "flashes of gold" in a white light that reminded them—this was perhaps the most common description —of a huge photographic flashbulb exploding over the city.

The duration of this curiously detached spectacle varied with the distance of the viewer from the point in mid-air where the two lumps of U-235 were driven together inside the bomb. It did not last more than a few seconds at the most.

For thousands in Hiroshima it did not last even that long, if in fact there was any moment of grace at all. They were simply burned black and dead where they stood by the radiant heat that turned central Hiroshima into a gigantic oven. For thousands of others there was perhaps a second or two, certainly not long enough for wonder or terror or even recognition of things seen but not believed, before they were shredded by the thousands of pieces of shattered window glass that flew before the blast waves or were crushed underneath walls, beams, bricks, or any other solid object that stood in the way of the explosion.

For everyone else in history's first atomic target, the initial assault on the visual sense was followed by an instinctive assumption that a very large bomb had scored a direct hit on or near the spot where they were standing.

Old Mr. Sakamoto, who a moment before had been lounging on the living-room floor with his newspaper, found himself standing barefoot in his back yard, the paper still in his hand. Then his wife staggered out of the house, and perhaps half a minute later his daughter-in-law Miho, who had been upstairs, groped her way out also.

Dr. Imagawa had just reached for his medical satchel to begin the examination of his patient. When the blackness lifted from his senses, he found himself standing on top of a five-foot pile of rubble that had been the sickroom. With him, surprisingly, were both the sick man and the patient's young son.

Mrs. Susukida, flat on the ground amid the pile of old roof tiles, was left all but naked, stripped of every piece of outer clothing and now wearing only her underwear, which itself was badly torn.

Mrs. Nukushina had just time to throw her hands over her eyes after she saw the blue flash. Then she was knocked insensible. When she recovered consciousness, she lay in what seemed to her to be utter darkness. All around her there was only rubble where a moment earlier there had been her home and her husband's bicycle and the bag of fresh tomatoes. She too was now without clothing except for her underwear. Her body was rapidly becoming covered with her own blood from dozens of cuts. She groped around until she found her four-year-old daughter Ikuko. She saw no trace of her husband. Dazed and terrified, she took the child's hand and fled.

But Michiyoshi Nukushina was there, and was still alive, though buried unconscious inside the wreckage of his home. His life had been saved because the blast blew him into a corner where two big, old-fashioned office safes, used in the family wine business, took the weight of the roof when it fell and thus spared him from being crushed. As he came to, raised his head and looked around, everything seemed strangely reddened. He discovered later that blood from cuts on his head had gushed down over his eyelids, forming a sort of red filter over his eyes. His first conscious thought was that the emergency water tank kept on hand for fire-bombing protection was only one-third full. As his head cleared, he called for his wife and daughter. There was no reply. Getting painfully to his feet—his left leg was badly broken—he found a stick for a crutch and hobbled out of the rubble.

Hold out your left hand, palm down, fingers spread, and you have a rough outline of the shape of Hiroshima. The sea is beyond the fingertips. The back of the hand is where the Ota River comes down from the hills to the north. The spot where the bomb exploded is about where a wedding ring would be worn, just south of the main military headquarters and in the center of the residential-commercial districts of the city. Major Ferebee's aim was nearly perfect. Little Boy was detonated little more than two hundred yards from the aiming point on his target chart, despite the fact that it was released from a fast-moving aircraft over three miles to the east and nearly six miles up in the air.

Dropped with such precision, the bomb performed better than its makers had predicted. Several factors combined by chance to produce even more devastation than had been expected.

First was the time of the explosion. All over Hiroshima, thousands of the charcoal braziers that were the stoves in most households were still full of hot coals after being used for breakfast cooking. Almost every stove was knocked over by the massive blast wave that followed the explosion, and each became an incendiary torch to set fire to the wood-and-paper houses. In addition, where Oppenheimer had estimated casualties on the assumption that most people would be inside their air-raid shelters, almost no one in Hiroshima was sheltered when the bomb actually fell. The recent all-clear, the fact that it was a time when most people were on their way to work, the mischance by which there had been no new alert when the *Enola Gay* approached the city, the fact that small formations of planes had flown over many times before without dropping bombs, all combined to leave people exposed. Thus more than seventy thousand persons instead of Oppenheimer's estimate of twenty thousand were killed outright or so badly injured that they were dead in a matter of hours.

The initial flash spawned a succession of calamities.

First came heat. It lasted only an instant but was so intense that it melted roof tiles, fused the quartz crystals in granite blocks, charred the exposed sides of telephone poles for almost two miles, and incinerated nearby humans so thoroughly that nothing remained except their shadows, burned into asphalt pavements or stone walls. Of course the heat was most intense near the "ground zero" point, but for thousands of yards it had the power to burn deeply. Bare skin was burned up to two and a half miles away.

A printed page was exposed to the heat rays a mile and a half from the point of explosion, and the black letters were burned right out of the white paper. Hundreds of women learned a more personal lesson in the varying heat-absorption qualities of different colors when darker parts of their clothing burned out while lighter shades remained unscorched, leaving the skin underneath etched in precise detail with the flower patterns of their kimonos. A dress with blue polka dots printed on white material came out of the heat with the dark dots completely gone but the white background barely singed. A similar phenomenon occurred in men's shirts. Dark stripes were burned out while the alternate light stripes were undamaged. Another factor that affected injury was the thickness of clothing. Many people had their skin burned except where a double-thickness seam or a folded lapel had stood between them and the fireball. Men wearing caps emerged with sharp lines etched across their temples. Below the line, exposed skin was burned, while above it, under the cap, there was no injury. Laborers working in the open with only undershirts on had the looping pattern of shoulder straps and armholes printed on their chests. Sometimes clothing protected the wearer only if it hung loosely. One man standing with his arm bent, so that the sleeve was drawn tightly over his elbow, was burned only around that joint.

The heat struck only what stood in the direct path of its straight-line radiation from the fireball. A man sitting at his desk writing a letter had his hands deeply burned because the heat rays coming through his window fell directly on them, while his face, only eighteen inches away but outside the path of the rays, was unmarked. In countless cases the human body was burned or spared by the peculiarity of its position at the moment of flash. A walking man whose arm was swinging forward at the critical instant was burned all down the side of his torso. Another, whose moving arm happened to be next to his body, was left with an unburned streak where the limb had blocked out the radiation. In scores of cases people were burned on one side of the face but not on the other because they had been standing or sitting in profile to the explosion. A shirtless laborer was burned all across his back—except for a narrow strip where the slight hollow down his spine left the skin in a "shadow" where the heat rays could not fall.

Some measure of the heat's intensity can be gained from the experience of the mayor of Kabe, a village ten miles outside the city. He was standing in his garden and even at that distance distinctly felt the heat on his face when the bomb exploded.

After the heat came the blast, sweeping outward from the fire-ball with the force of a five hundred-mile-an-hour wind. Only those objects that offered a minimum of surface resistance—handrails on bridges, pipes, utility poles—remained standing. The walls of a few office buildings, specially built to resist earth-quakes, remained standing, but they now enclosed nothing but wreckage, as their roofs were driven down to the ground, carry-ing everything inside down under them. Otherwise, in a giant circle more than two miles across, everything was reduced to rubble. The blast drove all before it. The stone columns flanking the entrance to the Shima Surgical Hospital, directly underneath the explosion, were rammed straight down into the ground. Every hard object that was dislodged, every brick, every broken timber, every roof tile, became a potentially lethal missile. Every window in the city was suddenly a shower of sharp glass splin-ters, driven with such speed and force that in hundreds of build-ings they were deeply imbedded in walls—or in people. Many people were picking tiny shards of glass from their eyes for weeks afterward as a result of the shattering of their spectacles, or try-ing to wash out bits of sand and grit driven under their eyelids. Even a blade of grass now became a weapon to injure the man who tended it. A group of boys working in an open field had their backs peppered with bits of grass and straw which hit them with such force that they were driven into the flesh.

Many were struck down by a combination of the heat and the blast. A group of schoolgirls was working on the roof of a build-ing, removing tiles as the structure was being demolished for a firebreak. Thus completely exposed, they were doubly hurt, burned and then blown to the ground. So quickly did the blast follow the heat that for many they seemed to come together. One man, knocked sprawling when the blast blew in his window, looked up from the floor to see a wood-and-paper screen across the room burning briskly.

Heat and blast together started and fed fires in thousands of places within a few seconds, thus instantly rendering useless the painfully constructed firebreaks. In some spots the ground itself seemed to spout fire, so numerous were the flickering little jets of flame spontaneously ignited by the radiant heat. The city's fire stations were crushed or burned along with everything else, and two-thirds of Hiroshima's firemen were killed or wounded. Even if it had been left intact, the fire department could have done little or nothing to save the city. Not only were there too many fires, but the blast had broken open the city's water mains in seventy thousand places, so there was no pressure. Between them, blast and fire destroyed every single building within an area of almost five square miles around the zero point. Although the walls of thirty structures still stood, they were no more than empty shells.

After heat, blast and fire, the people of Hiroshima had still other ordeals ahead of them. A few minutes after the explosion, a strange rain began to fall. The raindrops were as big as marbles —and they were black. This frightening phenomenon resulted from the vaporization of moisture in the fireball and condensation in the cloud that spouted up from it. As the cloud, carrying water vapor and the pulverized dust of Hiroshima, reached colder air at higher altitudes, the moisture condensed and fell out as rain. There was not enough to put out the fires, but there was enough of this "black rain" to heighten the bewilderment and panic of people already unnerved by what had hit them.

After the rain came a wind—the great "fire wind"—which blew back in toward the center of the catastrophe, increasing in force as the air over Hiroshima grew hotter and hotter because of the great fires. The wind blew so hard that it uprooted huge trees in the parks where survivors were collecting. It whipped up high waves on the rivers of Hiroshima and drowned many who had gone into the water in an attempt to escape from the heat and flames around them. Some of those who drowned had been pushed into the rivers when the crush of fleeing people overflowed the bridges, making fatal bottlenecks of the only escape routes from the stricken islands. Thousands of people were simply fleeing, blindly and without an objective except to get out of the city. Some in the suburbs, seeing them come, thought at first they were Negroes, not Japanese, so blackened were their skins. The refugees could not explain what had burned them. "We saw the flash," they said, "and this is what happened."

One of those who struggled toward a bridge was Nukushina, the wine seller turned fireman whose life had been saved by the big office safes in his house just over a half mile from "zero," the point over which the bomb exploded. Leaning on his stick, he limped to the Sumiyoshi bridge a few hundred yards away, where, with unusual foresight, he kept a small boat tied up, loaded with fresh water and a little food, ready for any possible emergency.

"I found my boat intact," he recalled later, "but it was already filled with other desperate victims. As I stood on the bridge wondering what to do next, black drops of rain began to splatter down. The river itself and the river banks were teeming with horrible specimens of humans who had survived and come seeking safety to the river."

Fortunately for Nukushina, another boat came by, operated by a friend who offered to take him on board.

"With his assistance, I climbed into the boat. At that time, they pointed out to me that my intestines were dangling from my stomach but there was nothing I could do about it. My clothes, boots and everything else were blown off my person, leaving me with only my loincloth. Survivors swimming in the river shouted for help, and as we leaned down to pull them aboard, the skin from their arms and hands literally peeled off into our hands.

"A fifteen- or sixteen-year-old girl suddenly popped up alongside our boat and as we offered her our hand to pull her on board, the front of her face suddenly dropped off as though it were a mask. The nose and other facial features suddenly dropped off with the mask, leaving only a pink, peachlike face front with holes where the eyes, nose and mouth used to be. As the head dropped under the surface, the girl's black hair left a swirling black eddy. . . ."

Here Nukushina mercifully lost consciousness. He came to five hours later as he was being transferred into a launch that carried him, with other wounded, to an emergency first-aid station set up on the island of Ninoshima in the harbor. There he found safety, but no medical care. Only twenty-eight doctors were left alive and able to work in a city of a quarter million people, fully half of whom were casualties.

When Hayano Susukida tried to get up off the ground onto which she and the other members of her tile-salvaging labor gang had been thrown, she thought she was going to die. Her whole back, bared by the blast, burned and stung when she moved. But the thought of her four-year-old daughter Kazuko, who had been evacuated from the city after Hayano's husband was sent overseas and the family home had been marked for destruction in the firebreak program, made her try again. This time she got to her feet and staggered home. The blast had not leveled her house, about a mile and a quarter from the zero point, and the fire had not yet reached it. Hurriedly she stuffed a few things—a bottle of vegetable oil, some mosquito netting, two quilts, a small radio—into an old baby carriage, and started wheeling it toward the nearest bomb shelter. After going a few feet, she had to carry the carriage, for the street was choked with debris. She reached the shelter and passed the oil around to those inside, using the last of it to salve her own burns, which had not blistered or peeled but were nevertheless strangely penetrating and painful. She wondered what time it was. Her wrist watch was gone, so she walked home again to get her alarm clock. It was still running; it showed a little after ten. Back at the shelter, she just sat and waited. At noon someone handed out a few rice balls. As the survivors ate, an Army truck miraculously appeared and carried them to the water front, just beyond the edge of the bomb's destruction. Then they were ferried over to the emergency hospital on Ninoshima Island.

Dr. Imagawa, a little further from the center of the blast, was not seriously injured, although he was cut by flying glass in a number of places. His first reaction was annoyance. His clothes were in tatters, and he wondered how he would find the new pair of shoes which he had left at his patient's front door. Helping the small boy down off the five-foot rubble pile that had been the sickroom, he asked the youngster to take him to the front door. Oddly enough, they could not even find where the front of the house had been. Imagawa, much to his disgust, was out a new pair of shoes. At an artesian well with a pump that was still operating, he washed as best he could and set out for suburban Furue where his wife and children should be. He stopped frequently in response to appeals for help from the injured. One was a woman who wandered aimlessly in the street holding her bare breast, which had been split open. She pleaded with him to tell her whether she would live. The doctor, although positive she could not survive, assured her that a mere breast injury would not be fatal. Later he drew water for a score of wounded from another well pump. Down the street, a trolley car burned briskly. Finally he got clear of the city and climbed the hill to Furue, where he found his family safe and uninjured. The walls of the house had cracked and in some places fallen, but his wife and the two little children had escaped injury, while the oldest girl had walked home from school without a scratch after the blast. The doctor ate, washed thoroughly, painted his cuts with iodine and worked till dark with his wife cleaning up their house. That evening the somewhat sybaritic physician sat down to dinner and then relaxed, as he had done the night before in Hiroshima—twenty-four hours and an age earlier—over a few cups of wine.

The doctor sipping his wine that night had one thing in common with Mrs. Susukida and Michiyoshi Nukushina, both lying injured and untended in the emergency hospital on Ninoshima Island. None of them knew what it was that had destroyed their city. Nor did they yet have either time or inclination to wonder.

But others, outside Hiroshima, were anxiously trying to find out what the *Enola Gay* had dropped on the city. The search for information was a frustrating one.

At first there had been no indication that anything unusual had happened in Hiroshima. A moment after 8:16 A.M., the

Tokyo control operator of the Japanese Broadcasting Corporation noticed that his telephone line to the radio station in Hiroshima had gone dead. He tried to re-establish his connection, but found that he could not get a call through to the western city.

Twenty minutes later the men in the railroad signal center in Tokyo realized that the main-line telegraph had stopped working. The break seemed to be just north of Hiroshima. Reports began to come in from stations near Hiroshima that there had been some kind of an explosion in the city. The railroad signalmen forwarded the messages to Army General Headquarters.

It was almost ten o'clock when Ryugen Hosokawa, managing editor of the *Asahi* vernacular newspaper in Tokyo, received a telephone call at his home. It was the office, reporting that Hiroshima had "almost completely collapsed" as the result of bombing by enemy planes. Hosokawa hurried to the office and sifted through the reports collected by *Asahi*'s relay room. Every one of them sounded to him like something quite different from any previous bombing. This must have been caused, he thought to himself, by very unusual bombs.

At about the same time Major Tosaku Hirano, a staff officer of the II Army Corps, was in General Headquarters in Tokyo. He had come up from Hiroshima a week earlier to report on the status of military supplies in the port city, and had been scheduled to fly back on Sunday. But he had put his departure off for a day or two and thus was still in the capital.

Now his telephone rang. It was a call from Central Command Headquarters in Osaka, an installation under the control of the II Army Corps in Hiroshima, reporting that its communications to Hiroshima and points west had failed.

Tokyo GHQ tried several times to raise the Hiroshima communications center, in the earth-and-concrete bunker next to the moat of the old castle, but could not get through. There was no explanation. The succession of reports from the radio network, from the railroad signal center, from *Asahi*'s newsroom and from Osaka indicated that something serious had happened, but no one could find out what it was.

Then, shortly after 1 P.M., General Headquarters finally heard from the II Army Corps. The message was short but stunning: "Hiroshima has been annihilated by one bomb and fires are spreading."

This flash came not from Corps Headquarters but from the Army shipping depot on the Hiroshima water front, which was outside the blast area and was not reached by the fire that followed. There was considerable damage at the shipping depot, something in the neighborhood of 30 per cent, but officers there were able to get a message out as far as Kure, where the naval station relayed it to Tokyo. There was no word at all from the II Army Corps Headquarters at the old castle in the northern part of town.

Reports continued to trickle in. By the middle of the afternoon, the Army knew that only three enemy planes had been over Hiroshima when the bomb exploded. It had been told that two of these did not drop any bombs. This information supported the startling assertion in the first flash that there had been only one bomb exploded. Something very big, and very frightening, had hit Hiroshima.

In mid-afternoon the managing editors of the five big Tokyo newspapers, plus their counterpart in the Domei news agency, were called to the office of the government Information and Intelligence Agency, which had charge of press and radio censorship. An Army press officer addressed the little group of newsmen:

"We believe that the bomb dropped on Hiroshima is different

from an ordinary one. However, we have inadequate information now, and we intend to make some announcement when proper information has been obtained. Until we issue such an announcement, run the news in an obscure place in your papers and as one no different from one reporting an ordinary air raid on a city."

In other words, the lid was on. The Army already had a strong suspicion that the Hiroshima bomb might be an atomic weapon. Japanese Naval intelligence had reported U.S. work on the bomb in late 1944, noting the interest of the American government in buying up all available pitchblende (uranium ore). Thus, although the best scientists in Japan had agreed that there was no chance of the United States producing a fission bomb in less than three to five years, there was now immediate suspicion that an atomic bomb had fallen. But the Army, anxious to keep the war going so it could fight a showdown hand-to-hand battle with the Americans on Japanese soil, was determined to withhold the news from the Japanese people as long as it could.

The editors protested mildly, but the decision stood. At six o'clock that evening, the radio gave the people of Japan their first hint that Hiroshima had been chosen for a place in history as the spot where man first proved he could tear apart the basic structure of his world. A listener, however, would have been hard put to deduce the true story from the first news item as it was read:

A few B-29s hit Hiroshima city at 8:20 A.M. August 6, and fled after dropping incendiaries and bombs. The extent of the damage is now under survey.

This cryptic item was repeated several times between six and nine o'clock without further explanation. On the nine o'clock program in Osaka, the sound of the musical chime that signaled the switch from national to local news was followed by this item:

An announcement by the Osaka railway bureau in regard to changes in various transportation organs and changes in handling of passenger baggage:

First of all, the government lines. Regarding the down train, trains from Osaka will turn back from Mihara on the Sanyo line. From Mihara to Kaitichi, the trains will take the route around Kure. . . .

Mihara was about halfway from Osaka to Hiroshima. Kaitichi was on the southeastern edge of Hiroshima. Trains headed there from Osaka on the main line ordinarily ran through the Hiroshima yards and station before swinging back to the smaller community.

The morning *Asahi* in Tokyo on August 7 carried a long front-page story with a sizable headline reporting "Small and Medium Cities Attacked by 400 B-29s." At the end of this story, there was a four-line item tacked on. It read:

Hiroshima Attacked by Incendiary Bombs

Hiroshima was attacked August 6th by two B-29 planes, which dropped incendiary bombs.

The planes invaded the city around 7:50 A.M. It seems that some damage was caused to the city and its vicinity.

Those who survived in Hiroshima still did not know what it was that had struck them so viciously the day before. They did not have much time for thinking about it. Merely keeping alive was a full-time job. Some thought, as they fled the burning city, that the Americans had deluged their homes with "Molotov flower baskets," as the unhappily familiar incendiary clusters were nicknamed. Others, sniffing the air and detecting a strong

192

"electric smell," decided that some kind of poison gas had been dropped. Another explanation was that a magnesium powder had been sprayed on the city, exploding wherever it fell on trolley wires and other exposed electrical conductors.

The prefectural government did what it could to bring order into the city. Somehow almost two hundred policemen were found for duty on August 7. They set to work, with whatever help they could commandeer, to clear the streets of bodies and debris. Police stations became emergency food depots, doling out hastily gathered supplies of rice, salt, pickled radishes, matches, canned goods, candles, straw sandals and toilet paper.

The governor of Hiroshima prefecture, Genshin Takano, issued a proclamation:

People of Hiroshima Prefecture: Although damage is great, we must remember that this is war. We must feel absolutely no fear. Already plans are being drawn up for relief and restoration measures. . . .

We must not rest a single day in our war effort. . . . We must bear in mind that the annihilation of the stubborn enemy is our road to revenge. We must subjugate all difficulties and pain, and go forward to battle for our Emperor.

But most people in Hiroshima, if they could overcome their pain on this second day of the atomic age, were more concerned with finding their loved ones than with battling for their Emperor.

Yuko Yamaguchi, waiting out the war in the rented suburban farmhouse while her husband served overseas in the Army, was unhurt. So were her three little children. But her father-in-law, who had driven into the city Sunday for the meeting of his gas company board of directors, and her mother-in-law, who had left early Monday morning to fetch more supplies from their requisitioned city house, had not been heard from since the bomb fell. Yuko had had no word, either, from her own parents.

So at 6:30 this Tuesday morning, she left her children and set out for the city, walking the whole way because the suburban rail lines were not running. It was a long walk. By the time she reached the Red Cross hospital, where she thought her in-laws might have been taken, it was noon.

Yuko did not find her husband's parents there. But, by sheerest chance, she found her own father, lying untended on the floor with an ugly wound in the back of his head. He begged his grief-stricken daughter for some water. When she did her best and filled a broken cup with stagnant water from a nearby pond, the delirious eye specialist was furious, insisting that ice and a slice of lemon be added to make it more palatable. Somehow, she found both in the wrecked hospital kitchen and made him as comfortable as possible. Then she started through the littered, jammed wards and halls to search for her other relatives. Again she found no trace of her in-laws, but at five o'clock she came on her own mother, lying unconscious, her face smashed almost beyond recognition and her intestines bared by a savage stomach wound.

Daughter dragged mother through the corridors to her father's side so the two could at least be together. There was little enough time. Near dusk the mother died, and Yuko had to carry the body outside, build a crude pyre and cremate it herself. At about dawn her father also died. This time, there were enough other corpses on hand so the hospital arranged a makeshift mass cremation, and Yuko left. She spent the day searching again for her husband's parents, but there was no trace of them, and she finally walked home to the hills to join her children. It was to be more than a month before she found any trace of her in-laws. Then she got only the stub of a commutation ticket bearing her mother-in-law's name, recovered from the wreckage of the train she had been riding at 8:16 A.M. Monday. A few charred bones uncovered still later in the burned-out office of the gas company president were the only trace ever found of her father-in-law.

Some who survived seemed to accept with stoicism the death of their loved ones. Miho Sakamoto, who with her husband's parents had escaped the blast and fire because their home was protected by the city's only high hill, was told on August 7 that her husband's military unit had been completely wiped out. She shed no tears and showed no emotion. Four days later, she visited the ruins of the building in which he had died, found a bent ash tray which she recognized as his and brought it home. That night, she seemed in good spirits when she went upstairs to the room she had shared with her Tsuneo. The next morning she did not come down to breakfast. Her mother-in-law found her lying in front of a little altar, the ash tray in front of her beside a photograph of her dead husband, the razor with which she had cut her throat still clutched in her hand. She left a note of apology to "My Honorable Father and Mother":

What I am about to do, I do not do on sudden impulse; nor is it due to temporary agitation. It is a mutual vow exchanged with my husband while he still lived. This is the road to our greatest happiness and we proceed thereon. Like a bird which has lost one wing, we are crippled birds who cannot go through life without one another. There is no other way. Please, do not bewail my fate. Somewhere both of us will again be living happily together as we have in the past. . . . My honorable Tsuneo must be anxiously awaiting me and I must rush to his side.

Sixteen-year-old Junichiro Susukida, at his factory-school dormitory in Otake, sixteen miles west of Hiroshima, had seen the fireball and the great cloud that rose over the city Monday morning. When the first refugees arrived with the news that the city had been badly hit, he was one of many students who demanded permission to go to their homes, and he was one of five finally allowed to go into the city to contact authorities at the main school building and seek news of the students' families.

By the time they reached Miya-jima, on the southwestern edge of the city, the students could see the fires still burning in the bright late afternoon. As they came closer, they began to realize the full extent of the calamity. It was dark before the boys reached their home neighborhood and began their search for relatives. Junichiro, though unable to find either his mother or younger brother, did at least encounter neighbors who told him his brother had survived, though wounded, and had been taken to the home of other relatives in Fuchu. He could learn nothing about his mother, however, and finally headed back to his dormitory in Otake. Dead tired when he arrived at 2 A.M., he was nevertheless too distraught to sleep. He sat in the school auditorium and incongruously played the piano until fatigue finally subdued his nerves just before dawn on Tuesday, August 7.

Junichiro was not the only one who did not sleep that night. In Tokyo, the truth about Hiroshima was beginning to be revealed in ways that made it clear that the facts could not be kept from the people of Japan much longer.

A little before midnight on the sixth, the Tokyo office of Domei, the quasi-governmental news agency that served the whole nation, much as the Associated Press or Reuters do in the west, received a bulletin from Okayama prefecture, just east of

Hiroshima. It was followed by a longer dispatch: the first eye-witness account of the bombing by a professional newsman.

Bin Nakamura, subchief of Domei's Hiroshima bureau, had been eating breakfast in his suburban garden when the bomb's explosion lifted him off the straw mat on which he was sitting and sent a wave of "immense" heat washing over his face. Once Nakamura discovered that the concussion and heat had not been caused by the nearby explosion of a "blockbuster"—his first re-action had been the typical one—he went to work as a reporter. On his bicycle and on foot, he spent the day in the city and talking to the refugees who streamed through his suburb. Then, at 10 P.M., like the experienced press-association man he was, he found communications at the suburban Haramura radio sta-tion and dictated a story to Okayama, the only point he could reach. In his dispatch, he said there was no way to tell what kind of a bomb had caused such havoc.

But before the night was much older the editors of Domei, and the leaders of Japan, had a way of telling much more about the bomb. In Saitama prefecture outside Tokyo, Domei operated a big monitoring station where nearly fifty workers, many of them Nisei girls born in the United States, listened to broadcasts from American stations. About 1 A.M. on the 7th of August (noon on the 6th in Washington, D.C.), Hideo Kinoshita, chief of the monitoring room, was awakened by the Japanese youth who had charge of the operation that night. The boy reported that U.S. stations were all broadcasting a statement by President Truman, describing the weapon that had been dropped on Hiroshima as "an atomic bomb." Kinoshita listened to the account and the boy's explanation of what "atomic bomb" might mean. Then he quickly called his own superior, Saiji Hasegawa, Domei's foreign news chief. Hasegawa was asleep in his hotel. When he was told of an "atomic bomb," he had no idea what it was, but although he was irritated at being awakened he hustled to his office. When he saw the text transcripts that were beginning to come through from the Saitama monitors, he was glad he had come to work. He reached for his telephone and called Hisatsune Sakomizu, chief secretary of the cabinet.

Sakomizu sleepily answered his bedside telephone, then came suddenly wide awake as he listened to the Domei executive. He already knew, from the first confused reports on the 6th, that the Americans had used some kind of new weapon. Now, learning that it was an atomic bomb, something the cabinet had discussed briefly almost a year earlier, he knew it meant just one thing: the war was over.

Sakomizu quickly called Prime Minister Suzuki, with whom he had been working in the effort to arrange a peace settlement by negotiation. They knew immediately, he said later,

. . . that if the announcement were true, no country could carry on a war. Without the atomic bomb it would be impossible for any country to defend itself against a nation which had the weapon. The chance had come to end the war. It was not necessary to blame the military side, the manufacturing people, or anyone else—just the atomic bomb. It was a good excuse.

The Army, however, was unwilling to accept this attitude, despite the urgings of the peace group that the bomb gave military leaders a chance to save face by blaming the "backwardness of scientific research" for Japan's inability to counter the new American bomb. The generals, sitting in an emergency cabinet meeting on the seventh, pointedly recalled an old Japanese legend about an Army commander who became a laughingstock because he mistook the fluttering of a flight of birds for the sound of an approaching enemy and fled. They argued that the bomb was not atomic but was merely a huge conventional projectile. They flatly refused Foreign Minister Togo's proposal to take up for immediate consideration the possibility of surrender on the terms of the Potsdam ultimatum, and insisted on keeping the Truman atomic statement from the Japanese people until the Army could conduct an "investigation" on the ground at Hiroshima.

The military had already started such a check. Major Hirano, the staff officer from the Hiroshima headquarters whose desire to spend a couple of extra nights in Tokyo had saved his life, called Yoshio Nishina, the nation's ranking nuclear scientist. He told him of the Truman claims and asked him to ride down to Hiroshima in his little liaison plane to investigate the matter. Nishina agreed to make the trip. The scientist was already pretty well convinced, on the basis of Hirano's report and further excerpts from the Truman statement given him a few minutes later by a reporter, that the bomb had indeed been the fission weapon which he and his colleagues had believed the United States could not manufacture so quickly. Truman's claim of a destructive power equal to twenty thousand tons of TNT coincided exactly with theoretical calculations made recently by one of Nishina's laboratory associates on the yield of an atomic bomb.

But the Army high command was keeping the lid on tight. When the Tokyo managing editors met again with the Information Agency censors that afternoon, they all had seen the text of Truman's statement. But they got nowhere with requests for permission to print it. The Army grudgingly allowed use of the phrase "a new-type bomb," but not the word "atomic." The editors argued hard this time, but to no avail. The end result of the wrangle was this communiqué from Imperial General Head-quarters at 3:30 P.M. on Tuesday, August 7:

1. A considerable amount of damage was caused by a few B-29s which attacked Hiroshima August 6th.
2. It seems that the enemy used a new-type bomb in the raid. Investigation of the effects is under way.

By evening, the newsmen were stretching the Army embargo as far as they could. A home service broadcast at 7 P.M. amplified the cryptic communiqué by adding that "a considerable number of houses were reduced to ashes and fires broke out in various parts of the city . . . investigations are now being made with regard to the effectiveness of the bomb, which should not be regarded as light." The broadcast went on to attack the Americans for "inhuman and atrocious conduct" and to urge Japanese not to be "misled" by "exaggerated propaganda" such as "an announcement regarding the use of a new-type bomb" by Truman.

One man who was not likely to be "misled" by any announcement that night was Major Hirano, who finally had started back to Hiroshima in his five-seater liaison plane late in the afternoon. He had arrived at the Tokyo airport with the hurriedly assembled team of investigators earlier in the day, but had been ordered to wait until afternoon to avoid the U.S. Navy fighter planes that were now operating over Japan daily. There was some top brass in the inspection group which apparently was not anxious to hasten the day of personal contact with American invaders. Thus it was almost seven in the evening when Hirano's plane came down over Hiroshima. It was still light, however, so he got the full picture with shocking suddenness:

The Face of Death

Being a soldier, my eye had been inured to the effects of bombing by that time. But this was a different sight. *There were no roads in the wastes that spread below our eyes:* that was my first impression. In the case of a normal air raid, roads were still visible after it was over. But in Hiroshima, everything was flattened and all roads were undiscernibly covered with debris.

When Hirano stepped from his plane, the first person he saw was an Air Force officer who came out on the runway to meet the team from Tokyo. His face was marked by a sharp dividing line right down the middle. One side was smooth and unhurt. The other, the one that had been toward the explosion, was burned, blistered, blackened. The investigators picked their way through the city to the wreckage of II Army Corps headquarters. Nobody was there. They finally found what was left of the head-quarters—a few officers holed up in a hillside cave. By the time they began their formal investigation the next morning, the men from Tokyo knew the truth anyway. Hirano, in fact, had known it the moment he caught sight of what was left of Hiroshima from his circling plane, just as Bob Caron had known it for the first time at 8:16 A.M. the day before, when he looked back from the *Enola Gay*.

CHAPTER TEN

Home Is the Hunter

WHEN Little Boy produced its split-second holocaust, none of the Americans in the bomber overhead could know that Hiroshima already was a missing city. The airmen wearing opaque goggles had sensed, rather than seen, a purple light of frightening intensity. It flashed through the three bombers in an instant and vanished as suddenly as it came.

Two of the B-29s, the *Enola Gay* and the *Great Artiste,* were eight miles from the point of explosion, rolling out of a tight downward turn to the northeast at an airspeed of 250 miles an hour. The planes were still almost five miles high after nosing down to gain speed. The third plane of the formation, George Marquardt's No. 91, was seventeen miles away, headed directly at the ballooning fireball with camera running.

In the moments after the explosion, men in the bombers were too busy to catalogue their feelings. Paul Tibbets ripped off his goggles and his eyes swept by long habit across the instrument panel. Co-pilot Lewis, with the turn being made to his side, had snatched off his goggles before the flash. It had been impossible for him to see the instruments through the dark glasses. Jeppson kept his eyes fixed on the bomb console, but regretted it at once, for with the bomb gone, there was nothing more for him to monitor. Ferebee had forgotten his goggles and had been momentarily blinded by what he could only compare to a photographer's flash bulb going off an inch in front of his face. He wondered if his sight had been impaired.

When the *Gay* completed its turn, Tibbets pulled the nose up again to gain altitude and slow the plane down. Scientists had warned that a shock wave probably would hit the plane about a minute after the bomb exploded. If the plane were climbing away at slower speed, the impact would be less, the aerodynamics experts calculated.

In the *Great Artiste,* where the windows of the after compartment had been taped over to make a dark room for the blast measuring equipment, the three scientists saw the flash shoot down the bomb-bay tunnel from the cockpit. It was as though a light bulb had been turned on and off in the thirty-foot tunnel. Alvarez, Johnston and Agnew were preoccupied with their film. Blast waves, telemetered from the parachuted transmitters, cut jagged lines on the film like a cardiogram. Chuck Sweeney and his co-pilot, Captain Donald Albury, leveled off after the downward escape run.

In No. 91 Bernard Waldman, the Notre Dame physicist, took pictures from the nose, flying straight toward the point of explosion. Waldman had less than a minute of film in his fast movie camera and he had counted out loud, beginning the instant the radio tone signal ceased. He was hunched in the bombardier's seat, using the camera in the same position where the bombsight usually operated. At forty seconds, or three seconds before the expected detonation, he started the camera, recording the first appearance of the fireball and smoke column. As No. 91 turned away from the debris over Hiroshima, First Lieutenant Russell E. Gackenbach, the twenty-two-year-old navigator, snapped some pictures from a little pocket camera. They turned out to be among the best taken. Waldman's pictures never panned out for a variety of causes, including dark-room troubles on Tinian.

Bob Caron, in the *Enola Gay*'s tail, saw a shimmering line rushing toward the plane. It had the appearance of a heat wave as seen far down an asphalt highway, but it extended in a long curve like a ripple from a rock tossed in a pond. Caron was see-ing the first rarefaction wave from an atomic bomb, caused by heavy compression of air followed by a vacuum in which vapor condensed instantaneously, forming a belt of speeding mist. The shock wave rushed at the plane at a speed of twelve miles a minute. Although its probable force had been stressed in brief-ings, the wave astounded occupants of the three planes with its violence. Caron felt as though some aerial monster had thumped the *Gay*'s tail with its paw. "Flak!" yelled Tibbets involuntarily. Parsons, who had been through air combat also, had a similar reaction. He felt as though a large anti-aircraft shell had burst twenty feet from the plane. But Parsons knew what it was. "No, no," he yelled at Tibbets. "That's not flak. That's it—the shock. We're in the clear now." The shock wave gave some the feel-ing that the bombers were being beaten with a telegraph pole. Marquardt had the sensation of a huge hand striking the fuselage immediately under his side cockpit window.

A second shock wave, this one a reflection of the blast from the ground, struck the bombers, but this time there was a warn-ing. "Here comes another one," said Caron on the intercom from his rear vantage point.

Once the peril to life and aircraft had passed, the planes flew south along the outskirts of Hiroshima and now, for the first time, the bomber crews observed what they had wrought.

"Holy Moses, what a mess," breathed Caron.

"My God," said Lewis, "what have we done?"

Dust boiled up from the entire city and long shafts of swirling gray matter rushed toward the center. A column of white smoke, incredibly tidy in form, stood straight up. At the base it was flecked with red and orange and at the top it spilled into an almost perfect mushroom. The stem of the strange cloud-flower reminded one man of an enormous grave marker. Within minutes the cloud mushroom pushed upward almost four miles. Then the mushroom split off from the column and began rising swiftly, finally to forty thousand feet. Two hundred miles away, the tail gunner of the *Jabbit III* saw the top of the cloud and told the crew that Hiroshima must be gone. To the three nearby planes, the picture of devastation had incongruities. While a wall of fire appeared to sweep the city beneath the smoke, dust and cloud, the big dock area stood out prominently, apparently unscarred.

Conflicting thoughts and emotions jostled one another in the minds of the airmen. Dutch Van Kirk was stunned at the scope of ruin, yet felt buoyant pride that the bomb had worked and relief that the peak of the mission had passed. Joe Stiborik was simply mystified at the extent of the explosion, but kept thinking how wonderful it would be if the turbulent mass of debris before him should end the war. Lewis thought: What fantastic thing has man brought forth? Jake Beser couldn't relate the scene to reality. It was as though the earth had vented some monstrous passion and the *Enola Gay* had just happened by. Marquardt heard someone say on his intercom: "It's nothing but fire and smoke." Then came a plea: "Don't fly so close to that mushroom." Expressions of awe mingled with yelps of exultation. "The war's over!" shouted one man. "Good God," said another, "could anyone live through that down there?" Jeppson found himself unable to comprehend what he saw. He felt a kind of numbness, a shock in which there was no joy. Waldman experienced a glow of elation, ignited by success, at first, but soon he thought of the people on the ground and was no longer happy.

Alvarez took one look at the sweep of boiling cloud, could see no evidence of a city anywhere and thought: "Ferebee has missed Hiroshima by miles and dropped the bomb somewhere in the country." He confided his speculation to Kermit Beahan, the *Great Artiste*'s bombardier. Beahan shook his head.

"Nope," he said. "You can't see a city because Tom hit the aiming point right on the nose. It was a beautiful job of bombing."

Parsons found calculations pushing his personal feelings aside. He knew that almost a year before Oppenheimer at Los Alamos had estimated that the first U-235 bomb would have a blast equivalent of ten thousand tons of TNT. It's at least that large, Parsons conjectured. The only question is—how much larger? Strangely enough, none of the technicians in the three planes was surprised at the fact of success. Although Little Boy, unlike Fat Man, had never been tested with its fissionable material, the scientists had been confident the U-235 projectile would work the first time. Only the scope of the havoc wrought was beyond the ken of their calculations.

As the planes flew a semicircle for observation, more cameras went into action. Johnston took color films from the *Great Artiste*. Caron used an Army K-20 in the tail of the *Enola Gay*.

"Better turn off, Colonel," Caron warned Tibbets. "That mushroom seems to be coming downwind at us."

Slowly the flight of three planes turned southeast and headed for Tinian Island. Several minutes before, as he straightened out from the escape run and the second shock wave passed, Tibbets had ordered a radio message sent in the clear. Tapped out by Nelson on his Morse key, it notified Tinian that the *Enola Gay* had bombed its primary target visually with good results; one-tenth cloud cover; no fighters, no flak.

Now Parsons wrote out a second message, using the code that he and Farrell had agreed upon. It read: "82 V 670. Able, Line 1, Line 2, Line 6, Line 9."

In the war operations room of the 313th Wing on Tinian, a knot of men, including Farrell, Purnell, Ashworth and Moyna- han, had been waiting restlessly for hours. Purnell had idly swung a golf club shaft used as a pointer by briefing officers. Farrell had fidgeted with his glasses and run his finger over his smudged copy of the code a dozen times, even though he had long since memorized the whole thing. An enlisted man brought the first strike message. The group huddled around it. Farrell was sur- prised. He hadn't counted on a dispatch in the clear. Besides, this told them little except that the bomb had been dropped. They were still arguing about it when the second message arrived. One glance told Farrell: Success. Without referring to his code sheet, he translated Parsons' message aloud:

"Clear cut, successful in all respects. Visible effects greater than Trinity [the New Mexico test]. Hiroshima. Conditions nor- mal in airplane following delivery, proceeding to regular base."

Farrell whooped with glee. They pounded one another on the back. After a few seconds of excited chatter, Farrell took a yellow sheet of Army Signal Corps dispatch paper and wrote this message in ink:

From: KKEE 060006 Z (Aug. 6, 10:06 A.M., Tinian time)
To: War
To Soso personal from Farrell for O'Leary:
    Table six line 25 [target] at table six line 17 [Hiroshima] attacked visually one-tenth cloud cover at 052315 Z. No fighters and no flak. Results by radio from Judge [Parsons] at 052330 Z as follows: Results clear cut, successful in all respects. Visible effects greater than Trinity. Conditions normal in airplane following delivery, proceeding to Papacy [Tinian]. Recommend you go all out with release program. Personal confirmation from Judge later. Congratulations from all.

This dispatch to Groves, addressed for security reasons to his secretary, Mrs. O'Leary, broke the long months of secrecy in the 509th Composite Group. The word quickly passed around the camp. Lou Schaffer of the M.P.s was sipping coffee in 509th headquarters when an officer burst into the hut.

"They did it," he shouted. "They wrecked Hiroshima. Tibbets is on his way home."

The word traveled to the air-conditioned bomb hut where scientists and men of the 1st Ordnance Squadron were hard at work on the second bomb, a Fat Man or plutonium weapon. Ramsey tuned a short-wave radio set to the Tokyo frequency. It wasn't long before the smooth and cheery voice of Tokyo Rose came on. She announced there had been a small raid by three airplanes on Hiroshima. An hour or so later, with no further reference to the raid, the station announced that train service to Hiroshima had been discontinued temporarily.

Homeward bound on what the airmen called the Hirohito highway, the *Enola Gay* and its escorts crossed Shikoku after flying over the inland sea. Far below the men could see heavily wooded mountains rolling to the Pacific, where little towns huddled near the shoreline. It was a scene of utter peace as though only nature was real and the war was a thing of dreams.

Near the coast Ferebee noted about twenty bursts of anti-aircraft fire, first of the day for the *Gay*, but the shells exploded haplessly about fifteen thousand feet below the plane and the white puffs drifted away in the morning sunlight like sticks of cotton candy tossed in a strong wind. The *Gay* had but one alarm. Caron had gone forward to the waist section for a sandwich.

"Fighter coming up behind," someone warned on the intercom.

Caron hurried back to the tail, wriggled into his gunner's seat and readied his twin .50s, scant protection against a cannon-firing Jap fighter. But there were no enemy planes. It was only Sweeney, closing from behind. The *Great Artiste* pulled abreast and settled down off the *Gay*'s wing for the long flight home.

Once the coast of Shikoku dropped away behind the bombers, tension evaporated. Everybody talked. Questions were on all lips. How many Japanese had been killed? How much of the city destroyed? Suppose the war will be over by the time we land? How many of these bombs do we have? Tibbets gave a brief history of the Manhattan project and the 509th's part in Silver Plate. Shumard wondered just how the bomb worked. Parsons was the only man aboard who knew and he wasn't talking about it. Beser told Shumard to think of it as a kind of airborne atom smasher. Lewis said he thought he could taste the fission, a kind of flat, metallic flavor. Ferebee wondered how much radiation they had absorbed and speculated whether it would make them all sterile. Parsons said there was little chance of that and explained that the radiation from an air burst was far less than from an atomic bomb exploding on the ground.

Some men philosophized. Lewis mused that man could not possibly continue wars with a weapon like this one in existence without blowing up the whole world. In the cockpit of the *Jabbit III*, Willie Wilson leaned across to his co-pilot, Carrington. Neither man was sure just what had happened, although their radio had picked up the successful strike report and their tail gunner had reported the top of a towering smoke column in the vicinity of Hiroshima.

"If this thing is as powerful as they say," said Wilson, "the nations will have to find some way of settling disputes without going to war."

Carrington had never considered the question before. He said he guessed so and wondered vaguely if their mission might indeed someday change the world.

In No. 91, crew members pressed physicist Waldman for an explanation of the atomic bomb. He reviewed the history of the effort and told of his own beginning in atomic research in 1938 when he had worked on a high voltage electrostatic generator at Notre Dame. He still carried radiation burns and showed them to the crew. There was scar tissue on fingers of his right hand and on the biceps of the right arm. He ended his story simply with a shake of his head.

"You boys made history today," he said.

Many men naturally thought of home: Sweeney of his Army nurse wife, Marquardt of the girl he had married only ten days before coming overseas, Jeppson of his baby daughter, Nancy, whom he had seen but once before flying to the Pacific. Alvarez thought of his wife, his four-year-old son, Walter, and his baby daughter, Jean. On a sudden inspiration, Alvarez began scribbling a letter to his son. In the upper right hand corner of a piece of tablet paper, he began, "August 6, 1945, 10 miles off the Jap coast at 28,000 feet." Then he wrote in part:

Dear Walter, This is the first grown-up letter I have ever written to you, and it is really for you to read when you are older. . . . Today the lead plane of our little formation dropped a single bomb which probably exploded with the force of 15,000 tons of high explosive. That means that the days of large bombing raids, with several hundred planes, are finished. A single plane disguised as a friendly transport can now wipe out a city. That means to me that nations will have to get along together in a friendly fashion, or suffer the consequences of sudden sneak attacks which can cripple them overnight.

What regrets I have about being a party to killing and maiming thousands of Japanese civilians this morning are tempered with the hope that this terrible weapon we have created may bring the countries of the world together and prevent further wars. Alfred Nobel thought that his invention of high explosives would have this effect, by making wars too terrible, but unfortunately it had just the opposite reaction. Our new destructive force is so many thousands of times worse that it may realize Nobel's dream. . . .

Caron reported to Tibbets when the top of the Hiroshima mushroom finally faded from sight. Van Kirk estimated that they were 363 nautical miles from Hiroshima. Talk faded with the cloud and a score of men in the bombers fell sound asleep. For some it was the first sleep in forty-eight hours. Below them submarines and PBYs circled on station, ready for rescue operations should any plane be forced to ditch. But the engines thrummed on with comforting monotony. Sweeney throttled back. He felt the *Enola Gay* should land first. It was Tibbets' hour, not his.

The *Enola Gay* touched down at North Field at 2:58 P.M., Tinian time, twelve hours and thirteen minutes after take-off. She was forty thousand pounds lighter after expenditure of fuel and bomb and she had traveled more than twenty-eight hundred miles. Her props formed glistening circles in the afternoon heat and the huge R on her tail seemed to quiver a little as Tibbets braked the plane. He was nine minutes ahead of Sweeney and thirty-seven minutes ahead of Marquardt. The *Gay* taxied to her hardstand, the last propeller turned to a halt and the men scrambled out behind the nose wheel.

Two hundred officers and enlisted men crowded under the *Gay*'s wings, including more generals and admirals than most of the plane's crew had ever seen before. The greeting delegation stood a bit self-consciously with hands on hips. They wore mussed khakis and only the collar bars and headgear differentiated them. The Air Force officers wore the floppy caps without the metal frame inside, "50 mission crush caps," the mark of the World War II flier. The Army officers retained the stiff top. Gold visor trim set off the ranking Navy officers. There were Tooey Spaatz, new Strategic Air Force boss; Lieutenant General Nathan F. Twining, new chief of the Marianas Air Force; Brigadier General John Davies, 313th Wing Commander; Farrell, Purnell, Ashworth.

"Attention to orders!" barked Davies.

Spaatz stepped forward and pinned the Distinguished Service Cross on the breast of Tibbets' dirty flight coveralls. Tibbets, his eyes red-rimmed from lack of sleep and his lower jaw hours overdue for a shave, was caught off guard. He hastily palmed his pipe in his left hand and tucked the stem under the sleeve of his coveralls. Spaatz shook Tibbets' hand and the crowd milled around again. Every man of the *Gay* was the center of a group of eager interviewers. Later every military man participating in the mission was decorated, although none of the four civilian physicists on the raid ever was.

Spaatz threw his arm around Beser's shoulders.

"How did it go, son?" the general asked the lieutenant.

Spaatz obviously was skeptical of the extent of the damage and he questioned Beser for ten minutes. Nolan, the M.D. and radiologist, examined the eyes of Ferebee and others who had failed to put on goggles when the bomb fell.

"It's not my eyes I'm worried about, Doc," said Ferebee. "It's my manhood."

Nolan assured all hands that they were in no danger of reproductive handicaps from radiation. This was an understatement. Ferebee later became the father of four children and Sweeney of eight.

At the official interrogation in the Quonset hut officers' club, Spaatz sat at the head of a long table and the crew of the *Gay* drew up chairs around it. Every man on the flight got a shot of bourbon whisky in a glass of lemonade and two more drinks for the asking. Hazen Payette, the rotund Detroit lawyer, conducted the questioning.

"Dutch," he asked Van Kirk, "what time was the drop made?"

Van Kirk consulted his pad. "At 091517 K (seventeen seconds past 9:15 A.M. Tinian time)," he said.

"Why were you late?"

The sally brought a roar of laughter. The first atomic bomb in war had been released exactly seventeen seconds after the time that had been scheduled days before. The interrogation lasted two hours. Occasionally a man would prop his head in his hands as fatigue got the best of him. Ferebee offered a story he repeated for months. He said he released the bomb thirteen and a half feet northeast of the assigned aiming point. Actually, as it was learned in Hiroshima later, the bomb exploded seven hundred feet from the bridge at which it was aimed, remarkable accuracy for a drop from six miles up. The mission had gone so smoothly that they could afford to joke.

The fruits of fame are perishable. After the interrogation, the *Gay*'s crew joined a hot-dog roast and beer party being given for all men of the 509th. When they arrived the last hot dog and can of beer had been consumed.

Although the news fanned quickly through the 509th, security prohibited mention of the atom to the thousands of other men on the island. When Jeppson returned to his tent, he found a boyhood friend from Nevada, Navy Lieutenant Jack Scott. Jeppson had played the piano and Scott the violin in a second-grade school show in Carson City, but it had been several years since they had seen each other. Scott was flying rescue missions, retrieving downed Air Force fliers from the sea off the coast of Japan.

"What you been up to?" asked Scott.

"We just won the war today," said Jeppson, deadpan.

Scott took his friend over to the Navy officers' club as a prize exhibit.

"Tell those guys what you told me," he ordered.

"Well," said Jeppson, hoisting a drink, "you fellows won't have to fly any more missions. The Air Force has just finished the war."

A profane and raucous outburst of disbelief greeted this announcement, which he declined to amplify. He did, however, make a mental note to revisit his Navy friends a few days later after the secret was out.

The photo planes returned to Tinian after nightfall. Interrogation plus the developing of the films only confirmed the information already furnished by the strike crews: Hiroshima was hidden under a mass of cloud and smoke. The pilots reported that upon arrival, four hours after the explosion, the cloud debris still reached to forty thousand feet. The top layer had a bluish cast, while smoke and dust gave a brownish yellow tint to the bottom of the ugly cloud. Only the seaward ends of the docks were visible.

The fact was that no American knew that night what had happened at Hiroshima. That the bomb had killed thousands of people and destroyed many blocks of buildings was taken for granted by Parsons, Farrell and others familiar with the Alamogordo test, but the evidence was all circumstantial. There was no certain way to know that an entire city had been devastated.

After developing their blast measurement films, Alvarez, Johnston and Agnew consulted with other scientists and concluded that the Hiroshima blast had been equal to about eight thousand tons of TNT, or slightly less than Oppenheimer had predicted and considerably less than Alvarez had guessed on the return flight. Later, however, they found an error in their calculations and finally pegged the explosive force at about seventeen thousand tons of TNT. When the White House statement was released a few hours later, it said twenty thousand tons, a figure based on the Alamogordo shot. This slight error of overstatement was never corrected publicly.

Farrell had slipped out of the interrogation of the *Enola Gay* crew before it ended to file a more complete report to Groves in Washington. It had been almost eight hours since his first bulletin. Now, at 5:50 P.M. Tinian time, he sent a message, addressed "O'Leary," which described details of the flight, then added:

Flash not so blinding as Trinity because of bright sunlight. First there was a ball of fire changing in a few seconds to purple clouds

and flames boiling and swirling upward. Flash observed just after airplane rolled out of turn. All agreed light was intensely bright. . . .
Entire city except outermost ends of dock areas was covered with a dark gray dust layer which joined the cloud column. It was extremely turbulent with flashes of fire visible in the dust. Estimated diameter of this dust layer is at least three miles. One observer stated it looked as though whole town was being torn apart with columns of dust rising out of valleys approaching the town. Due to dust visual observations of structural damage could not be made.

Judge and other observers felt this strike was tremendous and awesome even in comparison with Tr. Its effects may be attributed by the Japanese to a huge meteor.

Washington was fourteen hours behind Tinian. Farrell's first message, which should have arrived about 8:30 P.M., Sunday, August 5, was delayed in transit and did not reach Groves until shortly before midnight. He read it carefully at his desk in the new War Department building in Foggy Bottom after an officer courier had rushed it across the Potomac from the Pentagon message center. Groves decided not to disturb General Marshall and other authorities at that late hour, but to wait for amplification. He lay down on a cot in his office and went to sleep.

In the outer office, a dozen Manhattan headquarters aides, including Jean O'Leary, John Derry, Bill Consodine, John Lansdale and Fred Rhodes, kept an all-night vigil. Consodine and Derry had cots in an office across the hall. They hadn't been out of the building for three days, but now they couldn't sleep. Emergency quarters had been rigged for Mrs. O'Leary in a first-aid room down the hall, but she preferred to sit up too. Soon after midnight a poker game got under way on the top of an office desk. At 2 A.M. Fred Rhodes got a call from his sister. His father had just died and he went home after waking Groves and getting emergency leave. The poker game went on. Mrs. O'Leary gradually accumulated a winning stack of nickels, dimes, quarters and dollar bills.

At 4:15 A.M. an officer courier handed a plain War Department envelope to Jean O'Leary. It was addressed, "Major O'Leary." The Army decoding officer at the Pentagon hadn't the slightest idea who "O'Leary" was and added the title of rank as a guess.

Consodine woke up Groves. Around a pot of coffee, the general gave them the latest news from Farrell and then set to work drafting his official report for General Marshall and Secretary Stimson. Groves shaved and changed into a clean uniform. At 6 A.M. he called George Harrison, Stimson's atomic liaison man, and asked him to meet him at Marshall's office shortly before 7, the hour when Marshall began each working day. Groves and Harrison were waiting when the erect and neatly groomed Army chief of staff entered his office at 6:58 A.M.

The three men agreed that since the bomb had been an obvious success, there was no point in withholding a public announcement. Stimson was resting at his Long Island home after the long sessions at Potsdam. Marshall reached him on the scramble phone at 7:45 A.M., gave him the news and the recommendation. Stimson discussed the form of a message to President Truman, who was aboard the U.S.S. *Augusta,* returning from Potsdam. The message was sent and Harrison called Stimson back four times that morning to keep him abreast of developments.

More details arrived by radio from Farrell shortly before 9 A.M.:

Judge and Yoke [Tibbets] will visit Curfew [Guam] tomorrow to describe operations to Carve [Nimitz]. Yoke awarded DSC by Spaatz on stepping from airplane on return. Errant [Purnell] is still thrilled

217

by the operation which went from start to finish with clock-like precision. Judge's performance was outstanding, including his personal loading of the Pkun [the bomb] in flight to insure safety at take-off. The three air force crews with the primary mission all performed superbly. Our entire efforts are now directed to FM [Fat Man bomb] scheduled as you previously advised.

Marshall, Groves and Harrison decided to speak with Farrell directly on the telecon. At about 10 A.M. (the next midnight on Tinian) they ordered: "Please have General Farrell come to the teletype at the request of the Secretary of War. Please have him stand by there and tell us how long it will take him to get there."

Farrell was getting ready for bed at long last when the message reached him. He pulled his pants on again and drove three miles by jeep, back to wing headquarters. The three men at the Pentagon got Stimson on the scramble phone and this conversation took place, Long Island to Washington to Tinian:

Secwar on telecon. Have you any more information from interrogation of the F-13 [photo] crews? Another question. General Groves wants to know if you see any reason for not releasing information to the American public at once.

Min please.

General Farrell sees no reason why information of Hiroshima strike should not be released to American public at once and strongly recommends such release.

Farrell to Groves. The F-13 crews saw several fires near the dock area in the fringes of the cloud. Their magnitude could not be determined because of the density of the smoke cloud.

Farrell got to sleep at 3 A.M. on Tinian, but was up at six to fly to Guam with Purnell, Parsons, Tibbets and Moynahan. They went into conference with Nimitz, Spaatz and LeMay. Radio

Saipan was bombarding the Marianas with President Truman's announcement of the Hiroshima strike. War correspondents on Guam were boiling at being excluded from one of the biggest stories of all time. Some reporters lamented they would be fired for failure to file dispatches on a mission that had taken place right under their noses. The military officers bowed to shrill demands for an immediate press conference, but the affair was as chilly as truce negotiations between enemy forces. Not only did security restrictions hold down the amount of information, but the order requiring all copy to be cleared in Washington created an impossible log jam. It was hours before Washington acceded to Farrell's plea and permitted newspapermen to send dispatches direct to their own papers.

The military commanders on Guam reached three decisions on the next moves. First, they agreed the date for the second atomic bomb, a plutonium weapon, should be moved up to August 9 from the original plan of August 11. It was reasoned that a swift one-two punch would convince Japanese leaders that Hiroshima was not some freak of nature. Second, they decided to open immediately a propaganda campaign requested by General Marshall. Objective: Quick surrender. Third, Stimson, Marshall and Groves should be persuaded to let them atom-bomb Tokyo, for the psychological effect, and to permit them to waive the requirement for visual bombing. A message was sent at once to Marshall, emphasizing that Spaatz and LeMay agreed on a priority for Tokyo. No answer was received. Later the "Tinian Joint Chiefs" came to the conclusion that if a third atomic bomb was needed to end the war, it should be dropped on Tokyo at night, but the question remained unresolved in Washington.

The decision to move up the date for the second atom strike forced Ramsey's bomb scientists into three shifts, working around the clock. Only that day information arrived from the States, giving results of a dummy bomb test carried out simultaneously with the one off Tinian on the fifth. The electronic specialists had to alter the fuzing mechanism of the Fat Man bomb on the basis of evidence supplied by Alvarez and Parsons from the Hiroshima blast.

Farrell placed Moynahan in charge of the propaganda campaign in company with Navy Lieutenant Robert Morris, a New York lawyer who headed psychological warfare for Nimitz, and Colonel Crocker Snow, an Air Force intelligence officer. They laid plans to drop 16,000,000 leaflets on forty-seven Japanese cities, flood the empire with surrender invitations via Radio Saipan and fly planes equipped with loudspeakers at low altitudes over Japanese urban areas. The Office of War Information printing plant on Saipan could turn out 1,800,000 leaflets a day. Three Japanese prisoners helped with the translation of the propaganda blurbs and surprisingly one of the Japanese suggested that the story of Hiroshima would gain greater credence if printed in a Japanese-language newspaper. The suggestion was adopted and a two-page tabloid newspaper was dropped along with the leaflets. Page 1 of the newspaper carried a picture of the atomic debris cloud rising over Hiroshima as taken by tail gunner Caron of the *Enola Gay*. The leaflet was less subtle than the newspaper. It read:

To the Japanese people:
  America asks that you take immediate heed of what we say on this leaflet.
  We are in possession of the most destructive explosive ever devised by man. A single one of our newly developed atomic bombs is actually the equivalent in explosive power to what 2,000 of our giant B-29s can carry on a single mission. This awful fact is one for you to

ponder and we solemnly assure you that it is grimly accurate.

We have just begun to use this weapon against your homeland. If you still have any doubt, make inquiry as to what happened to Hiroshima when just one atomic bomb fell on that city.

Before using this bomb to destroy every resource of the military by which they are prolonging this useless war, we ask that you now petition the Emperor to end the war. Our President has outlined for you the thirteen consequences of an honorable surrender. We urge that you accept these consequences and begin work of building a new, better and peace-loving Japan.

You should take steps now to cease military resistance. Otherwise, we shall resolutely employ this bomb and all our other superior weapons to promptly and forcefully end the war.

Evacuate your cities now!

General Lauris Norstad in Washington Air Force headquarters added a suggestion in a message to Spaatz. He said Stimson was releasing a map of Hiroshima on which the aiming point was marked.

"It is believed here," said Norstad, "that the accuracy with which this bomb was placed may counter a thought that the CENTERBOARD project involves wanton, indiscriminate bombing. This may be a useful idea for the psychological warfare propaganda now emanating from Guam."

By August 8, two days after Hiroshima, Air Force commanders began to feel a bit heady with the tremendous new weapon for which the airplane was the obvious delivery instrument. Hap Arnold's headquarters sent Spaatz a message which said in part:

Atomic bombing story received largest and heaviest smash play of entire war with three deck banner headlines evening and morning papers, complete 1st page coverage and sidebars running through most pages 2 and 3. Radio networks gave national play with all commentators and newscasters highlighting . . .

It added fuel to the interservice rivalries when Air Force officers realized that General MacArthur, symbol of American land forces in the Pacific, was forbidden by Washington to release any information on the atomic show. Indeed MacArthur had none to give, having himself learned of the bomb's existence only a few days before.

The same day, August 8, thirty-two copies of orders for the second atomic raid on August 9 were mimeographed at Guam headquarters. Top Secret Field Order No. 17 listed but two targets: Primary, "Kokura Arsenal and City;" secondary, "Nagasaki Urban Area."

In the bomb assembly hut on Tinian, scientists permitted Farrell to hold plutonium for the Fat Man bomb in his hands. It felt strangely warm and Farrell wondered anew at this dawning atomic age when such a small and unlikely thing could tear a city from the face of the earth. Again Dr. Nolan called on Flight Surgeon Spike Myers to warn that in event of a take-off crash, he was not to rush in aid before testing for radioactivity. "Oh, no, not again?" said Myers.

This time the precautions were more thorough. Unlike the Little Boy bomb, the Fat Man could not be armed in flight. It had sixty-four detonators arranged in a circle for the "implosion" method of driving the pieces of plutonium into a critical mass. Should the plane crash on take-off, fire could set off the detonators causing an atomic explosion that would level half the island.

In the hours before take-off of the second mission, Alvarez, Phil Morrison and Robert Serber fell to discussing the probable state of atomic knowledge in Japan. These three scientists had known a Japanese physicist, Ryokichi Sagane, before the war. Sagane had studied with them under Lawrence at the University of California Radiation Laboratory in 1938, then returned to

Japan to help build his country's first cyclotron. They speculated that Sagane, now forty-one, would be in the University of Tokyo physics department, if still alive. Why not write him a letter? It was no sooner suggested than Alvarez took a sheet of paper and wrote, in ink:

> Headquarters
> Atomic Bomb Command
> August 9, 1945

To: Prof. R. Sagane

From: Three of your former scientific colleagues during your stay in in the United States

We are sending this as a personal message to urge that you use your influence as a reputable nuclear physicist to convince the Japanese General Staff of the terrible consequences which will be suffered by your people if you continue in this war.

You have known for several years that an atomic bomb could be built if a nation were willing to pay the enormous cost of preparing the necessary material. Now that you have seen that we have constructed the production plants, there can be no doubt in your mind that all the output of these factories, working 24 hours a day, will be exploded on your homeland.

Within the space of three weeks, we have proof-fired one bomb in the American desert, exploded one in Hiroshima and fired the third this morning.

We implore you to confirm these facts to your leaders and to do your utmost to stop the destruction and waste of life which can only result in the total annihilation of all your cities if continued. As scientists, we deplore the use to which a beautiful discovery has been put, but we can assure you that unless Japan surrenders at once, this rain of atomic bombs will increase many fold in fury.

The letter, with two carbon copies, was not signed. Alvarez addressed three plain envelopes: "Prof. R. Sagane, Physics Department, University of Tokyo." With the letters inside, the envelopes were fixed to the sides of the cylinders which would parachute down and transmit data back to the observation plane. Several layers of Scotch tape were used to plaster the envelopes tight to the cylinders so that wind could not blow under the corners and tear the letters away.

The second atomic bomb flight was jinxed almost from the start and, in the end, almost nothing about it went right. The pilot, Chuck Sweeney, could not fly his own plane, the *Great Artiste*. Instead, he flew *Bock's Car*, usually flown by Captain Frederick C. Bock, Jr. Sweeney was escorted by two observation planes, one flown by Major James Hopkins and the other by Bock. At the last minute, Serber was put off an observation plane for lack of a parachute, despite the fact that he was the only man skilled in operating the high-speed camera.

Marquardt's plane scouted weather over the prime target, Kokura, while McKnight's crew appraised weather over Nagasaki. Although Nagasaki was a harbor city with four big Mitsubishi aircraft plants, it was not ideal for an atom target; the city was broken by hills and valleys which would limit the blast effect. Also it had already been raided five times by American bombers. Kokura, an undamaged city with a huge Army arsenal, was the more logical target.

Scientists, fearful of a take-off crash with the armed bomb, lined the end of the runway with trucks and fire-fighters of the Tinian fire department. Although Sweeney got off without incident at 3:49 A.M., the risk of an atomic accident had greatly agitated the technicians. Ramsey went immediately to his quarters and penned an eloquent letter to Oppenheimer, stating that highest priority must be given to the job of inventing a take-off safety device for the plutonium bomb.

Instead of Deac Parsons, Sweeney carried Commander Ashworth as the bomb commander and weaponeer for Fat Man. Bock piloted the plane loaded with scientists to measure the blast while Hopkins' plane carried two British observers, Group Captain Cheshire and William Penney, a London mathematics professor who was to be knighted for his endeavors in the British atomic effort. *New York Times* reporter Bill Laurence, writing the official eyewitness chronicle for the Manhattan District, was also along.

Bad weather forced the planes to fly west of Iwo Jima, reducing the possibility of transferring the bomb should *Bock's Car* lose an engine. Then it was discovered that six hundred gallons of gasoline were trapped in the bomb-bay tank and could not be used. Sweeney decided to press on, calculating the fuel reserves as sufficient, if not reassuringly ample. At the rendezvous point off the south coast of Kyushu, Sweeney met Bock, but circled for forty-five minutes without catching sight of Hopkins. Sweeney headed for Kokura. It was closed in completely. He made three passes over the city, but Bombardier Beahan couldn't find the smallest hole in the cloud cover. After consulting with Ashworth, Sweeney flew on to Nagasaki. It too was hidden by cloud. Ashworth ordered a radar drop if necessary, taking it upon himself to countermand Washington's orders because of the shortage of fuel. The entire bomb run was made by radar, but at the last minute Beahan found a hole. He released the Fat Man, but missed the aiming point by three miles. After the escape run, five distinct and powerful shock waves slapped *Bock's Car.* Sweeney did not dally. He headed for Okinawa, several hundred miles closer than Tinian.

Things still continued to go wrong. The strike message was sent, but not received on Tinian until afternoon because of the delay in the mission. On Tinian, Farrell, weak with tension and worry for the crew, vomited his lunch. As Sweeney neared Okinawa, his voice radio wouldn't work and he could not warn of an emergency landing. *Bock's Car* shot off emergency flares and barreled through the traffic circle. When the plane braked to a halt at the very end of the runway, there was enough gasoline left to taxi to the apron—and hardly a gallon more. After refueling and after Ashworth reported to Farrell, *Bock's Car* finally landed at Tinian a few minutes before midnight.

Two more links in the chain of misfortune were added later. Some Dutch and British prisoners of war, only recently moved to the Nagasaki area, were killed in the atomic blast. And the day after the raid, in a grim error by the circulation department of the propaganda campaign, leaflets urging evacuation fluttered down on fire-and blast-ravaged Nagasaki.

The same day *Bock's Car* bombed Nagasaki, another preface to the atomic world of the future was written in the United States. Seymour Katcoff, a twenty-six-year-old physical chemistry Ph.D., and Jack M. Hubbard, a young meteorologist, headed a team that prepared to sample the atmosphere over America for radioactivity from the Hiroshima blast. The men placed large paper filters in the bomb bays of two B-29s at Wendover Field. Katcoff took off with a crew of ten to sample the air over the northwestern section of the United States, but all four engines of the plane failed over the Sierra Nevada mountains and an emergency landing at Bakersfield, California, burned out the tires. Katcoff tried again the next day in another plane with David H. Frisch, a young nuclear physicist from New York. They made two trips, one over British Columbia and another over the sea to the southern tip of Alaska. They found low levels of radioactivity in the filters, but were uncertain whether any of it had drifted across the Pacific from Hiroshima.

On Tinian Island, the men from private to general anticipated an hourly notice of surrender by Japan, especially when Russia's declaration of war dovetailed with the wrecking of Nagasaki. But Radio Tokyo said nothing of surrender. The war continued.

A photo mission returned from Hiroshima and reported that two large fires still burned in the west central part of the city. Lieutenant Colonel Classen, deputy commander of the 509th, flew color films of the Hiroshima bombing back to the States for developing. Three more plutonium bomb casings, FM-1, FM-2 and FM-5, were readied in the bomb assembly hut. The second Fat Man bomb was scheduled for testing, minus the fissionable material, on August 13. Enough plutonium for a third strike at Japan was expected from Hanford via Los Alamos within ten days.

Cardinal Spellman arrived to say mass on Tinian. The 509th flew daily bomb missions over Japan with practice bombs. Farrell and Parsons briefed the Air Force generals on the history and power of the A-bomb. Farrell circulated his copy of the Smyth report, the only copy in the Pacific of this official, semitechnical atomic story. Spaatz visited the bomb hut and shook his head in disbelief when shown the size of the fissionable material that could level a city. And then, suddenly and anticlimactically, it was all over on Tinian Island. On August 13 Colonel Kirkpatrick sent a laconic message, marking the end of man's first venture in atomic warfare, to Manhattan headquarters in Washington:

Recommend shipment Sixth Bowery be temporarily deferred.

CHAPTER ELEVEN

No High Ground

FRANKLIN H. GRAHAM was a captain in the United States Army, but he was not out of place in the wardroom of the Navy cruiser *Augusta* on August 6, 1945. He was one of the officers in the war room at the White House, and when the President went to sea the "map room" and the men who ran it went with him. Graham was watch officer today. He had come down to the officers' mess for lunch, leaving orders that any messages coming into the radio room should be brought to him at once.

He never finished his meal. A minute or two before noon, a yeoman hurried into the wardroom and handed him a code dispatch that had just come in over the special White House circuit. Graham took it at once to the first lieutenant's office, which had been turned over to the presidential party for the voyage. There he hurriedly decoded the brief flash. It was addressed to the President:

Big bomb dropped on Hiroshima August five at seven fifteen P.M. Washington time. First reports indicate complete success which was even more conspicuous than earlier test.

Graham stared for a second at the words he had translated from the jumble of numbers and letters in the coded dispatch. Then, like any good briefing officer, he grabbed a small map of Japan from among his papers. He located Hiroshima, circled it with a red pencil and took the map with him as he ran belowdecks to the after mess hall where Harry S. Truman was sharing a meal with the enlisted men. It was a hot day, for the ship had entered the Gulf Stream as it neared the end of a record run from Europe. With Truman at a small table were men from Connecticut, New York, California, New Jersey, Arkansas and Minnesota.

Graham excused himself, breaking into the conversation, and handed the President the message and the map.

Truman scanned the twenty-six-word bulletin, took a deep breath and said: "Captain Graham, this is the greatest thing in history." The President seemed both excited and deeply moved. The sailors at his table fell silent, but for the moment he said no more.

While Graham was carrying the dispatch to Truman, a second message from Washington rattled onto the teletype printer in the *Augusta*'s radio room. This time a naval officer, Lieutenant George M. Elsey, also attached to the White House staff, decoded the report and hustled down to the mess hall. He handed it to Truman, who read:

Following info regarding Manhattan received. "Hiroshima bombed visually with only one tenth cover at 052315Z. There was no fighter opposition and no flak. Parsons reports fifteen minutes after drop as follows: 'Results clear cut successful in all respects. Visible effects greater than in any test. Conditions normal in airplane following delivery.'"

229

The second message seemed to break Truman's silence. He jumped up and took the report to Secretary Byrnes, who was eating at another table. "It's time for us to get on home!" he said.

Elsey told Truman that he had heard, over the radio in the cabin where he had decoded the dispatch, a brief news flash from Washington saying that the President had announced the use of an atomic bomb against Japan. This meant that Stimson had released the statement prepared in advance for this moment. When Elsey told him of it, Truman knew he was no longer bound to silence.

The chief executive picked up a fork and banged it on the side of a water glass. The mess hall quieted quickly. Truman, in a voice that barely masked his excitement, asked the crewmen to listen for a moment. He said he had just received two messages telling him of the highly successful results of the first attack on Japan with a terrifically powerful new weapon which used an explosive twenty thousand times as powerful as TNT. It was called, he added, an "atomic bomb."

The crew cheered, but Truman did not wait to take a bow. He was out the door and down the passageway to officers' country like a boy headed home on the last day of school. He burst through the wardroom door and waved the surprised officers back into their chairs as they started to rise.

"Keep your seats, gentlemen. I have an announcement to make to you."

He paused for a moment, looking around as if to pick out the men with whom he had dined the night before, then simply added:

"We have just dropped a bomb on Japan which has more

power than twenty thousand tons of TNT. It was an overwhelming success. We won the gamble!"

The same news bulletins now pouring from the radios aboard the *Augusta* were also startling the entire world. For most, the news was impossible to comprehend. The world had changed in an instant, and not only was the change itself a shock, but few people had the slightest understanding of the way in which it had been accomplished. Yet somehow almost everyone who heard the news knew or sensed that it was of tremendous importance.

It came first from the White House, where Truman's statement was issued a few minutes before 11 A.M., eastern war time:

Sixteen hours ago an American airplane dropped one bomb on Hiroshima, an important Japanese Army base. That bomb had more power than 20,000 tons of T.N.T. It had more than two thousand times the blast power of the British "Grand Slam" which is the largest bomb ever yet used in the history of warfare.

The Japanese began the war from the air at Pearl Harbor. They have been repaid many fold. And the end is not yet. . . .

It is an atomic bomb. It is a harnessing of the basic power of the universe. The force from which the sun draws its power has been loosed against those who brought war to the Far East. . . .

It was to spare the Japanese people from utter destruction that the ultimatum of July 26 was issued at Potsdam. Their leaders promptly rejected that ultimatum. If they do not now accept our terms they may expect a rain of ruin from the air, the like of which has never been seen on this earth. . . .

Eight miles east of Hudson, Wisconsin, William P. Steven, managing editor of the Minneapolis *Tribune,* was driving along

U.S. Highway 12. He snapped on his car radio to check the late news. Steven had served a hitch in the Office of Censorship, and when he heard the words "atomic bomb" he suddenly recalled a briefing several years before when an Army officer had explained why certain scientific material, including stories on uranium research, must be kept out of print. He stepped on the gas and rushed to his office to telephone the paper's Washington bureau.

Newsmen in Washington were suddenly snowed under. Queries poured into the wire-service offices. Those papers which maintained their own bureaus in the capital ordered coverage of every angle, regardless of story lengths or wire tolls.

Sidney Shalett, Pentagon correspondent for the *New York Times,* had gone that morning to the office of General Jacob L. Devers, newly named commander of the Army Ground Forces. He had an assignment from his Sunday editor to write a story on the Army's plans for training the mass of foot soldiers needed for the final assault on Japan. As Devers described how the infantry would win the war, a secretary came in and told Shalett he was wanted on the telephone in the outer office. The caller was Luther Huston, the *Times* Washington bureau manager.

"Forget your infantry general," Huston ordered. "Get down to the press room and start writing about the atomic bomb we just dropped on Japan."

Shalett stepped back into Devers' office just long enough to apologize and explain why he had to leave. The general, whose infantrymen had become suddenly, permanently and vastly less important, blinked at him as he left.

There was plenty of grist for the reporters' mills that day. The Army put out a dramatic description of the test shot at Alamogordo, including eyewitness accounts. A statement by Stimson amplified the first presidential announcement. Another long release gave details on the "hidden cities" at Oak Ridge, Hanford and Los Alamos that produced the bomb.

Papers sold for a dollar a copy on the streets of Oak Ridge, where seventy-five thousand atomic workers grabbed at the chance to discover what they had been making. A Knoxville *Journal* vendor sold sixteen hundred papers in half an hour there. At Los Alamos, young physicists ran whooping and shouting down the hallways as they heard the first news on their radios.

The great secret was out. But for some men, the Manhattan security office provided a final taste of the melodrama in which it seemed to delight. Samuel Goudsmit, the naturalized Dutchman who had snared the German atomic scientists a few months earlier for ALSOS, was in Berlin. On the morning of August 6, he was searching for scientific material in the ruins of Heinrich Himmler's headquarters when an officer appeared with orders for him to fly to Frankfurt at once. Goudsmit could get no explanation from him, or from anyone else, but he obeyed and flew west.

After dinner in Frankfurt that night, Goudsmit escorted Mary Bohan, the secretary for the ALSOS team, to the WAC hotel where she was billeted. In the lobby, the sergeant at the desk had a little radio blaring. Midnight struck and the news broadcast, giving Goudsmit his first word of Hiroshima, suddenly made it clear why he had been spirited out of Berlin: Manhattan's security officers in Washington were afraid the Russians would kidnap him and try to force atomic secrets from him if he were still in Berlin, deep in the Soviet-occupied area, when the news broke.

In Britain there was a different tone to the announcement of Hiroshima. The news hit the United States with the impact of a fire siren, but it seemed to go out across war-weary England like the deep, somber tones of Big Ben. Clement Attlee, the new Prime Minister, announced the bomb with a formal statement, as befitted the head of a nation which had shared fully in unlocking the atom's mystery and power. But Attlee had been in office so short a time that he could do no more than add an introduction to the long announcement that Winston Churchill had prepared a fortnight earlier. It was the voice of Attlee that carried the news to the British Empire, but the words were unmistakably Churchill's:

. . . It is now for Japan to realize . . . what the consequence will be of an indefinite continuance of this terrible means of maintaining a rule of law in the world.

This revelation of the secrets of nature so long mercifully withheld from man should arouse the most solemn reflections in the mind and conscience of every human being capable of comprehension. We must indeed pray that these awful agencies will be made to conduce to peace among the nations and that, instead of wreaking measureless havoc upon the entire globe, they may become a perennial foundation of world prosperity.

Among those who learned of the bomb from Churchill's statement were the German scientists interned at Farm Hall. At first, these men who had worked for more than five years without even solving the theoretical problems could not believe it. But as further details came to them, their incredulity faded. They sat up far into the night working equations and debating how the Americans had done it, and they brooded over the new terror that the international fraternity of science had released on the world. One in particular, Otto Hahn, who had discovered in 1938 how to break the uranium atom, took the news hard. His depression was so deep that his colleagues took turns sitting up with him—to make sure he did not take his own life—until he finally fell asleep after 2 A.M.

Across the North Sea in Germany, General Dwight Eisenhower also mused on the news of Hiroshima. As he said later, he knew at once that his theories of warfare, which had enabled him to direct the greatest ground force in history to the defeat of Hitler's armies, were at once utterly outmoded. The whole idea of the bomb was repugnant to him. He had felt this way since first hearing of it in detail at Potsdam in July. But Eisenhower saw one ray of hope: that science might at last have produced "something so terrible and destructive that future wars may be impossible. . . . It may blackmail the world into peace." He had no idea on this night in 1945 how many times he would again have to contemplate this problem, not just as an interested professional kibitzer but as the man on whom would rest the ultimate responsibility for the security of his nation and the peace of the entire world.

Those who got their news from Radio Moscow had long been accustomed to seeing things through the wrong end of the telescope. Tonight was no exception. In mid-evening a special program extolled the progress of Soviet science. This was followed by an account of the decoration of a Russian scientist for his "contributions to victory." Then, after midnight, the bare text of Harry Truman's announcement was read at dictation speed for use in provincial papers the next day. There was no other comment from Moscow.

By now it was the morning of August 7 in the Pacific, and the crew of the destroyer escort *Cecil J. Doyle* was starting another day of searching for bodies in the area where the cruiser *Indianapolis* had been torpedoed. Then the news of Hiroshima reached the ship, transmitted by the Navy on its regular daily news broadcast to all ships. To the *Doyle's* crew, continuously at sea since February, it was good news. Even without full understanding, they knew this bomb would shorten the war. To the skipper, Lieutenant Commander W. Graham Claytor, it was more than merely good news. It meant that there was now a chance that the orders he had in his safe—orders that would send the *Doyle* to almost certain destruction as a radar picket ship in the invasion of Kyushu—would never be executed.

There was less optimism among the Marines who were winding up preparations for that invasion at their Hawaiian base. The news reached Major Bill Miller's 3rd battalion of the 13th Marines by radio, and it was received with satisfaction—but with extreme skepticism. These battle-wary men had met the Japanese hand-to-hand on beaches from Guadalcanal to Iwo Jima, and no report of a single bomb, no matter how big, could convince them that the enemy would quit without a lot more killing. There was no change in the regimental orders. Miller was to load his battalion onto an LST that week for the long voyage west toward the final rendezvous off Zephyr, Winton and Studebaker beaches on the west shore of Kyushu.

The news of Hiroshima meant change, in some form and to some degree, to all who heard it. To Claytor, it was a reprieve; to Miller, it was at least a glimmer of hope. To some others, for the most part young men who had not been blooded, it was an entirely different thing.

Private Ed Bushnell was hitchhiking into town from his family's home outside Williamstown, Massachusetts, shortly after noon on August 6. He was in uniform, and a passing motorist stopped to give him a lift. As the car started up again, the driver turned to Bushnell and asked him what he thought of "the news." When the young G.I. was noncommittal (he hadn't heard *any* news that day), the man explained: An "atomic bomb" had been dropped on Japan, and the war was all but over.

For Bushnell, who had wangled a last-minute transfer out of a unit bound for European occupation duty and into one headed for Pacific combat, the first reaction was a wash of disappointment. The war was over and the world had passed him by. He had decided, in the heat of his eighteen years, that his destiny lay in the Pacific. That was to be "his war." Now it was gone. The story of the world had changed, and in the new version his role was not to be that of a man at war but the far less exciting one of a boy back at school.

There were other portents of change that day in events that had no connection with the explosion over Hiroshima. Early on the morning of August 6, at the Bethesda Naval Medical Center outside Washington, Senator Hiram Johnson of California died in his sleep. Illness had kept the old man off the Senate floor during debate on ratification of the new United Nations charter; he could only send word that if present he would have voted "no." With Johnson's death the last bitter voice of die-hard isolationism was silenced. This man who helped lead the Senate fight against the League of Nations in 1919, who opposed the inevitable preparations for our entry into World War II, who fought with his final failing energy the creation of a new world organization, died on the very day that the scientists and soldiers of his own country destroyed the old framework of civilization and in so doing added new urgency to the search for a world order.

Another death the same day also marked, in a different way, the great change. Major Richard I. Bong, winner of the Congressional Medal of Honor for shooting down forty enemy planes in the Pacific, crashed to his death in a test flight in California. He was only twenty-four years old, and he was flying the latest thing in fighter aircraft, a P-80 jet. Yet in a sense both the flier and the plane he died trying to perfect were already obsolete. The vast destructive power of the atom would inevitably be wedded to the new ballistic missile, first used by the Germans in their V-2 attacks on England. It would require only a decade, a mere page in the new history whose writing began on August 6, for this robot partnership to make the finest manned aircraft a second-best weapon.

Man groped on August 6 for the shape of his future, and he saw many things.

A writer in London had a vision to fit his nation's maritime traditions. He saw "a day within measurable time when, in effect, the liner *Queen Mary* could be driven across the Atlantic on a teacupful of fuel."

But a writer for the Vatican newspaper *Osservatore Romano* spoke the fears of many religious leaders in many faiths: ". . .This incredible destructive instrument remains a temptation for posterity."

Some would not face the future at all. An ugly, bloated caricature of a man named Hermann Goering, in an American military prison in Luxembourg, said: "I don't believe it." Then, a little later: "I don't want anything to do with it. I am leaving this world."

The chairman of the peace commission of the Federal Council of Churches of Christ in America wrote a statement calling for at least a temporary suppression of the new weapon. "We pray that our authorities may, in this difficult matter, find and follow the way of Christian statesmanship." The writer was John Foster Dulles, who could not forsee that a decade later, as Secretary of

State, he would want to make this weapon the central instrument of American foreign policy.

The military specialist of the *New York Times* also looked ahead, and he did not like what he saw. "Now we have been the first to introduce a new weapon of unknowable effects which may bring us the victory quickly but which will sow the seeds of hate more widely than ever," wrote Hanson Baldwin. "We may yet reap the whirlwind."

For the present, though, victory was coming, and coming quickly.

In Tokyo the Japanese government could no longer hope to end the war before the ultimate calamity was inflicted on its homeland. The calamity had already come. Foreign Minister Togo wired his ambassador in Moscow on the afternoon of August 6 to move faster in his effort to procure Russian mediation: "Various circumstances require an immediate interview with Molotov." At 3:40 P.M. August 7, he wired again: "The situation has become more and more acute."

Togo also put more pressure on the stubborn Japanese militarists, who were so set on the idea of a death struggle on their own beaches that they were trying to pretend the atomic bomb was nothing new and were suppressing the news of the attack. Togo spent two and a half hours with War Minister Anami on the evening of August 7. For the first time, Anami conceded that Japan faced early and inevitable defeat. The next morning Togo conferred with Suzuki and then called on the Emperor. He explained the atomic bomb, drawing on the American broadcasts for his facts, and said he believed the only course left open was to surrender—using the bomb as an excuse. Hirohito replied that he agreed, and that any hope of securing advantageous conditions through negotiation was "wishful thinking." He told Togo he wanted measures taken to end the war "at the earliest possible date."

Togo's conversations with Anami and the Emperor seem to have settled the basic question. From the moment he left Hirohito's library on August 8, the process of surrender was in motion, and all that came after that followed the desires expressed by the Emperor that morning.

It was a full day, however, before all six members of the Supreme War Council could be collected for a meeting, and as a result there was another powerful spur to surrender when the "inner cabinet" met. Russia declared war on Japan on August 8, two days after Hiroshima, and sent her troops swarming into Manchuria in the first hours of August 9 to establish a claim on the spoils of war. The Japanese leaders convened at 10 A.M. For the first time, all six agreed that Japan must surrender, but now there was a new dispute over the terms of capitulation. Three members insisted not only that the Emperor must be retained (on that, all six agreed) but also that there must be no foreign occupation and no foreign war crimes trials in Japan.

On these points, the meeting was deadlocked for two hours, and at one o'clock the leaders broke up for lunch before carrying the debate to an emergency session of the full cabinet. When the cabinet convened at 2:30, there were new disasters, actual and threatened, to hasten matters. Sweeney's crew had dropped the second atomic bomb on Nagasaki, and War Minister Anami had a frightening report which he read to the group. It was the record of the interrogation of an American pilot captured the day before, who had told his captors:

... One atomic bomb is enough to devastate an area covering six square miles—an explosive power equivalent to the effects of a total

240

of bombs carried by 2,000 B-29s, each carrying thirty-six 500-pound bombs. . . .

Our next target after Hiroshima is Tokyo. The attack will inevitably come, because such an attack is considered to have a major propaganda effect. . . .

The rest of the pilot's statement consisted of imaginary and wholly inaccurate statistics on the bomb itself, but the Japanese did not know they were false. Their own professor Sagane could have given them a thorough briefing on the weapon if he had received the letter addressed to him by his former colleagues on Tinian and dropped with the recording instruments in the second atomic attack. But the one copy that had been picked up, about thirty miles north of Nagasaki, had been seized by the Japanese Naval Air Force, and he did not get it until six weeks later. Thus the captured flier's improvisations were unchallenged, and his remark about the "propaganda effect" was precisely correct. The idea of an atomic attack on Tokyo shook the Japanese leaders. The cabinet did not reach a decision in the afternoon, but agreed to send the question back to the six-man council, which was called to meet late that evening with the Emperor present.

All during this day of maneuvering, Lord Privy Seal Kido shuttled between the Emperor and his peace-minded ministers. Kido's diary noted when he saw Hirohito on August 9—9:55 A.M., before the first council meeting; 10:55 A.M., during the meeting; 3:10 P.M., during the cabinet meeting; 4:35 P.M., as it was ending; and twice in the evening, from 10:50 to 10:53 and again from 11:25 to 11:37, just before the climactic council session. Hirohito was prepared for his role when he joined the council a few minutes before midnight.

It was a lovely night, for once unspoiled by air-raid alarms, with the moonlight so bright that one of Togo's aides, waiting outside, "could count each pine needle on the ground." The council nevertheless met in the stifling heat of the Emperor's bomb shelter, an eighteen-by-thirty-six-foot concrete room sunk in a hillside behind the palace. There, beyond two massive steel doors, the rulers of Japan came to the end of the road.

They argued for more than two hours, the dispute over the conditions under which surrender would be acceptable still flaring. Finally, after 2 A.M., Premier Suzuki rose and asked the Emperor to "substitute the Imperial guidance for the decision of this conference."

It was a bold and stunning move. The Emperor never spoke at council meetings except to ratify decisions previously made without consulting him. But now, obviously expecting Suzuki's cue and prepared for his moment, he acted without hesitation. He said he agreed with Togo. He noted that the military's judgment had been proved misleading many times. To continue the war, he said, "means nothing but the destruction of the whole nation." Japan must accept the Allied ultimatum, he said, "bearing what is very hard to bear."

Suzuki was on his feet the moment Hirohito finished. "The Imperial decision has been expressed," he said. "This should be the conclusion of this conference." He had his way now. A hasty cabinet meeting ratified the decision and by morning the Foreign Ministry, whose officials had been waiting outside the bomb shelter in the moonlight and mosquitoes of the summer night, dispatched a message through Switzerland to the Allies. It agreed to accept the terms of the Potsdam ultimatum, with the "understanding" that the Emperor would remain in power.

The rest was merely a matter of time. The American government was now faced squarely with the Emperor question, which it had dodged earlier. But although some of Truman's top advisers were still dubious, the issue was now joined to a direct and forthright offer by the Japanese to surrender. It did not take long for the United States to find an acceptable answer: a masterful reply drafted by Byrnes proposed to allow Hirohito to stay, provided he was made "subject to the authority" of the Allied occupation commander and agreed to sign the surrender document himself. At the suggestion of the British, this second clause was modified to stipulate only that he be required to "authorize and ensure" the signature. The revised reply was sent off on the morning of August 11. Three days later, despite last-ditch objections from the military leaders and an abortive revolt by the palace guard, the Japanese surrendered.

World War II was over. But the instrument that brought it to such a sudden end had started a new conflict that would last much longer. This new war would be fought not on the beaches and in the chancellories, not even in the laboratories, but in the more intimate and troubled area of man's mind and conscience. Americans, and men everywhere, would ponder one question above all others: had it been right to use the bomb?

The man who ordered its use, President Truman, was blunt and positive in accepting responsibility and defending his action:

The final decision of where and when to use the atomic bomb was up to me. Let there be no mistake about it. I regarded the bomb as a military weapon and never had any doubt that it should be used. The top military advisers to the President recommended its use, and when I talked to Churchill he unhesitatingly told me that he favored use of the atomic bomb if it might aid to end the war.

Yet there were those who wondered how much choice Truman really had. By the time he learned of the project, two billion dollars had been spent in secret. The 509th was ready to go overseas. Franklin D. Roosevelt and Churchill had reached a tentative decision months earlier to use the bomb against Japan. General Groves, another who believed the decision to drop it was correct, would say years later that Truman entered the picture too late to change it. The President, he argued, "was like a little boy on a toboggan. He never had an opportunity to say 'we *will* drop the bomb.' All he could do was say 'no.' " Any political leader who refused to drop it, Groves said, would have been "crucified" if American lives had subsequently been lost in an invasion of Japan.

The atomic bomb was dropped to save lives which Allied leaders feared would otherwise be lost by the thousands on the beaches and in the rice paddies of Japan. Yet even some who faced death on those beaches were troubled. Navy Captain Arthur A. Ageton was in a San Francisco restaurant enjoying a final Stateside rest before flying out to take up his post as a beach control officer in one of the Kyushu landings. Ageton had handled a similar job at Okinawa and was under no illusions about the perils of his next assignment. But when a newsboy came running through the restaurant hawking an extra, and Ageton read the story of Hiroshima, he felt instant and inescapable revulsion.

There were troubled hearts in the high command too. Fleet Admiral William D. Leahy, chief of staff to both Roosevelt and Truman, liked the bomb even less after it fell than he did when he denounced it as "a fool thing" before it was tested. His postwar judgment would be a bitter one:

. . . The use of this barbarous weapon at Hiroshima and Nagasaki was of no material assistance in our war against Japan. The Japanese were already defeated and ready to surrender because of the effective sea blockade and the successful bombing with conventional weapons. . . .

My own feeling was that in being the first to use it, we had adopted an ethical standard common to the barbarians of the Dark Ages. I was not taught to make war in that fashion and wars cannot be won by destroying women and children. . . . One of the professors associated with the Manhattan project told me that he had hoped the bomb wouldn't work. I wish that he had been right.

Even those who had justified their decision to drop the bomb as one that would accomplish a net saving of lives now had to fight with their consciences. As a practical matter, if not in strict constitutional terms, Secretary of War Stimson had more to say about the bomb than any other man. He had helped father the Manhattan project, had exercised constant personal supervision, had supported the work. He had also seen, well before others, the problems ahead, and in fact had begun thinking and planning for the future control of the atom long before the first bomb was even assembled. He never swerved in recommending its use once he was convinced this was the right course. Later, examining his own actions, he had this to say:

I see too many stern and heart-rending decisions to be willing to pretend that war is anything else than what it is. The face of war is the face of death; death is an inevitable part of every order that a wartime leader gives. The decision to use the atomic bomb was a decision that brought death to over a hundred thousand Japanese. No explanation can change that fact and I do not wish to gloss it over.

But this deliberate, premeditated destruction was our least abhorrent alternative. The destruction of Hiroshima and Nagasaki put an end to the Japanese war. It stopped the fire raids, and the strangling blockade; it ended the ghastly specter of a clash of great land armies.

In this last great action of the Second World War we were given final proof that war is death. . . .

Who was right? Truman, who saw the bomb as a "military weapon" to end a war? Or Leahy, who was taught to make war in a civilized fashion? Or Stimson, who saw war as death itself? Few who knew as much as these three about the situation in 1945 would call themselves fit to render final judgment, then or later. The absolute verdicts came from people who knew less and who felt less keenly, if at all, the weight of responsibility and authority.

Yet verdicts were delivered, some quickly, some in the fullness of time. Within a few days after Hiroshima, Mrs. Jean O'Leary, Groves' secretary, was getting telephone calls from members of her family who now knew what her secret job was all about. How could she possibly be connected with such a horrible thing? Why did she let her name be used in the publicity? At the time, Jean O'Leary could not understand this attitude. To her, it was a job to do as part of the war. Later, she would have qualms about the use of the bomb.

A later expression came from former President Herbert Hoover. At the funeral of James Forrestal in 1947, Hoover approached Ralph Bard, the one Interim Committee dissenter, and told him he thought he had been right to demand a demonstration before the bomb was dropped on Japan.

One question that disturbed Americans later concerned not Hiroshima but Nagasaki. Some who acknowledged the military justification for the first atomic attack wondered what excuse there was for a repetition of the slaughter three days later, when the Japanese leaders were already moving to surrender and were frantically trying to arrange the means to do it. Those who asked this question found it hard to reach a clear-cut answer on the basis of the facts available *at the time*. The original order for the atomic bombing said flatly that "additional bombs will be delivered . . . as soon as made ready." If Truman and Churchill contemplated going through the decision-making process a second time, they gave no evidence of it, either then or later. The commanders on Tinian had no authority to withhold use of the second bomb, even if they had wished to. From their action in speeding the schedule for the Nagasaki bomb, it is clear they had no such desire. Neither the men on Tinian nor their superiors in Washington knew what was going on in Japan; there was no overt evidence that the shock of Hiroshima had produced the hoped-for decision to surrender. The first combat test of the plutonium bomb, then, went hand-in-hand with the first explosion of a uranium bomb. The high command, the generals in the field and the men who flew the missions all saw the new weapons as a way of ending the war, and they were prepared to use them until the war ended. That the war was, in fact, ending on August 9, 1945, is clear today; it was not at all clear at the time. Here again, men who pondered this question later found it hard to render absolute judgment.

Those most intimately involved, the men who flew the *Enola Gay* and *Bock's Car* and *Straight Flush* and *Jabbit III,* mirrored the differing reactions of other Americans. Major Charles Sweeney, who carried instruments over Hiroshima and dropped the bomb on Nagasaki, saw the killing of 115,000 civilians as balanced by the saving of many more lives, both American and Japanese, that would otherwise have been lost in an invasion of Japan. He found it hard to differentiate between the napalm that killed over 78,000 in Tokyo and the uranium that killed about the same number in Hiroshima. Yet Sweeney undertook a lecture tour, telling of the atomic bombings—and sending all the profits to an orphanage in Hiroshima.

Co-pilot Robert Lewis of the *Enola Gay* began pondering the matter on the way back to Tinian that morning. In the shadow of the mushroom cloud, and later, he reached the conclusion that it had to be done. Perhaps, he thought, the sacrifice of Hiroshima would not be in vain, because it showed that the new weapon's threat was so great that the world could not possibly afford another war. Lewis went on television, years later, to help raise money for the medical treatment of girls disfigured by the bomb he helped deliver.

More deeply affected than any other American who flew over Hiroshima was Major Claude Eatherly, pilot of the plane that signed the city's death warrant with its weather report. Twelve years later, Eatherly, his mind disturbed, was arrested for the robbery of two Texas post offices. He was found not guilty by reason of insanity. A Veterans Administration psychiatrist who testified at the trial said that Eatherly's "feeling of guilt" over Hiroshima had contributed to his mental troubles.

Reports of Eatherly's difficulties circulated widely over the years, and many people eventually gained the impression that he was the pilot of the plane that actually dropped the bomb. Some newspapers in other countries carried stories to this effect. They did not fit the facts. Colonel Paul Tibbets, still in the Air Force, was by 1960 commander of the 6th Air Division of the Strategic Air Command at MacDill Air Force Base in Florida. He remained what he had been in 1945: the epitome of cool stability.

John Abbott Wilson and Ellsworth T. Carrington were pilot and co-pilot in *Jabbit III*, the weather plane over the secondary target of Kokura on August 6. They learned what had happened to Hiroshima before they returned to Tinian, and they discussed it as they sat together in the cockpit of their B-29 that morning. After the war ended they went home separately, returned to college and lost touch with each other. It came as a surprise when they discovered later that each had found himself caught up in the undergraduate movement for World Federalism. For Carrington, the final verdict on the bomb was a harsh one: "Later it came out that the Japs had been trying to surrender but were afraid of nonsense about unconditional surrender. Since Japan was already beaten, it was a tragic U.S. flub to needlessly vaporize 140,000 people."

Not all the atomic warriors were so persuaded, either on August 6 or later. Dutch Van Kirk, the *Enola Gay*'s navigator, put it briefly: "What's the difference, one bomb or thousands?" Morris R. Jeppson, assistant weaponeer at Hiroshima, later became president of a firm manufacturing some of the complex machines used in the new world of atomic science at whose birth he assisted. His view: "One could question whether this was the best way to go about it tactically—this is purely academic—but I still think it would have made a delightful show to drop one on top of Mount Fujiyama, blow off the top of it. But when you have only two shots, I suppose the decision was to make them as effective as possible." Staff Sergeant Joe Stiborik, the twenty-nine-year-old radar operator of the *Enola Gay*, took part in many discussions among crew members about their mission. "It always ended that it was a job we had to do," he recalled later, "and that if the Japs had had an A-bomb they would have done the same thing to us." Physicist Luis W. Alvarez, who monitored the recording instruments in the *Great Artiste* at Hiroshima, believed that the shock of the bomb was required to end the war. Unlike Carrington, he did not believe that the complex maneuverings for negotiated peace could have succeeded.

Not many men on Tinian wrestled with ethical questions soon after Hiroshima, but some did. These sought out Chaplain Downey in the privacy of his quarters. What did he think about the morality of leveling a whole city with one bomb? The Lutheran preacher had no easy answer, but he gave it as his opinion, one he continued to hold afterward, that the quantity of killing was not an issue. The wrong was the killing, whether by fire bombs from hundreds of planes, by one atomic bomb or by a single rifle bullet. War itself, he believed, was the evil that man must conquer.

For physicist Alvarez there was a special surprise when he returned to the United States. He found a complete reversal of attitude at Los Alamos, the very birthplace of the weapon. When he left for the Pacific, everyone in the secret city had been enthusiastic about the bomb; now, he found the scientists "almost neurotic" in their post-mortem opposition. He noted that those who had carried the bomb out to the Pacific, and had thus seen the battle zone at first hand, seemed far less worried about the morality of using the bomb than those who had remained at home in the United States.

The scientists had good reason to be troubled. Perhaps more than any other group they were able to comprehend the magnitude of the change wrought by their handiwork. They had let the atomic genie out of the bottle in which it had been locked through the ages, and they knew not only that it would be impossible to bottle it up again, but also that everything it touched would be forever changed.

Those whose consciences kept them awake through the hot summer nights in 1945 thought primarily of the evil consequences. Among the worriers were some—scientists or privileged political leaders—who knew that the Hiroshima bomb, terrible as it was, could soon be dwarfed by another nuclear monstrosity. The few who knew of it called it simply "Super." For two years at Los Alamos, the brilliant and impatient Edward Teller had worked almost alone, in the only lab on the mesa that was not dedicated to the production of Little Boy or Fat Man. Teller had leapfrogged from the early theoretical work on fission to something the world would call "fusion," and which would make possible the hydrogen bomb.

There was no talk of Super in 1945, at least in public. But Stimson's statement on August 6 carried a veiled warning to the world. Discussing the power of the Hiroshima bomb, he said: "More important for the long-range implications of the new weapon is the possibility that another scale of magnitude will be evolved after considerable research and development."

Before Hiroshima, military men measured destructive power in tons of TNT. After Hiroshima, they needed a new unit of terror; they coined the word "kiloton" and calculated now in units of one thousand tons of conventional explosive. Teller's work was to make even this out-of-date within a few years. The jump from Little Boy in 1945 to Super in 1952 would be so great that still another yardstick—the "megaton," meaning the equivalent of *one million* tons of TNT—would have to be invented.

The world was beginning to hear, a few weeks after the bombing of Hiroshima, about people there who had survived heat, fire and blast but who were now strangely ill. Their hair fell out, their gums bled, their white blood cells disappeared, their skins were spotted with hundreds of pinpoint hemorrhages, and they died. The Japanese had a word for it: *genshibakudan-*

sho, the "sickness of the original-child bomb." Americans called it radiation sickness. It was the first disease in the case book of the changed world.

There would be others. Almost fifteen years later, Japanese doctors would begin to find thyroid cancer appearing in people who were young children in Hiroshima the day the bomb fell.

These victims had at least been under the fireball, so that they could be tagged in advance as susceptible to some misfortune, early or late, because of radiation. Indeed, some scientists forecast in 1945 that one or two or even more generations would have to be born and breed and reproduce themselves before the full effect of that one day's exposure to gamma rays could be measured.

But there would be another entry in the case book of atomic-age medicine that would be the more frightening because it could affect people who spent their entire lives half a world away from any atomic explosion. The new peril would be called strontium 90. This radioactive fission product could be carried into the upper air from a nuclear blast and fall to earth thousands of miles away. There it could be absorbed into the soil, then into growing plants, then into the systems of animals who ate the plants, then into humans who ate milk or meat from the animals. Finally it could concentrate, like calcium, in human bones. Once there, in sufficient quantities, it could cause cancer. There would be little consolation in the fact that learned men could argue over how much strontium 90 the human system might absorb without damage.

The visions of those who looked ahead in 1945 were not all gloomy. The energy of the atom had been released for war, but it could be used for peace—for commerce, for agriculture, for healing—as well.

In a controlled chain reaction, the atom could be made to give up its vast store of energy slowly and usefully. The British writer who foresaw a day when ships could cross an ocean on a "teacupful" of fuel was no blind optimist. In a decade, man would have developed the engines and built the vessels to travel for thousands of miles on the power released by a small lump of uranium.

If the heat of a chain reaction could drive a steam turbine in a ship, it could do the same thing to make electric power. This could bring electricity to areas where the cost of conventional fuel was prohibitively high or where there was no falling water to turn turbines. It could be used in a tiny "package" power plant carried in a truck or an airplane to remote locations. It could drive an apparatus to purify sea water and thus make arable desert lands which a booming world population would need for growing food.

Radioactive elements could be used in other ways, too. At Brookhaven National Laboratory on Long Island a strange garden would bloom under the invisible glare of radiation. Here scientists would expose plants to produce dozens of mutations in a year, where previously a decade or more of patient selection would have been required. In this way, man could keep up with the infinite proliferation of plant diseases, instead of always being a long step behind. Types of wheat and oats would be produced that were resistant to rust. Other mutations in the atomic garden would yield strains of plants and trees that bore larger fruits, or ripened in a shorter season, or gave produce that better withstood handling, marketing and processing.

Other men would learn to use radiation to preserve food and

seed, so that lack of refrigeration would not cause stored meat to spoil or seed potatoes to sprout and rot. Men would find ways to use radiation in the fight against insect pests. Within ten years after Hiroshima, scientists of the U.S. Department of Agriculture would be able to wipe out a cattle pest known as the screwworm fly by simply exposing male flies to radiation and thus rendering them sterile. Since the female fly mates only once, the process could not fail, once enough sterilized males were released. In 1959 the scientists started a similar attack on the much more widespread oriental fruit fly. The site of their first tests in this new effort was only a few miles from Tinian, on Rota Island, the isolated Japanese outpost on which Nimitz wanted a "small" atomic bomb dropped in 1945.

And if the atom added new diseases to the annals of medicine, it also furnished new cures. Doctors would be able to use radioactive substances to treat cancers that had previously been invariably fatal. They would be able to use radioactive "tracers" to explore the human system so that an injection of iodine would become a signboard telling them where to go to cut out sickness.

Fifteen years after Hiroshima, the annual U.S. government budget for atomic energy programs would reach $2,500,000,000, more than the cost of four years' work on the Manhattan project. And, in 1959, over three quarters of this spending would be for peaceful projects, not weapons.

The beneficent atom would serve vanquished as well as victors. Fifteen years after U.S. troops crossed the Rhine, the West German government would count the number of hospitals, laboratories and industries using radioactive isotopes in their daily work. The total for a single year was over one thousand.

In that summer of 1945, men with the requisite specialized knowledge could forecast the eventual coming of all these physical changes, good and bad. It was not so easy to forsee the political changes that were triggered at 8:16 A.M. on August 6 over Hiroshima. These would not be governed by the scientific method; the imprecise art of politics would determine the changes in the face of the world.

Of all the great powers, none was more concerned for its future in 1945 than Great Britain. Her empire, its fabric rotted by time and rising nationalism and ripped by war, was coming apart. Her leaders were searching for new ways to maintain her position in the postwar world.

To Winston Churchill, the atomic bomb seemed the ideal instrument. Here was the lever to keep England on a par with the new colossus of Russia. With the secret of the atomic bomb its exclusive possession, the West could use the threat of it to contain the already aggressive Soviets.

Churchill expounded this view enthusiastically to his Chief of Staff, Field-Marshal Sir Alan Brooke. But Brooke did not agree that the bomb solved England's problems. Instead, he believed that the fission of the atom had deeply undermined his nation's security, for the simple reason that Russia would never rest, nor agree to any kind of international controls, until she too had the bomb in her arsenal, ready to help her gobble up all of Europe. The atomic scientists were unanimous in their opinion that no secrecy curtain could keep the necessary knowledge from the Soviets for very long. Russia had already swept up all the German scientists she could lay hands on and hauled them off to work on this and other problems, including the ballistic missile that could eventually be used to deliver nuclear warheads. She had spared no energy to penetrate Manhattan's secrecy barriers. When Little

Boy exploded over Hiroshima, the Soviets intensified their drive for atomic secrets. When the Smyth report was released, the Washington correspondent for the Soviet news agency Tass was at the Pentagon within an hour—asking for six copies. On August 22, little more than a fortnight after Hiroshima, the director of military intelligence in Moscow sent a secret coded cable to the Russian military attaché in Canada:

Take measures to organize acquisition of documentary materials on the atomic bomb!
The technical process, drawings, calculations.

DIRECTOR
22.8.45

Both Churchill and Brooke, as it turned out, were right. Churchill's prediction that the atomic bomb would be the most powerful single weapon in the East-West struggle was accurate enough. But it was incomplete, because he did not see what his field-marshal saw. Russia would do just what Brooke predicted and would frustrate every attempt at international control of the atom while she rushed to build her own nuclear stockpile. The United States, bearing the responsibility for first using the bomb, would seek repeatedly to reach a control agreement. Stimson's early work was followed by intensive efforts to find a means of control under the United Nations. But the Russians repeatedly balked. The reason would become clear in August, 1949, when the world learned of "Joe One," the first Russian test explosion of the plutonium bomb. It had several times the power of the first U.S. atomic weapons.

From then on, the lexicon of world power politics would be changed. The decade of the fifties would be keyed to a series of new phrases: "nuclear stalemate," "mutual deterrence" and "massive retaliation." There would be frightening discussions, too, of bombs so "dirty" that poisonous fall-out could kill millions of civilians. Now both sides possessed the ultimate weapon, and the balance of terror put warfare back to its pre-Hiroshima state, so that the United States would fight a war for three years in Korea without using its most powerful weapons, while the Russian pilots who flew for the other side were likewise deprived of their most potent arm.

The hostility between East and West would become so bitter that there would even be talk of "preventive war" to heighten the tension caused by recurrent and ever-larger test explosions in the American desert, in the far Pacific and in Soviet Siberia. Finally both sides would come to the realization that, as Stimson said before he died, "there is no other choice" but to seek an end to the awful competition. There would then be a hiatus in the race, while scientists and diplomats from the U.S. and U.S.S.R. attempted first to define the problem and then to write a workable agreement that both sides could trust.

This was all in the future in that summer of 1945. But one exchange of messages between two perceptive Americans summed up man's fears and hopes within a week after the destruction of Hiroshima. Robert A. Lovett, Assistant Secretary of War for Air, and General Carl Spaatz, commander of the Strategic Air Force, were good friends. Many times the old soldier had cited a favorite West Point classroom maxim, "Seize the high ground," in explaining military tactics to his civilian superior. The line illustrated the first principle of infantry warfare: that terrain can control the outcome of a battle.

The phrase came back to Lovett on August 14, 1945. With formal Japanese surrender only a few hours away, he sent a personal note to Spaatz on the War Department telecommunications circuit to Tinian:

SPAATZ FROM LOVETT
I AM STUCK HERE WITH NO IMMEDIATE PROSPECT OF BREAKING LOOSE SO RELY ON YOU TO SEIZE ME HIGH GROUND. . . . CONGRATULATIONS TO ALL AND AFFECTIONATE REGARDS.

BOB

A few minutes later, the tough old flier who had led the pulverization of Germany from the air and then had supervised the dropping of the atomic bomb on Japan replied:

AUGUST 141310Z TELECON LOVETT FROM SPAATZ
PERSONAL. HAVE LOOKED AT GOOD PHOTOS OF HIROSHIMA TODAY. THE ATOMIC BOMB DISPOSES OF ALL HIGH GROUND.

Bibliography

AMRINE, MICHAEL, *The Great Decision,* New York, 1959, G. P. Putnam's Sons.

ARNOLD, H. H., *Global Mission,* New York, 1949, Harper & Brothers.

ASHWORTH, CMDR. F. L., *Atomic Bombings of Hiroshima and Nagasaki,* 1947, n.p.

BAXTER, JAMES PHINNEY, *Scientists Against Time,* Boston, 1952, Little, Brown & Co.

BRYANT, ARTHUR, *Triumph in the West,* New York, 1959, Doubleday & Co., Inc.

BUTOW, ROBERT J. C., *Japan's Decision to Surrender,* Stanford, Calif., 1954, Stanford University Press.

BYRNES, JAMES F., *Speaking Frankly,* New York, 1947, Harper & Brothers.

——, *All in One Lifetime,* New York, 1958, Harper & Brothers.

CHURCHILL, WINSTON S., *Triumph and Tragedy,* Boston, 1953, Houghton Mifflin Co.

CLINE, RAY S., *United States Army in World War II, The Operations Division,* Washington, 1951, Government Printing Office.

COMPTON, ARTHUR H., *Atomic Quest,* New York, 1956, Oxford University Press.

CRAVEN, WESLEY FRANK, and CATE, JAMES LEA, eds., *Army Air Forces in World War II, Volume Five, The Pacific—Matterhorn to Nagasaki,* Chicago, 1953, University of Chicago Press.

DANIELS, JONATHAN, *The Man of Independence,* Philadelphia, 1950, J. B. Lippincott Co.

EISENHOWER, DWIGHT D., *Crusade in Europe,* Garden City, N.Y., 1948, Doubleday & Co., Inc.

GOUDSMIT, SAMUEL A., *Alsos,* New York, 1947, Henry Schuman, Inc.

GREW, JOSEPH C., *Turbulent Era,* Vol. II, Boston, 1952, Houghton Mifflin Co.

HACHIYA, MICHIHIKO, *Hiroshima Diary,* Chapel Hill, N.C., 1955, University of North Carolina Press.

HERSEY, JOHN, *Hiroshima,* New York, 1946, Alfred A. Knopf.

HOUGH, FRANK O., *The Island War,* Philadelphia, 1947, J. B. Lippincott Co.

HULL, CORDELL, *The Memoirs of Cordell Hull, Vol. II,* New York, 1948, the Macmillan Co.

JANIS, IRVING L., *Psychological Effects of the Atomic Attacks on Japan,* Santa Monica, Calif., 1950, the RAND Corporation.

JUNGK, ROBERT, *Brighter Than a Thousand Suns,* New York, 1958, Harcourt, Brace & Co.

KARIG, WALTER, *Battle Report: Victory in the Pacific,* with Russell L. Harris and Frank A. Manson, New York, 1949, Rinehart & Co., Inc.

KASE, TOSHIKAZU, *Journey to the Missouri,* New Haven, Conn., 1950, Yale University Press.

KATO, MASUO, *The Lost War,* New York, 1946, Alfred A. Knopf.

LANDSTROM, RUSSELL, *The Associated Press News Annual: 1945,* New York, 1946, Rinehart & Co., Inc.

LAURENCE, WILLIAM L., *Dawn Over Zero,* New York, 1946, Alfred A. Knopf.

LEAHY, FLEET ADMIRAL WILLIAM D., *I Was There,* New York, 1950, McGraw-Hill Book Co., Inc.

MILLER, MERLE, and SPITZER, ABE, *We Dropped the A-Bomb,* New York, 1946, Crowell & Co.

MILLIS, WALTER, and DUFFIELD, E. S., *The Forrestal Diaries,* New York, 1951, The Viking Press.

MOYNAHAN, JOHN F., *Atomic Diary,* Newark, N. J., 1946, Barton Publishing Co.

NEWCOMB, RICHARD F., *Abandon Ship!,* New York, 1958, Henry Holt & Co.

OSSIP, JEROME J., et al., *509th Pictorial Album,* Tinian Island, 1945, n.p.

OUGHTERSON, ASHLEY W., and WARREN, SHIELDS, *Medical Effects of the Atomic Bomb in Japan,* New York, 1956, McGraw-Hill Book Co., Inc.

Bibliography

PARKER, LT. COL. DAVID B., ed., *The Atomic Bombings of Hiroshima and Nagasaki*, n.d., U.S. Army, Manhattan Engineer District.

SHERWOOD, ROBERT E., *Roosevelt and Hopkins*, New York, 1948, Harper & Brothers.

SMITH, MERRIMAN, *Thank You, Mr. President*, New York, 1946, Harper & Brothers.

SMYTH, HENRY DE WOLF, *Atomic Energy*, Washington, 1945, Government Printing Office.

SPECIAL COMMITTEE ON ATOMIC ENERGY, U.S. Senate, 79th Congress, *Hearings*. Washington, 1946, Government Printing Office.

STATE, DEPARTMENT OF, ed., *The Conference at Malta and Yalta*, Washington, 1954, Government Printing Office.

———, *The Potsdam Conference*, unpublished manuscript.

STIMSON, HENRY L., "The Decision to Use the Atomic Bomb," New York, 1947, *Harper's* Magazine.

———, *Diary*, May, 1945-August, 1945, unpublished ms., Sterling Memorial Library, Yale University, New Haven, Conn.

STIMSON, HENRY L., and BUNDY, MCGEORGE, *On Active Service in Peace and War*, New York, 1948, Harper & Brothers.

TASCHERAU, ROBERT, and KELLOCK, R. L., *The Report of the Royal Commission*, Ottawa, 1946, Controller of Stationery.

TRUMAN, HARRY S., *Year of Decisions*, Garden City, N. Y., 1955, Doubleday & Co., Inc.

TRUMBULL, ROBERT, *Nine Who Survived Hiroshima and Nagasaki*, New York, 1957, E. P. Dutton & Co., Inc.

TULLY, GRACE, *F.D.R. My Boss*, New York, 1949, Charles Scribner's Sons.

U.S. ARMY OFFICE OF MILITARY HISTORY, *Interview with Yoshio Nishina*, unpublished transcript, Tokyo, 1945.

U.S. ATOMIC ENERGY COMMISSION, *In the Matter of J. Robert Oppenheimer* (transcript of hearings before personnel security board), Washington, 1954, Government Printing Office.

U.S. STRATEGIC BOMBING SURVEY, *Reports, Pacific War*. Washington, 1945-1947, Government Printing Office.

    No. 2—*Japan's Struggle to End the War.*

No. 3—*The Effects of Atomic Bombs on Hiroshima and Nagasaki.*

No. 13—*The Effects of Atomic Bombs on Health and Medical Services in Hiroshima and Nagasaki.*

No. 14—*The Effects of Strategic Bombing on Japanese Morale.*

No. 60—*Effects of Air Attack on the City of Hiroshima.*

No. 72—*Interrogations of Japanese Officials* (2 volumes).

No. 93—*Effects of the Atomic Bomb on Hiroshima, Japan.*

WATERMAN, ALAN, ed., *Combat Scientists*, Boston, 1947, Atlantic-Little Brown.

Index

265

Index

Index

Index

Index

King, Adm. Ernest J., 87, 89, 90, 108, 120
"Kingman," 81
Kinoshita, Hideo, 197
Kirkpatrick, Col. Elmer E., 90, 147-148, 164-165, 227
Kistiakowsky, George B., 59, 117
Kitamura, Kojiro, 19, 20, 22, 23
Kokura, 52, 122, 125, 140-141, 142, 143, 155, 156, 168, 222, 224, 225
Konoye, Funimaro, 33, 34, 35
Korea, 20
Kyle, Col. William H., 111, 112, 120
Kyoto, 106, 121, 122
Kyushu, 7, 8, 9, 108, 236

Laggin' Dragon, 136-138
Lamont, Thomas W. II, 12
Lansdale, Col. John, Jr., 70, 72, 80, 132, 216
Laurence, William L., 6, 160, 225
Lawrence, Ernest O., 59, 102, 106, 113, 118
Lawrence, William L., 6
League of Nations, 237
Leahy, Adm. William D., 30, 31, 32, 73, 96, 97, 100, 106, 108, 118, 120, 123, 127, 128, 244-245, 246
LeMay, Gen. Curtis E., 4, 98, 106, 111, 126, 139-140, 142, 145, 218, 219
Lewis, Capt. Robert A., 79, 85-86, 156, 157, 158, 163, 164, 171, 202-203, 205, 210, 248
Leyte, 8
Life with Father, 13
"Little Boy," 61, 130*ff*., 158*ff*., 206
Los Alamos, 10, 60, 61, 67, 68, 71, 80, 83, 92
Lovett, Robert A., 127, 257-258
Lozovsky, Alexander, 34-35
Luce, Clare Boothe, 13
Luzon, 7, 108

MacArthur, Gen. Douglas, 11, 73, 89, 108, 122, 124, 141-142, 222
Madigan, Michael J., 74

Malik, Jacob, 27, 28, 32
Manchuria, 20
Manhattan Engineering District, 57*ff*.
Manila, 8
Marianas, 4
Marquardt, Capt. George W., 141, 148, 154, 157, 164, 165, 170, 204, 205, 210, 212, 224
Marshall, Gen. George C., 31-32, 74, 87, 96, 102, 103, 120-121, 123, 125, 216, 217, 218, 219
Martin, Joseph W., Jr., 74
Matsuo, Doctor, 45
MATTERHORN, 104
McCloy, John J., 108, 109, 123
McCormack, John W., 74
McFarland, Gen. A. J., 108
McKnight, Capt. Charles F., 157, 159, 165, 172, 224
McMorris, Adm. C. H., 90
McVay, Capt. Charles B., 133
megaton, 251
Miller, Maj. William, 7, 8, 236
"Misplay," 138
Molotov, Vyacheslav M., 24, 34, 239
"Morose," 138
Morris, Lt. Robert, 220
Morrison, Philip, 129, 130, 144, 222-223
Moynahan, Maj. John F., 139, 149, 207, 218, 220
Mussolini, Benito, 53, 56
Myers, Col. Harold A. (Spike), 129-130, 222

Nagasaki, 52, 124, 125, 142, 143, 155, 156, 168, 222, 224, 225-226, 240, 246-247
Nakamura, Bin, 197
National Defense Research Committee, 56
Nelson, Corp. Richard, 51, 156, 169, 207
New York Times, 239
Nicely, Gillon Truett, 156, 168
"Nicholas Baker," 60
Nichols, Col. Kenneth D., 64-65, 66, 67, 123

269

Index

Index

Index